ALOE VERA
A Scientific Approach

ALOE VERA
A Scientific Approach

Robert H. Davis, Ph.D.

VANTAGE PRESS
New York

All persons making use of the information and techniques contained within the pages of this book are reminded that the information and techniques are intended to provide guidelines only. Each individual should seek the advice of his or her own physician before starting any new medical program, and the opinions expressed herein are solely those of the author.

IASC — International Aloe Science Council.

FIRST EDITION

Published by Vantage Press, Inc.
516 West 34th Street, New York, New York 10001

Manufactured in the United States of America
ISBN: 0-533-12137-X

Library of Congress Catalog Card No.: 96-90679

0 9 8 7 6 5 4 3 2 1

To Jesus Christ and His Gospel

The Scripture says that all men are sinners and fall short of the 100 percent-perfection required to get into heaven. Man cannot save himself. God loves us and does not want to punish us for our sin, but because He is holy and righteous, He must punish our sin. The Word (Jesus) became flesh and dwelt among us. Jesus hung on the tree at Calvary, and God put every sin we ever committed from our birth to our death on Jesus. He forgave all our sins and purchased a place for us in heaven. We receive this gift by trusting in Jesus and what He did for us at Calvary. Jesus says, "But as many as receive me, I give them the right to become children of God." He also says, "Behold, I stand at the door of your heart and knock. If you open the door, I will come in and dine with you and to you I will give the victory." Right now, pray and ask Jesus to come into your heart and be your Lord and Savior.

Contents

	Foreword	ix
	Acknowledgments	xi
1.	Introduction	1
2.	The Aloe Leaf	8
3.	The Making of Aloe Vera	30
4.	The Biological Vehicle Effect of Aloe Vera	47
5.	The Gowda Experiment	85
6.	Improved Wound Healing by Aloe Vera	109
7.	Gibberellin: A Growth Factor in Aloe Vera	132
8.	Does Aloe Vera Have a Place in AIDS Therapy?	161
9.	Steroids, Sterols, and Aloe Vera	183
10.	Aspirin and Aloe	226
11.	Biological Standardization of Aloe Vera	263
12.	The Conductor–Orchestra Concept of Aloe Vera	290
13.	General Summary	310
	Index	319

Adulteration p 38 →

Foreword

There has been a significant evolution in our understanding of the science of aloe vera during the past decade. Research throughout the world, especially in the United States, Korea, Japan and Europe has revealed more of the basic biological mechanisms for the pharmacological activity of aloe, and new clinical indications for its use in the treatment of human disease and regulating metabolism of the human body. This "hard science" has been invaluable to the aloe industry and consumers alike by expanding the many uses for aloe and improving the efficacy of this phytomedicinal plant as a consumer product.

I am very pleased and honored that Dr. Robert Davis has taken on the enormous task of compiling the latest developments in the science of aloe. He is uniquely qualified for this task, having studied the biological activity and chemistry of aloe vera for more than ten years and being a key scientific advisor to the International Aloe Science Council, the aloe industry and consumers. Unlike many books in this field, this publication gives a balanced and rigorous analysis of the leading research on aloe largely due to the scientific objectivity of Dr. Davis and other authors. I am confident this book will be essential reading in the years to come for anyone interested in the production, use and research of aloe vera.

Nam Yang Aloe International is pleased to sponsor the preparation and publication of this book with the hope that it will advance the scientific understanding of aloe vera and promote the manufacture of aloe products that deliver the maximum healthful benefit to mankind. If this book stimulates further research and development of aloe vera, we will consider our efforts well-rewarded.

Mr. B. William Lee
President and CEO
Nam Yang Aloe International, Ltd.

Acknowledgments

No book results from the efforts of a single person. As I wrote the manuscript, I felt I was standing on the shoulders of giants. I wish to express my special thanks and appreciation to Mr. B. William Lee, president and CEO of Aloecorp, in Dallas, Texas. Mr. Lee's encouragement and financial support made possible the difficult task of writing this book. His friendship made the job much easier. My thanks also go to Mr. Bill C. Coats, president, of Coats Aloe International, Inc., of Dallas, who gave me the idea for the title. Since the book contains a great deal of scientific data on aloe, Bill Coats felt the title should stress the scientific approach to aloe vera. My thanks and appreciation go to Jess F. Clarke, Jr., president of Miracle of Aloe, at Westport, Connecticut, for his sound advice and support of my research. His great enthusiasm helped me to move my research forward when things got rough. I thank Mr. William J. Wylie, an attorney-at-law of Wheaton, Illinois, for his precious help in getting me through some difficult decisions pertaining to certain areas in the text. To James H. Leathem, Ph.D., professor of endocrinology at Rutgers University, my major professor (now deceased), goes my great appreciation for giving me the broad scientific background to tackle the huge spectrum of aloe vera.

Instrumental in the making of this volume were some of my students: G. M. Hartman, R. C. Haas, W. L. Parker, R. T. Samson, D. P. Murdoch, M. G. Leitner, J. M. Russo, M. E. Byrne, J. M. Kabbani, N. P. Maro, P. S. Agnew, E. Shapiro, E. N. Erlick, E. D. Engel, D. C. Hanley, W. A. Solomon, and B. Saffran. These students, now doctors, working in my laboratory won many awards doing research on Aloe vera. Thanks go to Joseph J. DiDonato, now a law student at Michigan State University, for helping me develop the many assays used to standardize aloe. Last, but not least, I wish to extend my appreciation to Mrs. Susan Shaughnessy for her help in editing and preparing the manuscript. Only she knows the labor of love required to write a book of this kind.

ALOE VERA
A Scientific Approach

1
Introduction

The healing power of aloe vera is well known to every mother who has an aloe plant on her windowsill. When she put aloe on the insect bites, burns, or wounds of her children, she was certain that it would stimulate the body to heal itself. Aloe vera gel softens skin, fades brown age spots, increases skin penetration, and improves circulation. Healing is a natural process in the body that can be enhanced by aloe vera. Today's traditional doctor is not interested in aloe vera and knows nothing about the *art* of healing. Modern medicine depends on technology, which is so expensive that it cannot be delivered to all people. As a result, traditional medicine is losing the health care system and hospitals are going bankrupt. Our hospitals and doctors have expensive methods that can handle trauma and crises but make no attempt to work with the body's healing mechanisms. Aloe vera can stimulate healing at a relatively lower cost than the expensive traditional treatments. Plant substances (herbs), like aloe vera, stimulate, protect, and modulate the immune system. Definite proof has been presented that aloe gel protects the damage of the immune system caused by the sun. People want better health care that is inexpensive. This is why they are using aloe vera and other plant products.

Inflammatory disorders demonstrate a worldwide distribution ranging from swelling to severe crippling rheumatoid arthritis. Well-known research attests to the effectiveness of cortisone, prednisone, dexamethasone, phenylbutazone, and acetylsalicylic acid in reducing inflammation. Nevertheless, these compounds have major toxicity problems. For example, aspirin at high doses causes blood clotting, hypersensitivity, anemia, upper gastrointestinal disturbance, and microbleeding problems. Steroids block the release of cell enzymes and decrease antibody production. Over a long period, steroids cause

Cushing's syndrome, electrolyte imbalance, fluid retention, diabetes, arteritis, and osteoporosis. I grew up watching the development of cortisone into decadron. The phenanthrene ring was built into a powerful anti-inflammatory compound, but with significant side effects. I, therefore, began to search for natural substances that had good anti-inflammatory activity, such as vitamin C and amino acids. In fact, certain amino acids were found to have the same activity as certain hormones but without the toxicity. One morning in my laboratory, my students and I were evaluating a thymus extract we were working on for anti-arthritic activity. By accident, we used an aloe extract from a leaf as a treatment control. It turned out that the aloe extract produced the best response we had ever seen with a natural substance. The literature revealed to us that it contained many of the compounds I had been working with over the years. This observation was in the middle to late 1970s. My laboratory has been working with aloe vera ever since. In the early days processors of aloe made miraculous therapeutic claims that aloe vera could do almost anything. The claims were anecdotal, with biblical references going back to ancient times. When a beneficial effect was recorded for aloe vera, it was usually a "one-shot" deal. The patient or animal was given aloe for a certain condition at one dose, and a response was observed. No real scientific design was presented, so no conclusive proof about the efficacy of aloe vera could be obtained. My laboratory has clearly shown that when you increase the dose of aloe vera, there is a corresponding straight-line increase in response in a number of biological activities. This principle of standardization proves that aloe vera works and that products of aloe vera are reliable ones in which the consumer can have confidence. No longer can anyone say that "aloe vera is a myth or the result of magic," because the efficacy is based on scientific dose-response curves. This has been clearly demonstrated, for example, on anti-inflammation, wound healing, and analgesia. However, aloe products that contain little or no aloe, as well as aloe products that are poorly processed, will be therapeutically inert. People buy aloe vera because of its amazing healing powers. If these therapeutic properties are missing, people will not continue to use aloe to heal their hurts. The International Aloe Science Council (IASC) now has a solid certification process that will guarantee that consumers get the pure aloe vera that they are paying for. I ask the question: "What is good aloe?" It is aloe that has all the desirable qualities it is supposed to have so that the active components are preserved with all their biological benefits.

Not only does aspirin deliver powerful pain relief, but the recent news reveals its ability to reduce the risk of heart attack, stroke, and colon cancer. Aspirin is a great drug, but to ensure effectiveness it must be given at relatively high doses and sometimes over a long period of time. Under these conditions aspirin can cause gastrointestinal bleeding and liver damage. The principle holds true, therefore, that more aspirin is not necessarily better, because aspirin can cause stomach problems that are dose-related. Nevertheless, people reap cardiovascular benefits if they take small amounts of aspirin each day. Aspirin works by inhibiting the body's synthesis of prostaglandin, which is released at the site of pain or inflammation. Prostaglandins promote pain but also cause blood vessels to constrict and platelets to become sticky and gum up blood vessel walls. When aspirin blocks the synthesis of prostaglandin, it opens up blood vessels and inhibits the stickiness of platelets. When we gave aloe vera with aspirin to reduce pain, a synergistic analgesic response was recorded. A similar response was obtained for anti-inflammation. This proves that aloe vera enhances the biological activity of aspirin so that a smaller dose of aspirin can be used to get the same response. Using aloe vera as a "biological vehicle" for aspirin, one can improve the therapeutic effectiveness, lower the dose, and reduce the side effects. Most of the truly great drugs, such as digitalis and aspirin, have significant toxicity problems. The more good a drug can do, the more bad it can do. This is a valid principle in pharmacology. Possibly by using aloe as a "biological vehicle" for active compounds one can maintain the biological activity and reduce the dosage of the active agent. Aloe vera may contribute activity to the test agent in an additive or synergistic fashion while, at the same time, increasing drug penetration. This finding may be of great value to medicine for arthritis, cancer, and heart disease.

Aloe vera was effective in reducing inflammation over a broad spectrum of irritants in experimental animals. It also prevented and regressed adjuvant induced arthritis. Aloe vera was able to prevent the infiltration of polymorphonuclear leukocytes (PMNs) into an induced area of inflammation. Possibly, aloe blocks leukotrienes, which is a mediator responsible for attracking PMNs. Since aloe vera inhibits irritant-induced edema, it probably blocks prostaglandin. In the acute inflammatory response, the inflammatory stimulus produces a tissue insult that releases vasoactive substances that act on venule endothelial cells. Macrophages and PMNs adhere to the inner wall surface and escape by the endothelial cell junctions. When these cells act back on the tissue insult, there is a respiratory burst and a release of oxygen radicals that prolong and exacerbate the inflammatory process. Interleukins released from the macrophage are involved in the inflammation. Aloe vera inhibits these mediators of inflammation as well as "mopping up" the oxygen radicals. Vitamin C and E found in aloe are excellent anti-oxidants. When we placed a cotton pellet under the skin of an animal, we found that aloe vera was unable to inhibit the growth of granuloma tissue. it has no antifibrosis activity over a large dose range. However, we wondered if aloe vera, acting as a biological vehicle, could improve the anti-fibrosis activity of hydrocortisone. In wound healing, aloe vera stimulates fibroblasts to produce collagen necessary for wound tensile strength. This is not a chronic inflammatory response but a stimulation of fibroblasts that is necessary for healthy wound healing. Aloe vera is a modulator capable of blocking the immune system observed in the adjuvant arthritic animal and can block the mediators responsible for inflammation. It also has a stimulatory system that can stimulate cellular and antibody immunity as well as stimulating wound healing by means of growth factors such as gibberellin, auxin, and mannose phosphate. The isolation of the wound healing and anti-inflammatory activities using the 50 percent ethanol extraction of aloe vera revealed that the supernatant contained 78 percent of the anti-inflammatory activity, whereas the precipitate had only 32 percent. On the other hand, the supernatant had 0 percent wound healing activity, whereas the precipitate had 160 percent wound healing activity in reference to the original aloe vera. This shows that the anti-inflammatory activity in aloe is masking some of the wound healing effect seen in the original aloe vera.

All of our studies seem to indicate that aloe vera is both orally and topically active on wound healing and inflammation, even in the diabetic. It can improve wound healing in the diabetic in a dose-response fashion over a dose range of 1 to 100 mg/kg. Mannose phosphate is a significant constituent in the 50 percent aloe vera extract. Mannose phosphate binds to the insulin-like growth factor receptor to exhibit biological activity. The inhibiting effect of mannose phosphate on topical croton oil–induced inflammation was dose-related. Glucose phosphate had no effect and served as a control. Mannose phosphate improved wound healing in a dose-response straight-line manner. We feel that mannose phosphate of aloe vera activates the insulin-like growth factor receptor of the fibroblast cell to increase the production of collagen. Collagen is needed to strengthen wounds. The aloe vera polysaccharide molecule consists of protein at one end and mannose 6 phosphate at the other end. The polysaccharide chain contains one glucose, which is covalently (strongly) linked to the protein, and six mannose sugars. The end mannose is a mannose phosphate that fits into the insulin-like growth factor receptor of the fibroblast. We feel the protein part of the aloe vera molecule acts to guide the polysaccharide chain into the receptor. The polysaccharide can stimulate the macrophage to produce a variety of effects. The polysaccharide (conductor) modulates the biological activity of the surrounding molecules (orchestra). The polarity of water and its ability to dissolve active agents help the conductor communicate with the orchestra to produce a harmony of biological activity.

Diabetes mellitus is a metabolic disorder characterized by a high blood sugar, thirst, hunger, and weakness. Peripheral vascular disease is a major factor in diabetes. Renal failure, coronary heart disease, blindness, infections, and atherosclerosis are also seen in the disease. We found that aloe vera could inhibit inflammation and improve wound healing in streptozotocin-induced diabetes. The free oxygen radicals produced in inflammation can be inhibited by aloe. The oxygen radicals play an important role in destroying beta cells and the production of diabetes. Aloe vera also contains important fractions that lower blood sugar. One wonders if aloe vera can contribute to the prevention of diabetes. Can the sugars present in aloe vera have a protective action by scavenging free radicals? Certainly aloe vera can play a role in blocking the arachidonic acid cascade in inflammation. The anti-oxidant status of aloe vera needs further study in regard to the impaired respiratory burst seen in diabetic PMNs.

Hydrocortisone is a most effective treatment for inflammation. However, while inhibiting inflammation, hydrocortisone blocks wound healing. This situation presents a conflicting dilemma for physicians. How can one improve wound healing and, at the same time, reduce inflammation? Aloe vera, given alone, has both biological activities. When given with hydrocortisone it improves penetration and it blocks the anti-wound properties of the steroid. Sterols in aloe have the same properties as hydrocortisone in inflammation and wound healing. The ability of aloe to inhibit inflammation comes in part from sterols. The plant growth factor gibberellin plays a major role in the ability of aloe vera to heal wounds. Gibberellin buffers sterols when wound healing is needed. When anti-inflammation is required, gibberellin probably works with sterols on inhibiting inflammation. Aloe vera's watery consistency exerts a major effect by increasing epithelial cell migration of wounds. Desiccation retards wound healing because the wound drops and prevents movement of cells. Aloe vera, unlike steroids, does not cause connective tissue breakdown, nor does it inhibit connective tissue formation while exhibiting acute anti-inflammatory activity. Steroid activity is clearly seen in diabetic patients who have too much circulatory steroid, which tends to prevent collagen formation and wound healing. Aloe vera may be an appealing steroid substitute. Aloe vera stimulates the entire process of wound healing. It normalizes connective tissue and epithelial elements as it prevents inflammation without inhibiting connective tissue. Aloe vera bridges the gap between inflammation and wound healing, which should contribute to the treatment of patients.

Researchers have had a disappointing thirteen years in their research with AIDS. No curative treatment has been found, and people are still dying of AIDS. This is a tragic time for research because researchers continue to hang onto traditional thinking. The AIDS epidemic is worldwide, and the full extent of its explosive impact is yet to be seen. Global AIDS may be out of control. There seems to be a complacency because there is no effective treatment for AIDS. I have reviewed the AIDS problem and have asked the question: "Does aloe vera have a place in AIDS therapy?" Aloe vera has had a positive immune response under laboratory conditions. Co-factors associated with AIDS may provide a good therapeutic target in which aloe vera might participate. The biological vehicle effect of aloe may help effective vaccines and medicines fight against the AIDS co-factors. Some of the deficiencies seen in AIDS that impair cellular and antibody immunity might be helped by aloe vera. The ability of aloe vera to stimulate the macrophage with the release of valuable growth factors and mediators should lead to important new insights in the treatment of AIDS.

Most people around the world have experienced or heard of the miraculous benefits of aloe vera. However, these miracles of aloe have not been explained or proven from a strong scientific basis. All the benefits are known, but the scientific foundation for the benefits has always been needed. In this book I show "how aloe vera works" from a scientific viewpoint. I show how aloe vera eliminates pain, inflammation, arthritis, and wounds. The "conductor-orchestra concept of aloe vera" takes into account all the biologically active components working synergistically to produce the maximum desired benefits with little or no toxicity. This concept helps the aloe industry understand the relationship of the polysaccharide with the other active components. I believe it is the standard by which the industry operates. Our ongoing research now has all the data by which to standardize and identify aloe vera so that it can attack the entire spectrum of human conditions.

2

The Aloe Leaf

Little attention has been given to the direct use of the aloe leaf as an estimate of the production of aloe vera. The leaf is triangular and stiff. The leaves are arranged in a radial alternate formation around developing "pup leaves."[1] The plant can be grown in almost any type of soil.[2] If the weather becomes dry, the leaves turn brown. Aloe plants do well in partial shade but return red on excessive exposure to the sun. Aloe leaves do well in heat but not in cold.[3] An acre of ground can yield eighty tons of leaves.[1] F. R. Bharucha and G. V. Joshi reported that alternating periods of light and darkness cause fluctuation of acid and carbohydrate content in aloe. Prolonged darkness of 186 hours at 9°C caused maximum acid formation due to an increase in malic acid.[4] Malic acid is formed from the "active" carbon in the formation of aloe. Freezing causes the rupture of leaf tubules and a disruption of gel flow within the transport system.[5] The brownish-red color formation is due to the formation of the anthraquinones.[6]

The purpose of this chapter is to discuss: the anatomy of the leaf; the aloe leaf assay in regard to water, solids, gel, and specific activity of glucose; the importance of mucilage to aloe vera; and the influence of wind on the transport and production of aloe vera. Some attention will be given to the aloe vera cell and how aloe is made within the leaf.

The Anatomy of the Leaf

Aloe plants exhibit radial arrangement of four rows of leaves alternately arranged. The outer two rows are fully developed whereas the inner two rows are not fully grown. The inner "pup leaves" receive nourishment from the outer leaves. Our low-amp faxitron X ray observed long tubes running from the leaf tip to the base of the leaf that carry nourishment to the young "pup leaves." The wind moves the leaves and provides the momentum to move the gel inward. Wind increases the movement and production of aloe vera in the leaf. We have dissected the leaf and have observed the long tubules seen by the faxitron.

A cross section of the leaf reveals an outer epidermis containing guard cells forming stomata through which CO_2 enters the rind.[7] The epidermis is covered with a "waxy coat" to prevent the escape of water (figure 2.1). The rind is the "manufacturing plant" where carbohydrate, fat, and protein are made. One wonders if the aloe gel could be removed from the leaf, and then, if the leaf was completely sealed, would it continue to manufacture aloe under suitable conditions? Carbon dioxide combines with water in the presence of chloroplasts (which provides green color), which forms an "active carbon."[8] The "active carbon" can form carbohydrates, proteins, fatty acids, and vitamins. The vascular bundles consist of xylem, which transports water, minerals, and nitrogen from the roots to the fifteen-cell thickness in the green rind. The phloem transports synthesized materials to other parts of the leaf. The vascular bundles connect with the long tubules running lengthwise toward the leaf base that nourishes the "pup leaves." The gel fillet consists of large parenchyma cells that store water and large amounts of carbohydrate (figures 2.2 and 2.3). Mucilage consists of long chain polysaccharides, which act as a container for the enclosed aloe gel. We thought, in the past, that mucilage functioned to move aloe from the rind to other parts of the leaf. However, this movement is caused by the wind and not mucilage. The polysaccharide of mucilage has good biological activity in regard to wound healing and anti-inflammation.

The Aloe Vera Cell

Figure 2.4 shows the aloe vera cell seen by electron microscopy at 40,000 magnification stained with Ruthenium Red or Periodic Acid Schiff stains that are specific for mucopolysaccharides. The nucleus is clearly visible, surrounded by two cell membranes that contain mucopolysaccharides that are being transferred into the cell lumen for storage. Some of this long chain polysaccharide is transferred to

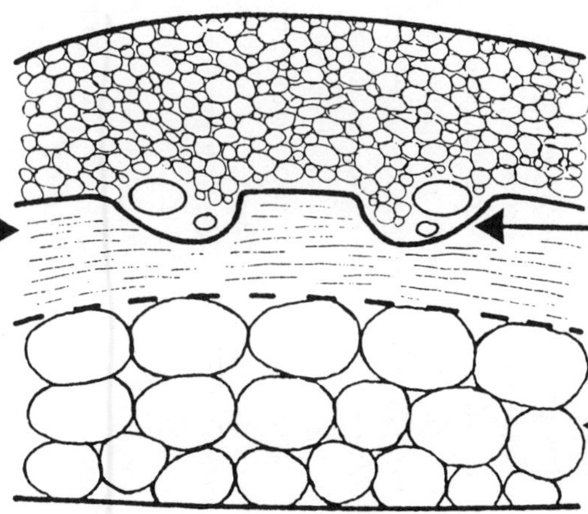
CROSS SECTION OF ALOE LEAF
RIND – 15 CELLS
(SYNTHESIS)
MUCILAGE
(CONTAINER)
XYLEM AND PHLOEM
(TRANSPORT)
PARENCHYMA
OR GEL FILLET
(STORAGE)

Fig. 2.1.

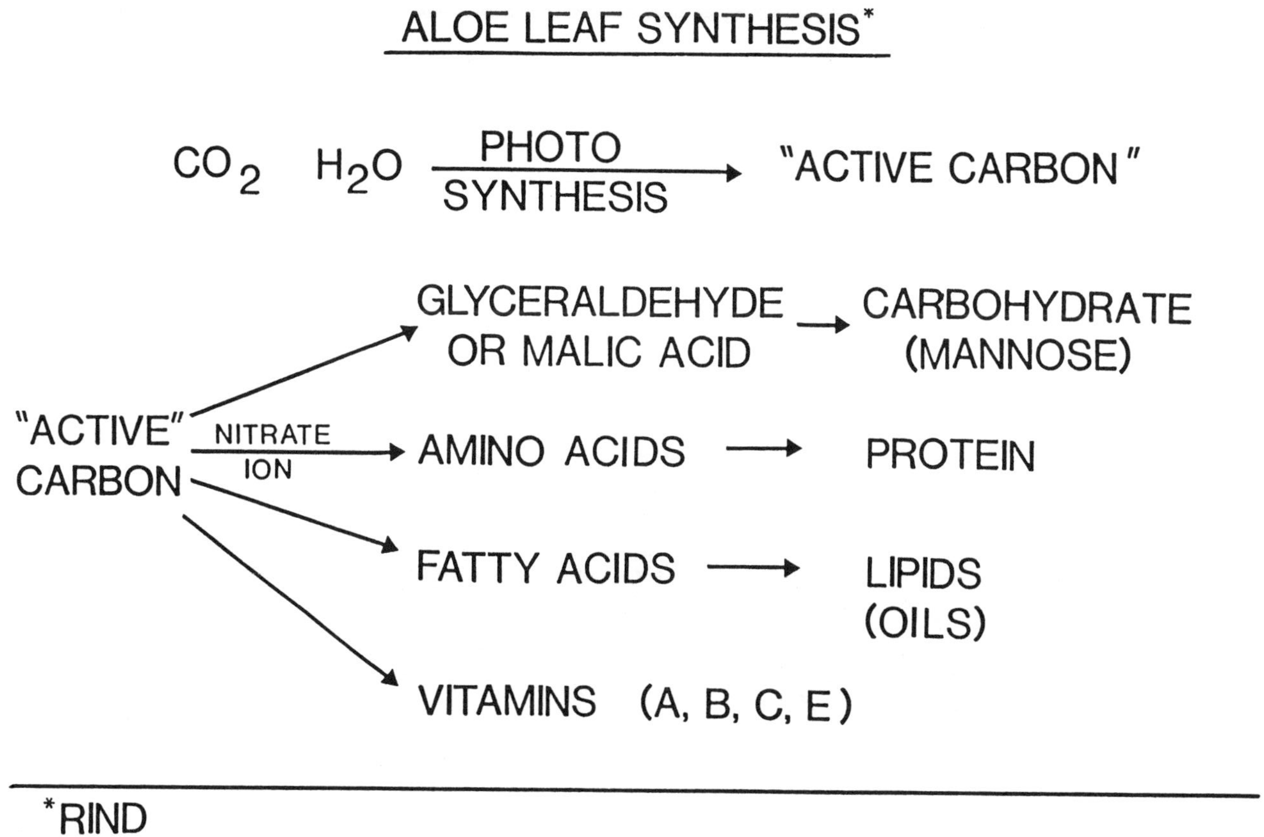
ALOE LEAF SYNTHESIS*
CO2
H2O
PHOTO
SYNTHESIS
"ACTIVE CARBON"
"ACTIVE" CARBON
NITRATE
ION
GLYCERALDEHYDE OR MALIC ACID
CARBOHYDRATE (MANNOSE)
AMINO ACIDS
PROTEIN
FATTY ACIDS
LIPIDS (OILS)
VITAMINS (A, B, C, E)
*RIND

Fig. 2.2.

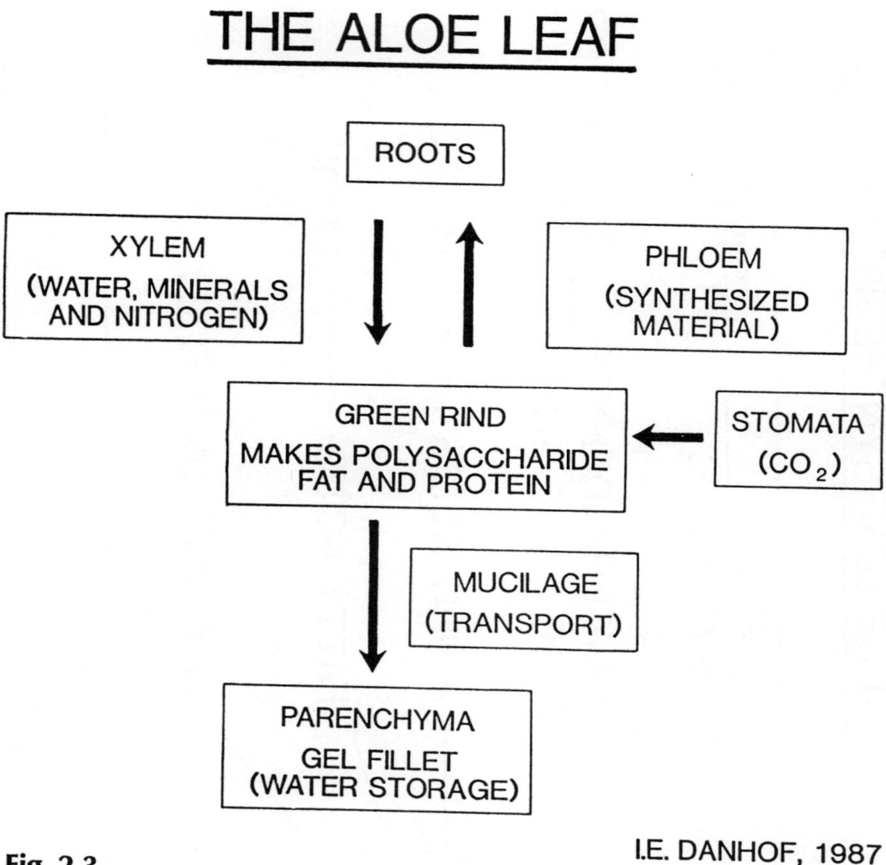
THE ALOE LEAF
ROOTS
XYLEM
(WATER, MINERALS
AND NITROGEN)
PHLOEM
(SYNTHESIZED
MATERIAL)
GREEN RIND
MAKES POLYSACCHARIDE
FAT AND PROTEIN
STOMATA
(CO_2)
MUCILAGE
(TRANSPORT)
PARENCHYMA
GEL FILLET
(WATER STORAGE)
I.E. DANHOF, 1987

Fig. 2.3.

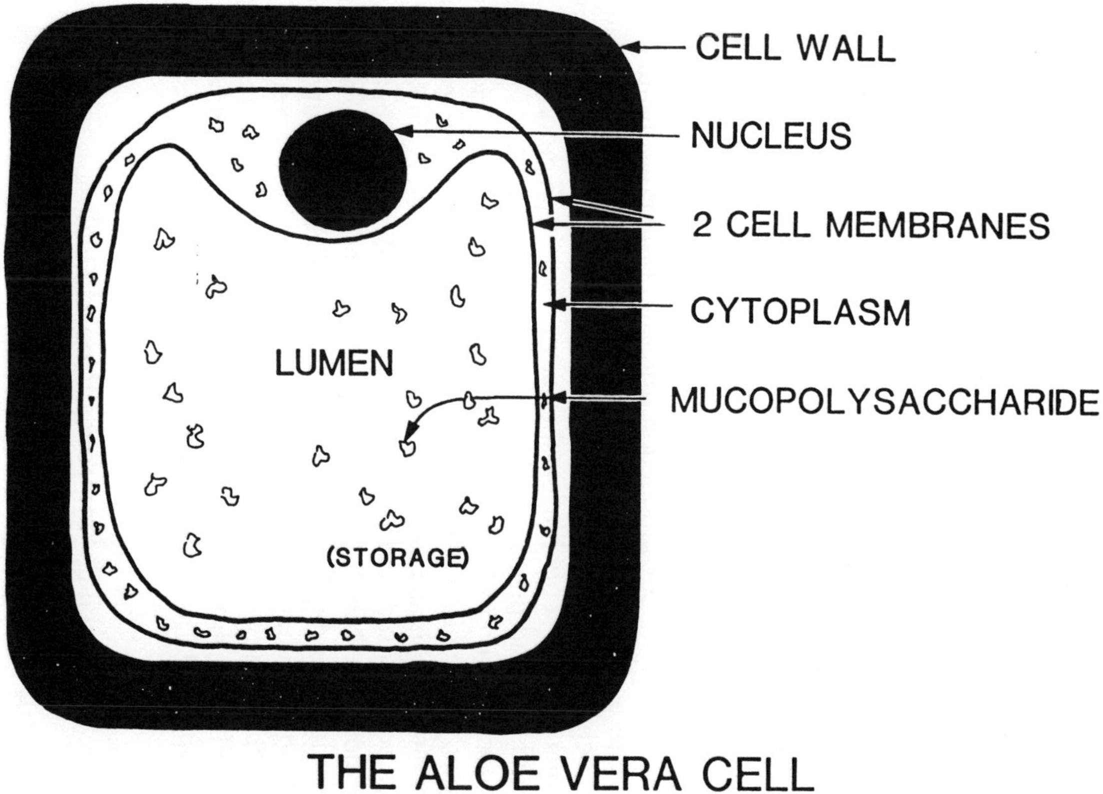
CELL WALL
NUCLEUS
2 CELL MEMBRANES
CYTOPLASM
MUCOPOLYSACCHARIDE
LUMEN
(STORAGE)
THE ALOE VERA CELL

Fig. 2.4.

mucilage under the rind. Since mucilage is bioactive, mucopolysaccharide is active. Mucopolysaccharides have a ratio of one glucose to six mannose molecules.[9] The glucose molecule is attached to the protein by a covalent bond. We have attempted to separate the protein from the polysaccharide so that we can characterize its biological activity. However, we failed to do so, because the bond was stronger than we thought. Possibly some of the growth factor characteristics could be coming from the protein. Anabolic or repair effects are usually associated with proteins. The polysaccharide chain has protein at one end and mannose phosphate (not glucose) at the other end. The mannose phosphate fits into the insulin-like growth factor receptor of the fibroblast to cause cell growth and repair.[10] Stimulation of the fibroblast by aloe vera forms collagen and proteoglycans to improve wound repair.

When we measure the metabolic activity of fresh aloe vera leaf at 1, 3, and 9 grams, we obtained a dose-response relationship of O_2 consumption and CO_2 production using the Columbus Institute O_2/CO_2 respirometer. This instrument is similar to the "old Warburg" but much more sensitive (figure 2.5). The biological activity of the "starting" aloe gel could reflect the activity of the end product manufactured. The end-product biological activity should have a straight-line function with O_2/CO_2 recorded in the initial aloe gel. However, if bacteria or fungus is present, an O_2/CO_2 response will be recorded, depending on the amount of bacteria or fungus present. In fact, this assay could be used to evaluate the anti-bacterial or anti-fungal activity of aloe vera. The degree of contamination in the Alaskan oil spill was evaluated using this assay method. The biological activity of aloe vera to inhibit fungus or bacteria could be tested using the respirometer in a dose-response relationship. Possibly the respirometer could be modified to show the effect of aloe on infected skin, which has great application in foot care medicine.

Mucilage Improves Wound Healing

Our electron microscope observations and the "fern reaction" suggest that mucilage is a long chain mucopolysaccharide. If the water is removed from the mucilage, what is left feels and looks like a bandage. It follows that when mucilage is placed over a wound,

METABOLIC ACTIVITY IN FRESH ALOE VERA LEAF GEL

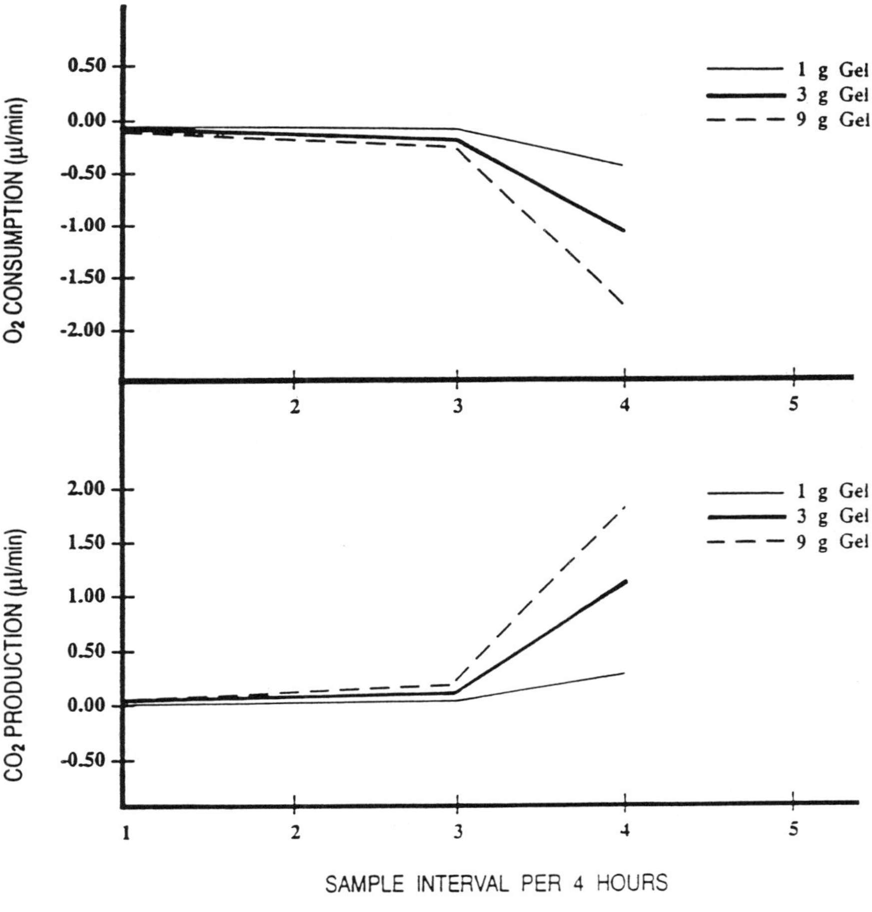

Fig. 2.5.

the wound area remains moist and does not drop, as seen in dry wounds. As a result, the epidermal and fibroblast growth factors come from the mucilage to stimulate the fibroblasts and epidermal cells for growth and repair. The cells migrate in a proper manner to increase wound healing. We allowed the wound to be exposed to the open air to get oxygen. However, this dries the wound and slows repair. The occlusive nature (cover) of mucilage increases wound healing from a mechanical and an endocrine viewpoint. Also, mucilage has good anti-inflammatory activity.

When an animal bites into the aloe leaf a hole in the leaf is produced, so there is the opportunity for the gel fillet to leak to the outside. However, this does not occur. The mucilage hardens and acts as a container that seals the hole and repairs it so that the gel does not become contaminated. The transformation of the mucilage from a liquid (sol) to a gel we call a sol-gel transformation. The sol-gel transformation of aloe is a significant discovery when the concepts are transferred from the aloe leaf to wound healing. Many parallels can be drawn between the healing of a wounded aloe plant and the needs of wounded animal tissue. The ability of aloe to conserve the water of burned animal tissue, in addition to its anti-inflammatory and analgesic ability, makes it a tremendous natural treatment. The transfer of energy from a sol (in which molecules are in random motion) to the fixed gel may go to the wound or inflammation to produce a natural therapy. Our electron microscope observations as well as the "fern reaction" suggest that mucilage is a long chain polysaccharide. The nature of the polysaccharide is not known; however, it probably relates to the protein in a manner similar to the plastic bristles attached to the wooden handle of a brush. It would be a major discovery if we could transfer the sol-gel transformation from the leaf to the wound. More work needs to be done on this aspect of aloe vera to make it a valuable product for health care. Transformation from a sol to a gel can be brought about by changes in temperature, ph, salt concentration, pressure, and agitation (figure 2.6).

The Aloe Leaf Assay

Samples of the aloe leaf (18mm diameter) were taken at constant intervals from the lateral tip to the base and weighed. A sample

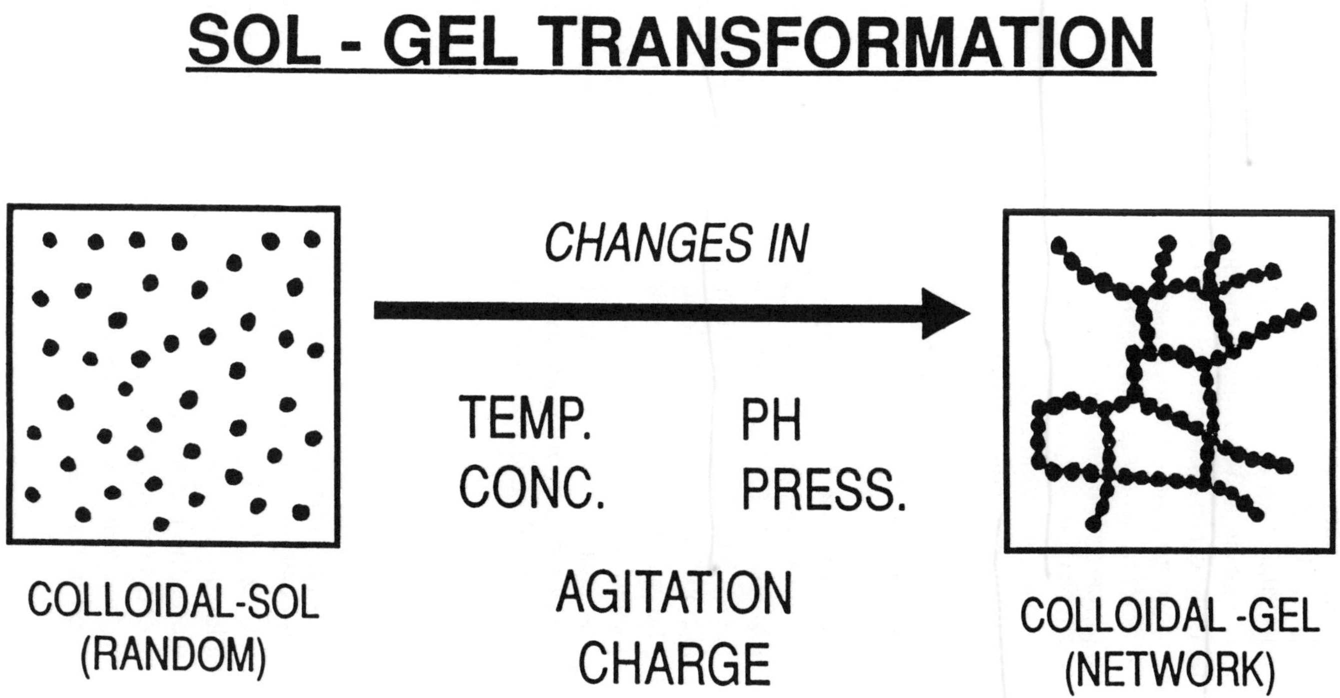
SOL - GEL TRANSFORMATION
CHANGES IN
TEMP.
CONC.
PH
PRESS.
AGITATION
CHARGE
COLLOIDAL-SOL
(RANDOM)
COLLOIDAL -GEL
(NETWORK)

Fig. 2.6.

weight (gm) to length (cm) relationship was obtained (figure 2.7). A straight-line relationship was recorded over the entire leaf. The slope, least squares, and "no evidence of a plateau" make the leaf assay ideal for comparing leaves and the production of aloe by plants per acre. The assay is fast, economical and easy to perform. As the fillet increases in weight, the rind decreases. The mean value for rind was 37.9±2.7 percent whereas the mean for fillet plus mucilage was 60.2±2.6 percent. The relationship between rind and fillet is shown in figure 2.8. Wind increases the gel from 49.1±1.8 percent to 70.02±2.3 percent. Wind also increases the percentage of water in relation to solids as evidence that wind decreases the viscosity so as to transport the gel from tip to leaf base to nourish "pup leaves" in the inner circle of leaves (figures 2.9, 2.10, and 2.11). In fact, the gel per leaf was increased from 208–241 to 269–305 gm by wind. These ranges represent the 95 percent confident limits for the assay. We feel that wind increased the amount of aloe vera in the leaf greater than 100 percent (figure 2.12 and 2.13). We should also mention that soil is a variable to this point, as the leaves were grown in two different places. Nevertheless, the wind increased the relative glucose from 351.5±69.7 ug/mg in controls to 696.2±114 ug/mg in leaves grown in the wind ($P<0.05$) (figure 2.14). When all the variables were controlled similar results were recorded in figures 2.15 and 2.16. The increase in aloe production by the wind could range from 100 to 2,300 percent. In our opinion, assaying the amount of glucose per mg of solid presents a good estimate of the amount of aloe vera in the leaf.

Summary

These results indicate that we can assay the amount of aloe vera accurately by weight as well as by using specific activity of glucose or the O_2/CO_2 relationship in the gel. The latter can be used to assess contamination as well as antibacterial/fungal activity of aloe vera. Wind increases the production of aloe vera 100 to 2,300 percent. If fans are placed strategically in a "greenhouse" or in a field, one can significantly increase the production of aloe. The aloe leaf assay could be used to compare the activity of leaves as well as show the

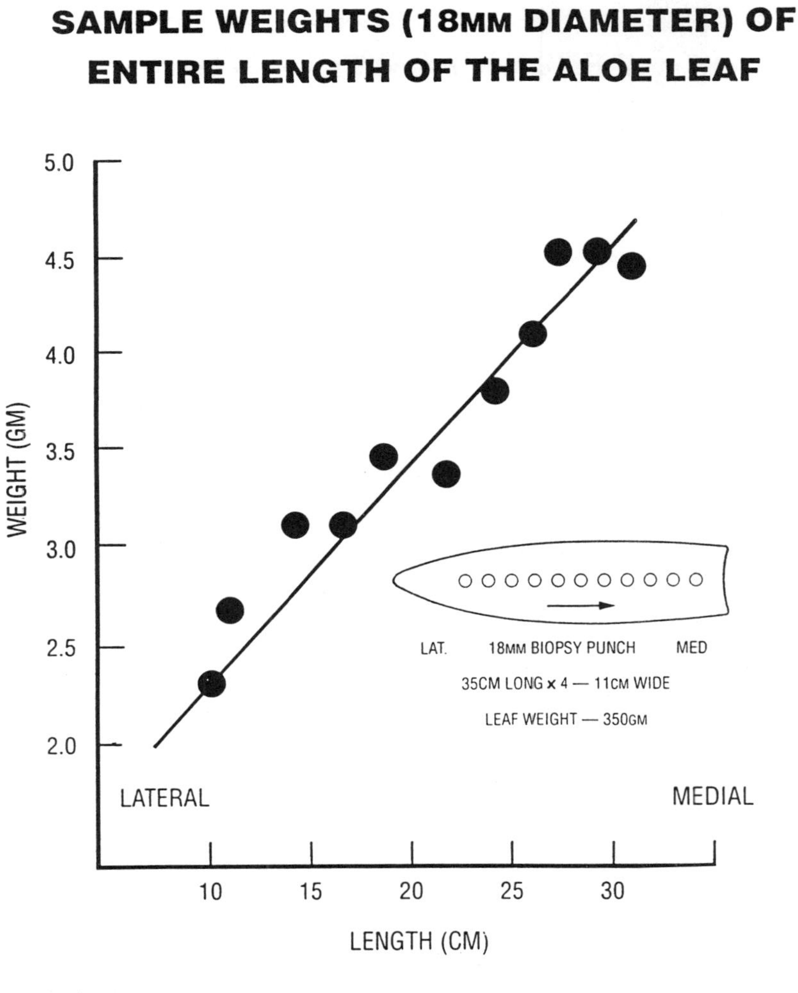
SAMPLE WEIGHTS (18MM DIAMETER) OF
ENTIRE LENGTH OF THE ALOE LEAF
5.0
4.5
4.0
3.5
3.0
2.5
2.0
WEIGHT (GM)
LAT.
18MM BIOPSY PUNCH
MED
35CM LONG x 4 — 11CM WIDE
LEAF WEIGHT — 350GM
LATERAL
MEDIAL
10
15
20
25
30
LENGTH (CM)

Fig. 2.7.

PERCENT COMPOSITION OF THE ALOE LEAF BY WEIGHT

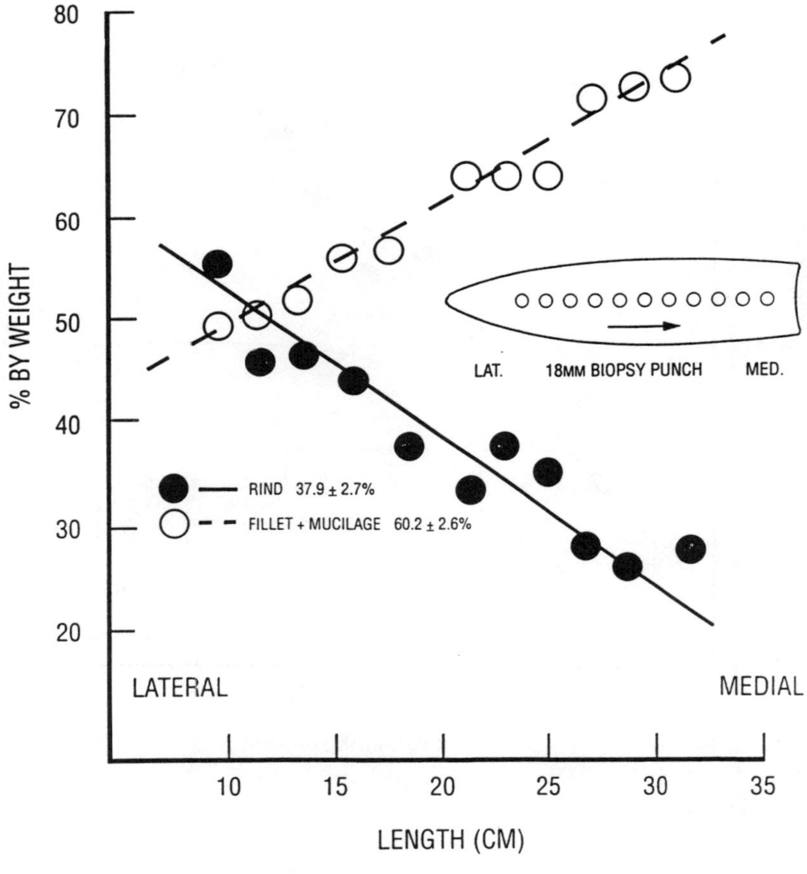

Fig. 2.8.

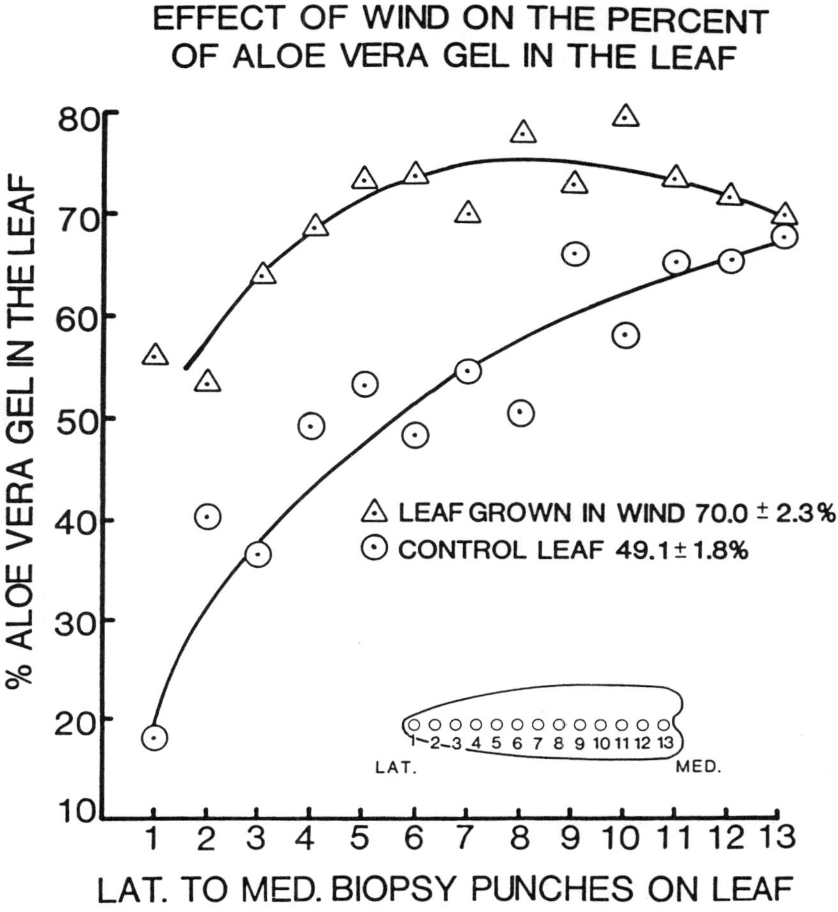

EFFECT OF WIND ON THE PERCENT
OF ALOE VERA GEL IN THE LEAF
% ALOE VERA GEL IN THE LEAF
80
70
60
50
40
30
20
10
LEAF GROWN IN WIND 70.0 ± 2.3%
CONTROL LEAF 49.1 ± 1.8%
1 2 3 4 5 6 7 8 9 10 11 12 13
LAT.
MED.
1 2 3 4 5 6 7 8 9 10 11 12 13
LAT. TO MED. BIOPSY PUNCHES ON LEAF

Fig. 2.9.

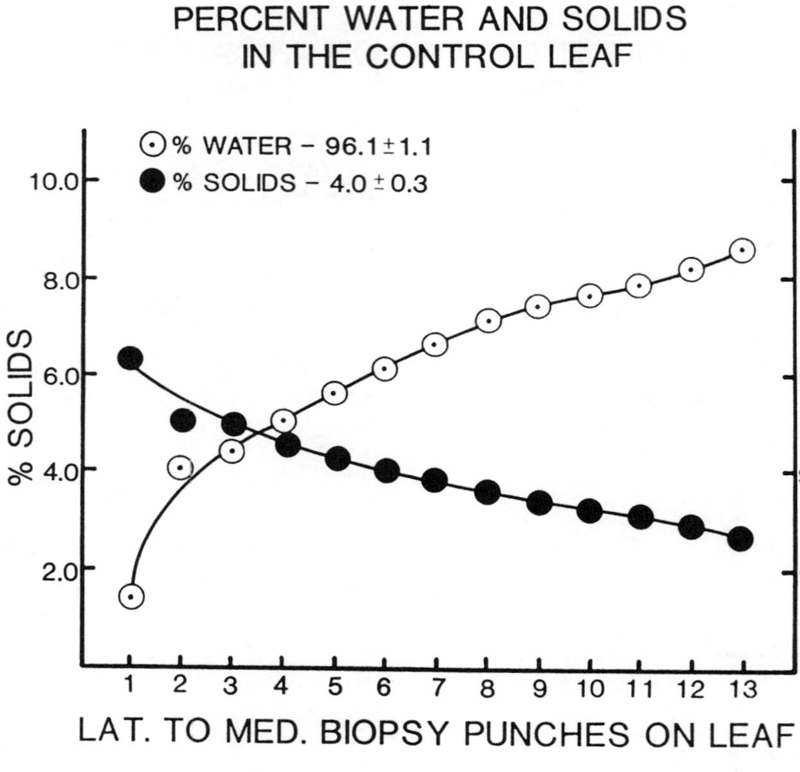
PERCENT WATER AND SOLIDS
IN THE CONTROL LEAF
% WATER - 96.1 ± 1.1
% SOLIDS - 4.0 ± 0.3
% SOLIDS
% WATER
10.0
8.0
6.0
4.0
2.0
98
97
96
95
94
93
1 2 3 4 5 6 7 8 9 10 11 12 13
LAT. TO MED. BIOPSY PUNCHES ON LEAF

Fig. 2.10.

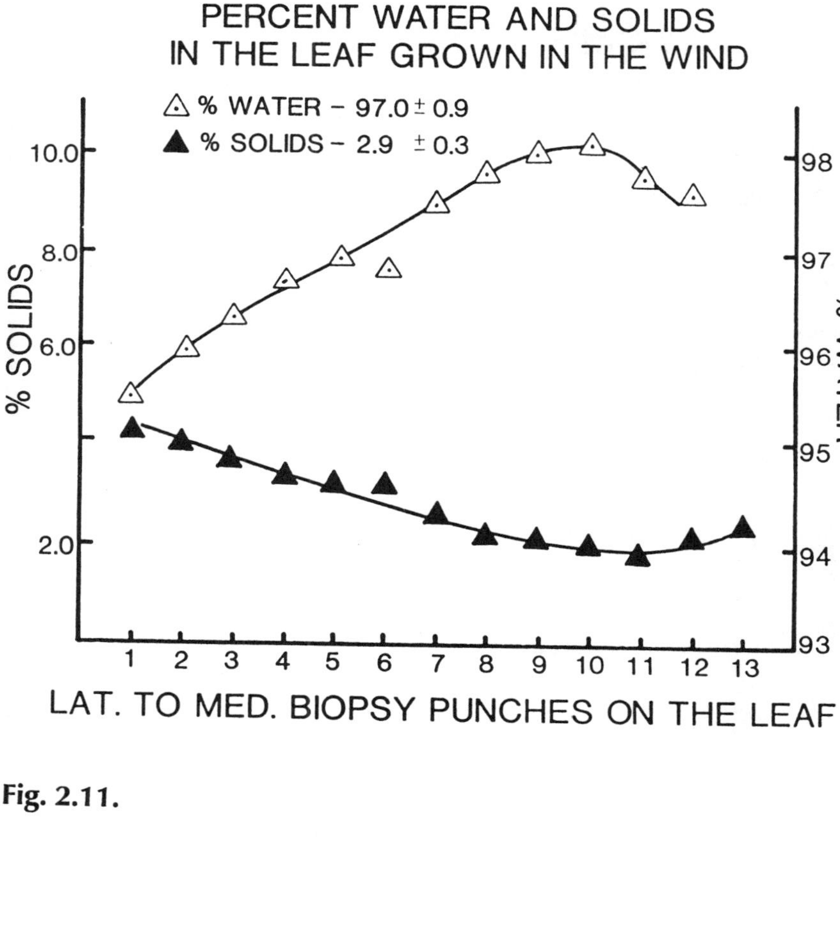

PERCENT WATER AND SOLIDS
IN THE LEAF GROWN IN THE WIND
% WATER - 97.0 ± 0.9
% SOLIDS - 2.9 ± 0.3
% SOLIDS
% WATER
10.0
8.0
6.0
2.0
98
97
96
95
94
93
1
2
3
4
5
6
7
8
9
10
11
12
13
LAT. TO MED. BIOPSY PUNCHES ON THE LEAF

Fig. 2.11.

Effect of Wind on the Amount of Aloe Vera Gel in the Leaf

	CONTROL LEAF	LEAF GROWN IN WIND
Leaf wt (gm)	457.0	410.0
Sample wt (gm/18mm)	2.6 ± 0.2	4.3 ± 0.3
Rind (%)	45.8 ± 3.8	29.1 ± 2.1
Gel (%)	49.1 ± 1.8	70.0 ± 2.3
Solid (%)	4.0 ± 0.3	2.9 ± 0.3
Water (%)	96.1 ± 1.1	97.0 ± 0.9
Gel / Leaf (gm)	224.4 ± 8.2	287.0 ± 9.0
	(208 - 241)	(269 - 305)

13 sample wt / leaf. Soil chemistry is a variable.

Fig. 2.12.

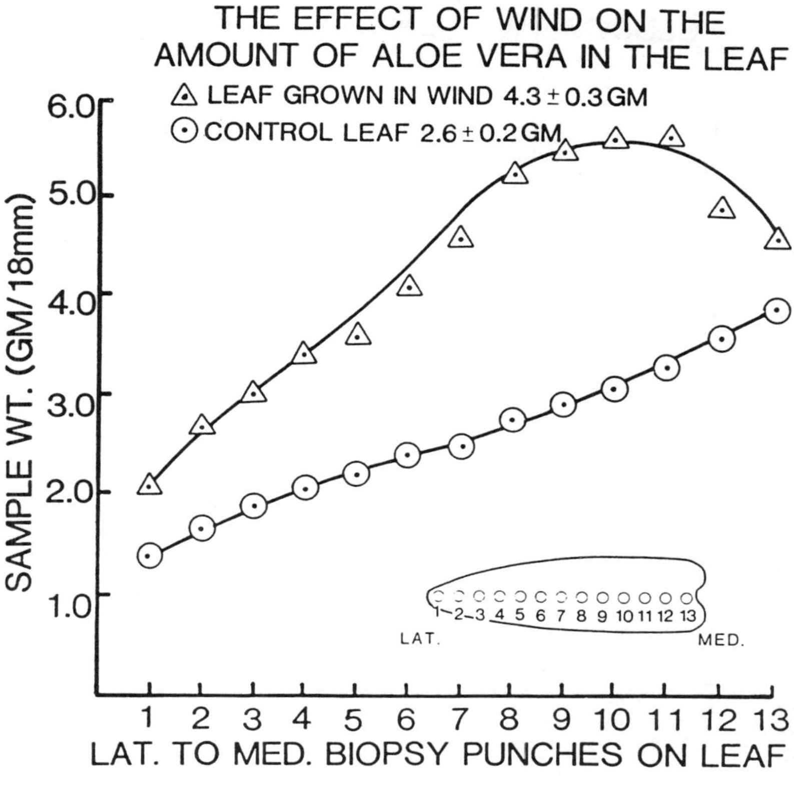
THE EFFECT OF WIND ON THE
AMOUNT OF ALOE VERA IN THE LEAF
LEAF GROWN IN WIND 4.3 ± 0.3 GM
CONTROL LEAF 2.6 ± 0.2 GM
SAMPLE WT. (GM/18mm)
6.0
5.0
4.0
3.0
2.0
1.0
1 2 3 4 5 6 7 8 9 10 11 12 13
LAT. TO MED. BIOPSY PUNCHES ON LEAF
LAT.
MED.

Fig. 2.13.

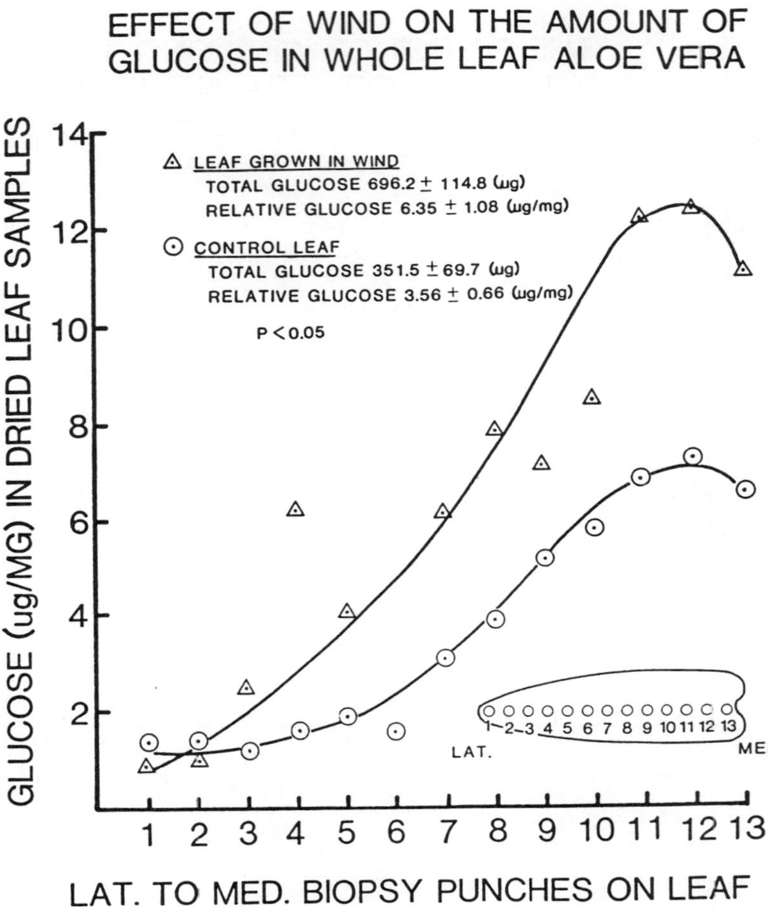

EFFECT OF WIND ON THE AMOUNT OF GLUCOSE IN WHOLE LEAF ALOE VERA
LEAF GROWN IN WIND
TOTAL GLUCOSE 696.2 ± 114.8 (ug)
RELATIVE GLUCOSE 6.35 ± 1.08 (ug/mg)
CONTROL LEAF
TOTAL GLUCOSE 351.5 ± 69.7 (ug)
RELATIVE GLUCOSE 3.56 ± 0.66 (ug/mg)
P < 0.05
GLUCOSE (ug/MG) IN DRIED LEAF SAMPLES
14
12
10
8
6
4
2
1 2 3 4 5 6 7 8 9 10 11 12 13
LAT.
MED.
1 2 3 4 5 6 7 8 9 10 11 12 13
LAT. TO MED. BIOPSY PUNCHES ON LEAF

Fig. 2.14.

PERCENT INCREASE IN ALOE VERA GEL BY WIND IN LEAVES FROM LAT. TIP TO MED. BASE OF LEAF

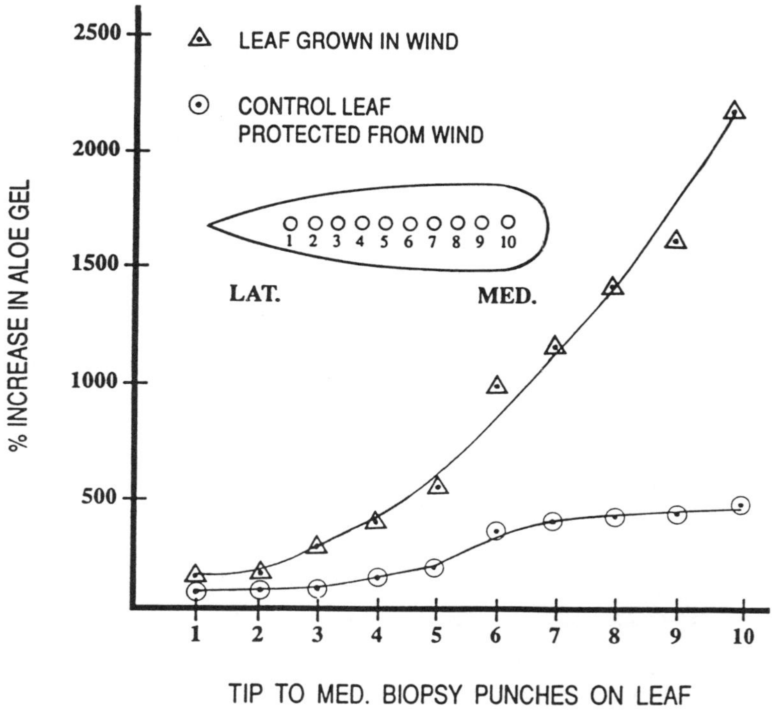

Fig. 2.15.

EFFECT OF WIND ON THE AMOUNT OF GLUCOSE IN WHOLE LEAF ALOE VERA

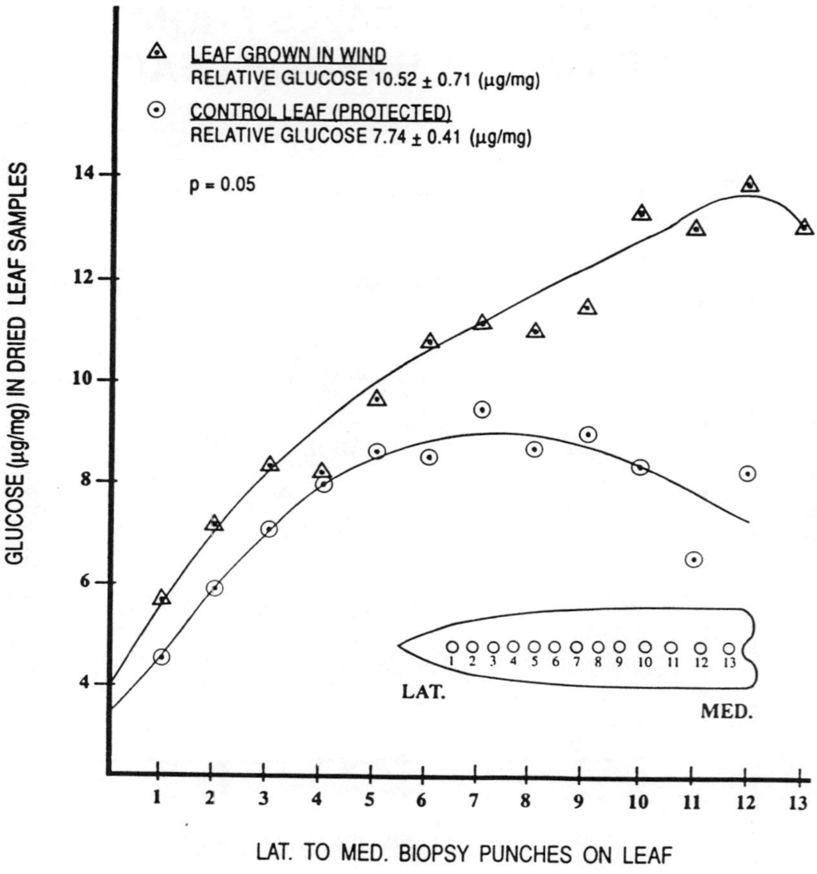

Fig. 2.16.

various influences on aloe vera production. The transfer of the healing of the aloe leaf to the healing of a wound will change the way medical personnel address the wound care problem. The mechanism in which the healing gel works must be analogous to the regular mechanism of action of aloe. The properties of the gel are such that it can act as a seal to prevent the escape of water and growth factors from the wound, which contributes to its "healing powers."

References

1. I. E. Danhof, *Remarkable Aloe: Aloe through the Ages,* vol. 1 (Grand Prairie, Tx: Omnimedicus Press, 1987).
2. P. Moroni, "Aloe in Cosmetic Formulation," *Cosmetic Technology,* September 1982, 42.
3. W. B. Day, "The Botany of Aloe," *Journal of the American Pharmacological Association* 11 (1992): 620.
4. F. R. Bharucha and G. V. Joshi, "Effect of Prolonged Darkness on Acid Metabolism in the Leaves of Aloe Vera Linnaeus," *Science and Culture,* 22 (1957): 389.
5. H. T. Blackhurt, A. F. De Werth, and B. A. Perry, *Aloe's Departmental Information Report,* Department of Soil and Crop Sciences, Texas A&M University, College Station, Texas, 1970.
6. Danhof, *Remarkable Aloe.*
7. R. H. Davis, "Comments on the Aloe Leaf," *Aloe Today* (Galveston, TX: Aloe Research Foundation, 1992).
8. S. P. Bartakke "Photosynthesis in Aloe vera var. indica," *Indian Science Congress Association Proceedings,* 62 (1975): 99.
9. D. Gowda, B. Neelisiddaiah, and Y. Anjaneyalo, "Structural Studies of Polysaccharides from Aloe Vera," *Carbohydrate Research,* 72 (1979): 201.
10. R. H. Davis, J. J. DiDonato, G. M. Hartman, and R. C. Haas, "Mannose-6-Phosphate: Anti-Inflammatory and Wound Healing Activity of a Growth Substance in Aloe Vera," *Journal of the American Podiatric Medical Association* 84 (1994): 77.

3

The Making of Aloe Vera

Early Medical Uses of Aloe

Aloe was listed in the Ebers papyrus (1500 B.C.) as an established cathartic. Alexander the Great, who died in 323 B.C. mentioned the virtues of aloe. Greek physicians wrote about their success in treating wounds, hemorrhoids, and hair loss (A.D. 75). In fact, Dioscorides, who accompanied Nero's army, mentioned aloe in his writings. Dioscorides stated that aloe could be used to treat wounds, heal skin infections, cure chapping, reduce hair loss, and eliminate hemorrhoids. In the Orient, aloe was used for eczema (A.D. 700). Aloe was primarily used as a cathartic, since some of the early applications are not well substantiated.[†] These applications include: dermatitis, burns, acne, ulcers, lacerations, colds, tuberculosis, dysentery, and headaches. In 1935, C. E. Collins and C. Collins published the first credible medical report on the use of aloe vera.[2] A woman received a significant dose of X ray on her scalp causing her to experience a radiodermatitis. For months she was unable to experience relief by the traditional forms of treatment. She applied the inner gelatinous fresh aloe vera leaf directly to her scalp wound. Within a day or so, she noted relief from itching and burning. In a few weeks her dermatitis was completely healed. Other studies reported, since then, have verified the Collins report. In China, aloe vera has been used as a common household remedy for centuries. In Mexico, aloe is used to treat skin problems. In the United States, aloe is used in herbalism and homeopathy. Madis Laboratories listed over one hundred medical disorders that have been treated by aloe. Some people feel that aloe vera is some kind of miracle drug. The skyrocketing sales of aloe vera cosmetics make many believe that they have found the fountain of youth in the aloe vera plant. The association of aloe vera with life has made its way into modern advertising. A plant that can heal its own wounds is certainly worth a try on man's wounds. While these early results with aloe vera revealed positive results, much of the work suffered from poor experimental design and small test samples. As a result, this early data was conflicting and inconsistent. However, the new experimental studies showed important and distinct physiological effects that were repeatable.

Significant Research Reports

Beginning with the early research of Collins and Collins in 1935, aloe vera was placed on a more sound foundation because investigators began to move from simple observation to experimental design. In the 1960s and '70s men like Farkas, Davis, Fujita, Waller, and Gowda began investigating the individual components of Aloe. Then, more recently, men like Danhof, McAnalley, Heggers, and Davis began to investigate the physiology and mechanism of action of aloe vera. From these important research reports have come many valuable concepts that have great therapeutic potential. The following reports are worth noting:

Collins and Collins, 1935—the first significant clinical use of aloe vera gel. They treated roentgen dermatitis with whole-leaf aloe vera gel. They split the leaf and macerated the gel. The aloe was then put in place with a bandage.[3]

Crewe, 1937—successfully used fresh aloe vera to treat eczema and ulcers. There was a cessation of pain and healing by aloe.[4]

Rowe, 1941—healing of radiation burns in rats were improved by aloe vera. Rowe found that 64 percent of the rats treated with gel showed an increased rate of healing. Complete healing in rats was recorded in six days.[5]

Farkas, 1963—reported on the amount of glucose and mannose as well as uronic acid in aloe vera gel.[6]

Fujita, 1976—showed bradykinase and carboxypeptidase activity in aloe arborescens.[7]

Waller, 1978—analyzed an acetone extract of macerated whole-leaf aloe for polysaccharide components, amino acids, and sterols. This is a landmark report.[8]

Gowda, 1979—presented important structural findings of polysaccharides in aloe vera. Gowda showed the linkage between sugars was 1–4. The molar ratio of mannose to glucose was 6:1. A great deal of research has this study as its foundation.[9]
Winters, 1981—found that fresh aloe vera leaves contained lectin-like compounds that increased the growth of normal human cells in tissue culture but not tumor cells.[10]
Yagi, 1982—reported on calcium isocitrate, which acted as a potent cardiac stimulant, and on a glycoprotein with antibradykinin activity.[11]
Danhof and McAnalley, 1983—obtained a dose-response relationship by increasing the dose of fresh aloe gel on human fibroblast growth in tissue culture. Yellow sap caused death of fibroblasts.[12]
Heggers and Robson, 1983—observed that aloe vera had antibacterial and anti-prostaglandin activity. Aloe prevented the vascular supply to the dermis in burned animals.[13]
Bland, 1985—evaluated the effect of oral aloe vera on gastric ph, stool specific gravity, protein digestion/absorption, and stool microbiology. The results showed that aloe has a beneficial influence on the gastrointestinal tract.[14]
Labadie, 1988—obtained two functionally and chemically distinct immunomodulatory compounds in the gel of aloe vera.[15]
Davis, 1991—separated the inhibitory anti-inflammatory system from the stimulatory wound healing system in aloe vera.[16]

Chemical Composition of Aloe Vera

The chemical components of aloe vera have been divided into sixteen groups. I counted some 100 compounds (table 3.1). However, if all the compounds in aloe vera were identified and counted, it is estimated the number would be greater than two hundred. This is a reasonable estimate of those ingredients that are responsible for the biological activity in aloe vera.[17] Anthraquinones have a laxative function, but they also have other important pharmacologic properties. They have anti-viral and anti-bacterial as well as anti-tumor activity. Certain anthraquinones are viricidal for both RNA and DNA envelopes. Working with three anthraquinones, our laboratory found

CHEMICAL COMPOSITION OF ALOE VERA

ANTHRAQUINONES (12)	STEROIDS (?)
INORGANIC IONS (9)	STEROLS (3)
SACCHARIDES (5)	LIGNINS (?)
ENZYMES (5)	URIC ACID (1)
AMINO ACIDS (19)	GIBBERELLIN (30)
CHOLESTEROL (1)	LECTIN LIKE SUBSTANCES (?)
TRIGLYCERIDES (?)	SALICYLIC ACID (1)
VITAMINS (8)	SAPONINS (?)

( ) = NUMBER OF COMPOUNDS.

Table 3.1.

that these anthraquinones had anti-inflammatory activity, but this activity was obtained by working through inflammation.[18] The inorganic minerals are well represented in aloe. Calcium is necessary for growth of bone. If calcium is deficient, poor growth results. Zinc is very important for wound healing. Mice fed zinc-deficient diets had poor wound healing. If zinc is supplemented in the diet, wound healing is improved.[19] Copper is also present in aloe. Copper works with oxidative enzymes for proper metabolic functions of the body. There are five saccharides in aloe. Mannose phosphate has good wound-healing and anti-inflammatory activity.[20] Mannose is the principal monosaccharide in the polysaccharide polymer of aloe vera. Vitamin B complex and vitamin C play a role in stress and inflammation. Our laboratory found that the B complex could maintain adrenalectomized rats and vitamin C reduced the inflammation in adjuvant-induced arthritis.[21] The lignins are involved in the pulp fibers of the leaf with cellulose. The saponins are glycosides that have cleansing and antiseptic actions. Some twenty amino acids are present in aloe vera. At least eight amino acids have anti-inflammatory activity. Some of these amino acids are effective against burns. Some five enzymes have been identified, but I am certain there are many more in aloe vera leaf gel. Three sterols in aloe vera have anti-inflammatory activity. B-sitosterol, also, had mild estrogenic activity.[22] Gibberellin, a growth factor in aloe, buffers these actions so that aloe's wound healing action can be expressed.[23] Salicylic acid has both analgesic and anti-inflammatory activity. Amino acids and sterols can be synergistic in some of these actions.[24] From an evaluation of the biologically active components in aloe vera, the total biological activity comes from a synergistic modulation of the compounds involved rather than from a single "magic bullet."[25] In any event, one sees the great potential for healing in aloe vera. The polysaccharide (conductor) in aloe synergizes with the surrounding two hundred or so active compounds by means of water. The end result is the fine array of biological activities. When this balance is disturbed, the therapeutic value of aloe vera is harmed.

The efficacy of aloe vera may be due to its miracle components, plus the fact that aloe is 95 percent water. Aloe vera makes water available to wounds in an occlusive manner. Water must be added to the lyophilized aloe vera to obtain the biological activities of aloe vera. Water plays a major role in the relationship between the polysaccharide and the two hundred estimated active compounds in aloe. The interaction between the conductor and the orchestra arises from water's polarity. Water has a positive and negative charge at either end of the molecule. The orchestra molecules and the conductor polysaccharide possess both polar and non-polar parts. The polarity of water molecules aligns their negative ends with the positive ends of other molecules. The polarized water molecules connect the conductor polysaccharide with the orchestra molecules in aloe vera. The water thus allows the polysaccharide to communicate with the surrounding biologically active molecules.[26]

What is "Good Aloe?"

"Good aloe" means that it has positive or desirable qualities. It means that it is complete and of high quality suitable for public use. Danhof was asked: "What is the best aloe vera?" He answered, "What do you want to use the aloe for?" The best aloe depends on the biological actions the final product contains. It should not contain materials that produce a negative effect. Since aloe vera contains more than two hundred constituents in less than 1 percent of solid, it follows that aloe should be processed in such a way as to make sure that all the components are present in satisfactory amounts and not altered by the processing. The active components must be preserved with all their biological actions and benefits.[27]

The basic procedure for processing aloe begins when the leaves are harvested. The leaves require adequate water but not too much. Aloe plants survive well in shade. Aloe leaves tolerate heat but do not do well in the cold. In fact, freezing produces many injurious effects to aloe leaves. When the leaves are harvested they are transported to a processing facility where they are washed and sanitized. After cleansing, the inner gel is separated from the rind. The gel is then freed from the cellulose pulp. The two major processing procedures used in the aloe industry to give us aloe are:

1. *Fillet method:* The rind is removed by a large knife or equivalent mechanical method. The yellow sap containing the

irritating anthraquinones is removed. However, the mucilage, which once was left on the meat table, is now carefully collected for product development. Since 12 percent of the total solids come from the rind, the total solids are less than that recorded for the whole-leaf method.

2. *Whole-Leaf Method:* The leaf is chopped into small pieces, and the rind particles are removed by passing the aloe through filters of various pore sizes. The anthraquinones are removed by charcoal filters. However, glycoproteins and other constituents may be removed by the charcoal. This method produces an aloe higher in carbohydrates and minerals. Preservative techniques include cold or heat methods with preservatives such as sodium benzoate or potassium sorbate. Each method had advantages and disadvantages in the making of aloe vera. Controlling the temperature and sanitation conditions during the manufacturing process preserves the chemical makeup, preventing loss of biological activity.

Why make pure aloe vera? Pure unadulterated aloe vera is needed to retain all the biological properties coming from the many ingredients in aloe. Adulteration is a major concern to the aloe industry.[28] It is believed that some of the aloe producers have used maltodextrin to make up for the lack of real aloe. Diluting aloe with water, adding calcium, and adding maltodextrin to powders are ways in which aloe vera can be adulterated. Sometimes the only ingredients found in aloe liquid are the preservative and water. Adulterating the aloe is a way to increase profits and cheat the customer. Claims made by the supplier will not be true, and the consumer is mislead into thinking he is buying pure aloe, with all its therapeutic benefits. As a result, the benefits to the consumer are not there, so the customer moves away from aloe vera. When aloe is pure, all the biologically active ingredients present in the orchestra synergize together in relationship to the polysaccharide (conductor) to produce a wonderful harmony of biological activities that have important therapeutic properties. The aloe industry expects the consumer to receive aloe products that provide all the benefits present in the leaf gel. If these biological benefits are not present, the consumer loses confidence in

ADULTERATION

aloe vera. Adulteration prevents aloe vera from becoming one of the greatest products sold in the country.

The IASC has developed standards for aloe vera and has implemented a certification program that guarantees the purity of aloe vera. The solids, calcium, magnesium, and HPLC profile have provided a good base upon which to evaluate the condition of a particular aloe vera. More recently, the percentage of polysaccharide, the alcohol-precipitable total hexose, the E peak, and the ionic conductivity have been added to the arsenal so as to give us a "fingerprint" of what is good aloe vera.[29] For example, the standard ARF preparation has 7.0 percent polysaccharide, 35 mg total hexose, and a nice "E peak" on the HPLC. When maltodextrin is added to the aloe vera in adulteration, the percentage of polysaccharide increases to 50 and the total hexose measures some 250 mg. The croton oil–induced edema assay shows a good dose-response curve on anti-inflammation. Excellent results have also been obtained on wound healing and PMN infiltration to provide an excellent biological standard for aloe vera. No longer can suppliers make claim to the purity of their aloe when they are at the same time adulterating their aloe product. The IASC can now guarantee the purity of aloe vera and, at the same time, warn consumers of unscrupulous suppliers who are making fraudulent claims. The suppliers of raw aloe material must provide customers with purity information for safety and labeling compliance. The FDA prohibits adulteration of aloe, and as a result persons responsible may be subject to severe fines and long prison terms.[30] Also, the labeling act requires that the label list each ingredient in the aloe product. If the label does not include the added maltodextrin, the product is mislabeled and there is intent to defraud.

The Fact Sheet on Aloe Vera

Aloe vera is a natural substance that contains many biologically active molecules. The molecules harmonize with the polysaccharide, according to our conductor-orchestra concept, to produce a beautiful spectrum of biological activities that give us many therapeutic benefits. Many of these active agents have been isolated, identified, and fractionated. The numerous biological activities of aloe can be used to characterize and discover new factors as well as to standardize aloe vera. A well-defined unit can be obtained for each biological activity so that new factors can be discovered and aloe vera can be put on a standard unit basis. In this way aloe vera can be standardized on a biological as well as a chemical basis. When aloe vera is put on a burn or wound, the many biologically active substances do not act in a random fashion but rather in a specific beneficial direction. Aloe vera with all its components, rather than a single component, should be the standard for aloe vera research.

Current evidence suggests that aloe vera contains a large polysaccharide molecule, which we have called the conductor. This molecule leads the many biologically active substances into a symphony of biological events to heal wounds, reduce inflammation, and eliminate pain. The conductor molecule fits into the fibroblasts, similar to a lock and key mechanism, so as to set in motion a cascade of important biological events, supported by aloe substances, which are part of the orchestra. The polarity of water is needed for the polysaccharide to communicate with the active substances to synergistically achieve the maximal desired benefits. I oppose the prevailing theory that there is only one active molecule in aloe (a polysaccharide) responsible for all its beneficial effects. In fact, all the biologically active substances in aloe vera are necessary to achieve the maximum end-benefit. This does not mean that we should not look at the individual ingredients in aloe for specific applications. Aloe vera can be used to attack an entire spectrum of human conditions when specific synergisms are brought into sharper focus. The research that is going on with aloe vera can potentially change many of the pharmacologic-endocrine concepts in the future.[31]

Aloe vera acts by inhibiting pain and inflammation as well as by stimulating wound healing in a dose-response fashion. Increasing the dose of aloe increases the biological response.[32] Mediators in aloe vera are believed to be responsible for these beneficial effects. Aloe vera improves the healing of open wounds and increases the wound tensile strength of incisional wounds. In both cases, aloe vera forms a straight-line dose-response curve, which can be used to standardize aloe preparations. The growth factors (gibberellin) stimulate fibroblasts to improve wound healing by increasing collagen and proteoglycans.[33] The sterols present in aloe vera contribute to the anti-inflammatory activity but inhibit wound healing. Gibberellin blocks the sterol inhibition of wound healing but enhances the anti-inflammatory response.[34] Growth factors modulate the anti-inflammatory and wound-healing effects such that aloe vera possesses both beneficial responses in a balanced way.

Aloe vera prevents and regresses adjuvant-induced arthritis with its inflammation.[35] The infiltration of PMNs induced by irritants can be blocked by aloe vera, suggesting that Aloe inhibits leukotrienes.[36] Irritants can release vasocative substances from mast cells, which cause vasodilation and edema. Our laboratory investigated the entire spectrum of irritants to produce acute inflammation by the release of mediators such as prostaglandin and histamine. The inhibition of these irritants by aloe tells us something about "how aloe works" because each irritant works through a different biochemical pathway. Both stimulatory and inhibitory components have been identified in aloe.[37] This means that aloe can act as a modulator of both immune and inflammatory reactions. Aloe can suppress the immune response in adjuvant arthritis but can also act as a stimulator of wound healing and antibody production. Aloe acts as an immune-modulator by influencing the production of lymphocyte and macrophage-derived mediators. Oxygen radicals can be picked up by vitamin C in aloe vera to reduce inflammation.

Compounds that are poorly absorbed through the stratum corneum of the skin require a vehicle to help them penetrate. Only 1 percent of steroids are absorbed, and the rest are wasted. Our data suggests that aloe vera aids in the absorption of hydrocortisone and adds to its biological activity. Aloe helps solubilize compounds and hydrates the stratum corneum in aiding compounds to penetrate the skin. Aloe can add or even synergize its biological activity with agents in producing their biological response. Thus aloe vera is a "biological vehicle."[38] Compounds that inhibit inflammation we have made part of the inhibitory system of aloe vera. Substances in aloe that improve wound healing and stimulate antibody production are called the stimulatory system. When a cell is stimulated, it selects an appropriate response, which is referred to as modulation. Modulation in aloe vera involves the interplay of many compounds rather than the action of a single "magic bullet."[39] R. P. Labadie found in aloe two substances. One substance stimulated antibody production, and another inhibited antibodies.[40] A similar story can be told in regard to cellular immunity. The antagonism between the anti-inflammatory or the inhibitory system on the stimulatory wound-healing system represents the synergy-antagonism of aloe components in modulation.

Some Thoughts on Government Regulation

The Food, Drug, and Cosmetic Act is the basic food and drug law of the United States. It is the most extensive law of its kind in the world. Many of the states have laws similar to the federal law or have added provisions to the federal requirement. This law assures the consumer that foods are pure, safe to eat, and produced under sanitary conditions. This law by itself tells us why we must make pure aloe. The law further states that foods, drugs, and devices must be safe and effective for their intended use. For example, cosmetics must be safe and must have the appropriate ingredients. The labeling and packaging must be truthful, informative, and not deceptive. The term *adulterated* includes products that are defective, unsafe, filthy, or produced under unsanitary conditions. *Misbranded,* includes statements, designs, or labelings that are false or misleading. Failure to register a drug, food, or device is a crime. The act provides that foods, drugs, or cosmetics are adulterated if they contain a color additive that has not been proven safe by the FDA. The color additive can be a dye, pigment, or some substance that imparts a color to the food.[41]

The FDA defines foods as articles used by man and animals as food. A food is adulterated or illegal if a harmful substance is added that may render the food injurious to a person's health. Food additives must be safe before they can become part of the food. A food is illegal if it is prepared, packed, or held under unsanitary conditions that can render it harmful to health. Aloe vera must be prepared and processed under the best conditions to provide the maximum benefit to a person's health. It is true that we are what we eat. The ingredients in a food must be listed by their common name in their order by weight unless the food is standardized. The label must include those ingredients. The ingredient does not refer to the chemical composition but rather the food components. Supplying a special dietary need such as a vitamin or mineral to the diet must comply with the FDA act. The label must provide all the information pertaining to the supplement. Aloe vera falls under the category of a food or nutritional supplement. The total processing falls under the category of food, additives, or nutritional supplements. Herbs or spices may be used for drug purposes and then become subject to the drug provision. If no therapeutic claims are made on the label or promotional material such herbs are regarded as foods and subject to food laws.[42]

The FDA is needed and does an outstanding job in not allowing harmful drugs on the market. However, the FDA discourages any new good drugs from coming on the market. The FDA, nevertheless, plays an essential role for evaluating the safety and efficacy of new medical treatments. The FDA in its enthusiasm precludes potentially innovative contributions from physicians, scientists, and small pharmaceutical companies that do not have the money to complete the FDA approval process. The medical profession is outstanding in treating emergency or crisis situations, but they treat all diseases in a manner that contributes to the high cost of health care. Our modern doctor knows nothing about the art of healing diseases. He relies on big, expensive equipment for crisis management. In an attempt to find inexpensive treatment, patients have had success in alternative treatments such as aloe vera and herbs.

The Access to Medical Treatment Act S-2140" would allow an individual to be treated by any licensed health care practitioner with any method of medical treatment the individual desires, so long as: 1) the treatment is not dangerous; and 2) the patient is fully informed of its side effects. The bill regulates the circumstances under which claims can be made with respect to the efficacy of the treatment. The FDA's role would not be changed. It would still have the responsibility for certifying treatments as safe and effective. The act attempts to open up the system to the use of new alternative treatments. This legislation establishes a "bypass" for the FDA approval process. Consumer protection is an essential element of this bill. It would follow that if a health care practitioner desired to treat a willing patient with aloe (virtually nontoxic at very high doses) for a condition in which there were ample proven therapeutic claims, he could do so consonant with the FDA. This is a major step forward for aloe vera and herbs.

The Hatch Amendment (table 3.2) was enacted into law on October 25, 1994, to establish standards with respect to nutritional supplements.[43] Congress found that nutrition and dietary supplements

PUBLIC LAW 103-417 - AN AMENDMENT TO THE FDA AND COSMETIC ACT TO ESTABLISH STANDARDS WITH RESPECT TO DIETARY SUPPLEMENTS AND OTHER PURPOSES (THE HATCH AMENDMENT)

---

1. PURPOSE - DIETARY SUPPLEMENTS ARE A BENEFIT TO THE HEALTH OF OUR PEOPLE.

2. DEFINITION - VITAMINS, MINERALS, AMINO ACIDS, HERB AND OTHER BOTANICALS, CONCENTRATES, EXTRACTS.

3. LABELING - TRUTHFUL AND NOT MISLEADING. AMOUNT OF EACH INGREDIENT.

4. GOOD MANUFACTURING PRACTICES - EXPIRATION DATE.

5. COMMISSION - 7 MEMBERS APPOINTED BY THE PRESIDENT. OFFICE OF DIETARY SUPPLEMENTS WITHIN NIH.

6. EFFECTIVE - DECEMBER 31, 1996

Table 3.2.

promoted health and prevented disease. They also found that there is a link between ingesting certain nutrients and preventing chronic disease such as cancer and heart disease. Fifty percent of Americans consume dietary supplements such as botanicals to improve their nutrition. This nutritional industry is an important part of the economy of the United States. A dietary supplement includes vitamins, minerals, herbs or botanicals such as aloe, concentrates, and extracts. A dietary ingredient must provide adequate information to give reasonable assurance that the ingredient will not present a significant risk of illness or injury. The name and amount of the ingredient must be determined and placed on the label in such a way that it is not misleading. Since aloe vera has over two hundred ingredients, each major category of ingredients could be identified and the amount assayed so that it is acceptable to the FDA. Aloe vera is processed differently by the different supplier companies. Thus the composition may vary slightly. Identifying the various categories of ingredients will help us to identify aloe vera.

Summary

I have traced back to the early Greeks and Egyptians the medical uses of aloe vera. Beginning with the work of Collins and Collins in 1935, the use of aloe vera in cosmetics has flourished. I also have cited some of the most significant research reports starting from the beginning. These are kind of Hall of Fame reports that show us how we got where we are in the research and development of aloe vera. These and other studies have stood the test of time. The chemical composition of aloe vera was presented to show the great potential of aloe vera. Water plays a major role in the therapeutic biological activity of Aloe. I asked the question: "What is good aloe?" The question of purity and why it is important was addressed. Standards have been developed by the IASC to guarantee purity of aloe vera. Adulteration of aloe does not have to be tolerated. This will save the aloe industry a great deal of money. A fact sheet on aloe vera gives us a "bird's-eye" view of the present status of aloe vera. Some thoughts were presented on government regulation of aloe vera. The

Hatch Amendment and the Access to Medical Treatment Act are of particular interest to the aloe industry.

References

1. B. C. Coats, and R. Ahola, *Aloe Vera the Silent Healer: A Modern Study of Aloe Vera* (Dallas, TX: Bill C. Coats, 1979), 1–288; H. N. Cole and K. K. Chen, "Aloe Vera in Oriental Dermatology," *Archives of Dermatological Syphilology,* 47 (1943): 250; K. Gottlieb, *Aloe Vera Heals: The Scientific Facts* (Denver, CO.: Royal Publications 1–31, 1980).
2. C. E. Collins and C. Collins "Roentgen Dermatitis Treated with Fresh Whole Leaf of Aloe Vera," *American Journal of Roentgenology* 33 (1935): 396.
3. Ibid.
4. J. E. Crewe, "The External Uses of Aloe," *Minnesota Medicine* 20 (1937): 670; J. E. Crewe, "Aloes in the Treatment of Burns and Scalds," *Minnesota Medicine* 22 (1939): 538.
5. T. D. Rowe, "Effect of Fresh Aloe Vera Gel in the Treatment of Third-Degree Roentgen Reactions on White Rats," *Journal of the American Pharmacological Association* (1940) 29:348; T. D. Rowe and L. M. Parks, "Phytochemical Study of Aloe Vera Leaf," *Journal of the American Pharmacological Association* (1941) 30:262; T. D. Rowe, B. K. Lovell, and L. M. Parks, "Further Observations on the Use of Aloe Vera Leaf in the Treatment of Third-Degree X-ray Reactions," *Journal of the American Pharmacological Association* 30 (1941): 266.
6. A. Farkas, "Topical Medicament including Polyuronide Derived from Aloe. U.S. Patent 3,103,466," *Chemical Abstracts* 60 (1963): 378.
7. K. Fujita and R. Teradaira, "Bradykininase Activity of Aloe Extract," *Biochemical Pharmacology* 25 (1976): 205; K. Fujita, I. Shasike, R. Teradaira, et al., "Properties of a Carboxypeptidase from Aloe," *Biochemical Pharmacology* 28 (1979): 1261.
8. G. R. Waller, S. Mangiafico, and C. R. Ritchey, "A Chemical Investigation of Aloe Bardadensis Miller," *Proceedings of the Oklahoma Academy Science* 58 (1978): 69.
9. D. C. Gowda, B. Neelisiddaiah, and Y. U. Anjaneyalu, "Structural Studies of Polysaccharides from Aloe Vera," *Carbohydrate Research* 72 (1978): 201.
10. W. D. Winters, R. Benavides, and W. J. Clouse, "Effect of Aloe Extracts on Human Normal and Tumor Cells Invitro," *Economic Botany,* 35 (1981): 89.
11. A. Yaki, N. Harada, H. Yamado et al., "Antibradykinin Active Material in Aloe Saponaria," *Journal of Pharmacological Science,* 71 (1982): 1172; A. Yaki, S. Shibata, I. Nishioka et al., "Cardiac Stimulant Action of Constituents of Aloe Saponaria," *Journal of Pharmacological Science* 71 (1982): 739.
12. I. E. Danhof and B. H. McAnalley, "Stabilized Aloe Vera: Effect on Human Skin Cells," *Drug Cosmetic Industries* 133 (1983): 52.
13. J. P. Heggers, and M. C. Robson, "Prostaglandins and Thromboxanes," in J. Ninnemann, Ed., *Traumatic Injury: Infection and Other Immunological Sequelae* (Baltimore: University Park Press, 1983), 79.
14. J. Bland, "Effect of Orally Consumed Aloe Vera Juice on Gastrointestinal Function in Normal Humans," *Preventative Medicine,* March/April 1985.

15. L. A. Hart, P. H. Van Enckevort, H. Van Dijk, R. Zaat, K. T. D. DeSilva, and R. P. Labadie, "Two Functionally and Chemically Distinct Immunomodulatory Compounds in the Gel of Aloe Vera," *J. Ethnopharmacology* 23 (1988): 61.
16. R. H. Davis, "Inhibitory and Stimulatory Systems in Aloe Vera," *Aloe Today,* Winter 1992.
17. R. M. Shelton "Aloe Vera: Its Chemical and Therapeutic Properties," *International Journal of Dermatology* 30 (1991): 679.
18. R. H. Davis, P. S. Agnew, and E. Shapiro, "Antiarthritic Activity of Anthraquinones Found in Aloe for Podiatric Medicine," *Journal of the American Podiatric Medical Association* 76 (1986): 61.
19. R. H. Davis, "Effect of Zinc Deficiency and Alloxan Induced Diabetes on Mouse Wound Healing," *Pennsylvania Academy of Science,* 41 (1983): 9.
20. R. H. Davis, J. J. DiDonato, G. M. Hartman, R. C. Haas, "Anti-inflammatory and Wound Healing Activity of a Growth Substance in Aloe Vera," *Journal of the American Podiatric Medical Association* 84 (1994): 77.
21. R. H. Davis, K. Y. Rosenthal, L. R. Cesario, G. R. Rouw, "Vitamin C Influence on Localized Adjuvant Arthritis," *Journal of the American Podiatric Medical Association* 80 (1990): 14; and R. H. Davis, Pennsylvania College of Podiatric Medicine, *Influence of Nutrition on the Growth and Survival of Cortisone Maintained Adrenalectomized Rats,* Ph.D. thesis, Rutgers University, 1958.
22. R. H. Davis, J. J. DiDonato, R. W. S. Johnson and C. B. Stewart, "Aloe Vera, Hydrocortisone and Sterol Influence on Wound Tensile Strength and Anti-inflammation," *Journal of the American Podiatric Medical Association* 84 (1994): 614.
23. R. H. Davis, J. J. DiDonato, G. M. Hartman, R. C. Haas, "Growth Factors in Aloe Vera," *Pennsylvania Academy of Science,* 66 (1993): 181.
24. R. H. Davis, "Biological Activity of Aloe Vera," *SOFW Journal* 119 (1993): 646.
25. R. H. Davis, "The Conductor-Orchestra Theory," *Aloe Today,* Spring 1995, 10.
26. Ibid.
27. I. E. Danhof, "Aloe Leaf Handling and Constituent Variability," *Aloe Today* Autumn/Winter 1988, 12.
28. T. A. Waller, F. M. Strickland, R. P. Pelley, *Quality Control and Biological Activity of Aloe Barbadensis Extracts Useful in the Cosmetic Industry* (London: Martin Caine, Aston 1994); N. F. Schmidt and H. Cutler, "The Comparative Purity of Commercially Available Aloe Vera," *Cosmetics and Toiletries* (in press).
29. Waller, Strickland, and Pelley, "Quality Control," *Requirements of Laws and Regulations, Enforced by the U.S. Food and Drug Administration,* (Washington, DC: U.S. Department of Health and Human Services, Public Health Service, Food and Drug Administration, 1988).
30?
31. R. H. Davis, "The Conductor Orchestra Theory," 10; "Biological Standardization of Aloe Vera," *Aloe Today,* Fall/Winter 1993, 12.
32. Ibid.
33. Davis, DiDonato, Hartman, and Haas, "Growth Factor," 181.
34. Davis, DiDonato, Johnson and Stewart, "Aloe Vera," 6th.
35. R. H. Davis, "A Natural Influence on Adjuvant Induced Arthritis in Rats," *Pennsylvania Academy of Science* 56 (1982): 112.
36. R. H. Davis, M. G. Leitner, J. M. Russo, and M. E. Byrne, "Anti-inflammatory Activity of Aloe Vera against a Spectrum of Irritants," *Journal of the American Podiatric Medical Association* 79 (1989): 263.

37. R. H. Davis, "Inhibitory and Stimulatory Systems."
38. R. H. Davis, W. L. Parker, and D. P. Murdoch, "Aloe Vera: A Biological Vehicle for Hydrocortisone," *Journal of the Pennsylvania Academy Science* 63 (1991): 209.
39. Davis, R. H. "Inhibitory and Stimulatory Systems."
40. Hart, VanEnckevort, Van Dijk, Zoat, DeSilva, and Labadie, "Two Functionally and Chemically Distinct Immunomodulatory Compounds." 61.
41. *Requirements of Laws and Regulations.*
42. Ibid.; Public Law 103:47, *103d Congress Congressional Record* 140 (1994): 99; "Food Labeling; General Requirements for Nutrient Content Claims for Dietary Supplements," *Federal Register* 60 (1995): 7711.
43. Public Law 103-417.

4
The Biological Vehicle Effect of Aloe Vera

Aloe vera contains 99.5 percent water and 0.5 percent solids. Water tends to move from the skin surface through the stratum corneum barrier to the vascular dermal layer. Aloe contains water-soluble compounds such as amino acids, enzymes, and carbohydrates as well as oil-soluble compounds such as vitamins, sterols, and anthraquinones. The water-soluble characteristics of aloe vera possibly originate from the leaf's gel, while the ability to solubilize oil and hydrophobic compounds probably comes from the outer rind. Possibly pharmacological agents of both solubilities can be placed in aloe and carried through the skin to blood vessels. By definition, a vehicle is a medium or carrier that carries an endocrine or pharmacological agent through a biological system. Most times, the vehicle has no biological activity of its own. It merely carries the pharmacological agent to the site where the biologic effect is to take place. Our earlier studies with vitamin C activity with aloe vera (topical and systemic), while not designed to show the "vehicle effect," support the effectiveness of aloe vera as a vehicle for water-soluble compounds.[1]

A "biological vehicle" is one that acts as a physical or physiological carrier for active biological agents but also adds biological activity to the test agent, no matter what the pharmacological agent under consideration is. In effect, it is a physical carriage plus added aloe vera activity. It must be remembered that the "orchestra" surrounding the "conductor" (the polysaccharide) contains many active compounds.[2] Thus aloe vera can add to the biological activity of most test agents. In our evaluation of aloe vera, many fractions of aloe vera show biological activity. Can we synergize these activities and then put them in aloe vera for a "vehicle effect?" Can we, on the other hand, supplement aloe vera with different sizes of polysaccharide to increase the combined aloe vera impact on a given biological activity? The polysaccharide chain is absorbed by the intestine and carried in the blood attached to blood protein (globulin). Possibly acid-alcohol will free the aloe from the blood protein. The polysaccharide is probably carried through the cell membrane (length perpendicular to membrane) by way of the protein moieties on the cell membrane. It is then metabolized within the cell. The size of the polysaccharide within the cell will determine its biological activity. For ten to fifteen years we have known that aloe vera is orally active on inflammation and wound healing.[3] However, we did not have any idea how it got from the intestine to the cell. It would be of value to label aloe vera and see where it goes after oral administration. We wonder if we can trace aloe vera from the intestine to the site of inflammation or tissue wound. These biological concepts with aloe vera must be considered in any project involving "the vehicle effect."

Skin Penetration of Mucilage and Aloe Vera

The penetration of topical agents may be influenced by the drug, the vehicle, and the skin. The vehicle may affect drug and skin penetration, thereby altering the biological activity. Little attention has been given to the influence of aloe vera and mucilage on the penetration through the skin. The stratum corneum acts as a barrier to drug penetration through the skin but also acts as a reservoir for molecules when the drug is applied on the skin. The methods, animal species, skin location, and drug concentration, as well as the experimental conditions, must be well defined to produce the best results. Poor penetration of hydrocortisone is recorded on the palms and soles, whereas the best penetration is recorded at the scrotum. In general, most of the hydrocortisone fails to penetrate the skin stratum corneum and is wasted. Aloe enhances penetration and adds to the biological activity of hydrocortisone. Aloe vera has anti-inflammatory activity and blocks the steroid's wound-inhibiting response. We feel that aloe vera increases the penetration of skin by water hydration, occlusiveness, and increase of compound solubility. This work attempts to prove that aloe vera increases the penetration through skin and can be used as a vehicle for drugs. Mucilage, on the other hand, is a seal forming a firm cover to keep moisture in wounds. In the aloe leaf, the mucilage seal produced by an animal bite prevents the leakage of gel to the outside and keeps the gel fillet sterile, thus acting as a gel sealant container.

The Trypan Blue Penetration Assay

Adult male ICR (Institute Cancer Research) mice (30 gm; 15 animals/group) were divided into four groups: 10 percent aloe in saline with 5 percent trypan blue; 10 percent mucilage in saline with 5 percent trypan blue; 5 percent aloe vera; 5 percent mucilage and 5 percent trypan blue, as well as 5 percent trypan blue as a control. Each animal was anesthetized with ether and identified with an ear punch. Control mice were injected intradermally with 0.01 ml 5 percent trypan blue using a Hamilton microsyringe and a 26-gauge x 3/8″ needle. Animals were given an intradermal injection of either 0.01 ml 10 percent aloe vera with 5 percent trypan blue, 10 percent mucilage with 5 percent trypan blue or the combination of 5 percent mucilage with 5 percent trypan blue. An initial penetration reading was made by holding the animal up to a bright light source such that the intradermal injection spot can be seen clearly and measured anterior to posterior with a caliper. Readings were taken at one, three, and six hours after the initial injection. The trypan blue assay is a simple immediate method to monitor cell membrane permeability.[4] This method was modified to measure tissue penetrability of aloe vera and mucilage. Standard errors of the mean values were calculated as well as the student's "t" test to determine if the differences were real.[5]

Aloe as a Biological Vehicle

Since aloe vera is 99.5 percent water, it is able to move through the surface of the skin (stratum corneum) to the vascular dermal area. Aloe contains water-soluble and insoluble compounds, which makes it a good carrier for all kinds of drugs—water- and lipid-soluble compounds. The water-soluble characteristics probably originate in the gel, and the insoluble characteristics probably come from the rind. Thus agents of both solubilities can go through the epidermal barrier to the dermal blood vessels. Aloe vera hydrates and covers the surface of the skin to increase the skin penetration. The absorption of steroid through the skin is different parts of the body varies depending on the thickness of the stratum corneum. For every gram of steroid applied to the skin 99 percent is wasted. More hydrocortisone is absorbed through genital skin that the soles of the feet. Aloe vera is an excellent vehicle for hydrocortisone.

The penetration of 5 percent trypan blue through the skin was 9.5± 0.7 mm in six hours (table 4.1). Aloe vera (10 percent) increased the penetration to 11.8 ± 1.2, a total of + 24.2 percent over trypan blue controls (figure 4.1). Ten percent mucilage, on the other hand, inhibited skin penetration—22.1 percent. Mucilage thus acts in an occlusive manner. A combination of 5 percent aloe vera and 5 percent mucilage inhibited penetration—34.7 percent. This data suggests that aloe vera acts to increase skin penetration and could be used to aid drugs to penetrate the skin. Mucilage probably acts as a cover to prevent the escape of fluid. Mucilage and aloe would be important in improving wound healing.

Skin is composed of polypeptide chains that form aggregates of collagen fibrils. The fibrils vary in diameter and length. The fibril bonding influences the swelling and water uptake by the skin.[6] Fibrils interweave to form fibers. The space between the fibers contains "ground substance." The most important constituents of ground substance are proteoglycans or the older term mucopolysaccharides. The skin structure has similarities that help us to understand the chemistry and action of aloe vera. Skin acts as a reservoir for receiving excess water and making water available for the entire organism. A considerable amount of water accumulates in the skin. In dehydration, the skin acts as a reservoir to supply other organs around the body. A large proportion of water in skin is found in ground substance. Skin proteins and mucopolysaccharides play an important role in controlling the water content of skin. Most of the water in skin is in the free form and not the bound form.

Stratum Corneum and Absorption

The diffusion of water through the skin is limited and controlled by the stratum corneum, which offers resistance to water transport. The greater the amount of water in the outer skin, the greater the permeability of the skin. Mucilage merely acts as a cover to prevent water from escaping from the skin. Water in the stratum corneum is in equilibrium with the atmosphere and the underlying tissue. The decreased absorption through the skin depends on morphology and

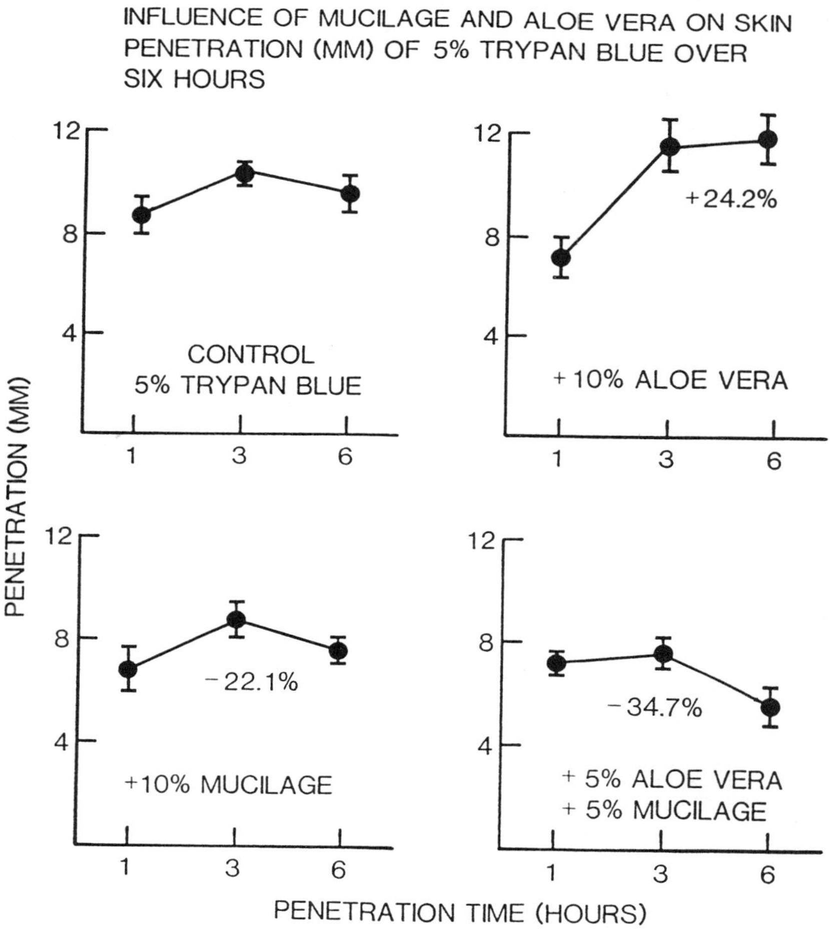
INFLUENCE OF MUCILAGE AND ALOE VERA ON SKIN PENETRATION (MM) OF 5% TRYPAN BLUE OVER SIX HOURS
PENETRATION (MM)
12
8
4
CONTROL
5% TRYPAN BLUE
+24.2%
+10% ALOE VERA
−22.1%
+10% MUCILAGE
−34.7%
+ 5% ALOE VERA
+ 5% MUCILAGE
1
3
6
PENETRATION TIME (HOURS)

Fig. 4.1.

INFLUENCE OF MUCILAGE AND ALOE VERA
ON SKIN PENETRATION (MM) OF
5% TRYPAN BLUE OVER SIX HOURS

	PENETRATION (MM)		
	1	3	6
5% TRYPAN BLUE	8.5 ± 0.9	10.0 ± 0.3	9.5 ± 0.7
+10% ALOE VERA	7.3 ± 0.9	11.5 ± 1.2	11.8 ± 1.2 ●
+10% MUCILAGE	6.9 ± 1.0	8.8 ± 0.7	7.4 ± 0.6 ■
+5% ALOE VERA 5% MUCILAGE	7.2 ± 0.5	7.8 ± 0.7	6.2 ± 0.6 ▲

15 MICE/GROUP ● $P=0.05$; ■ $P>0.05$, $P<0.001$; ▲ $P>0.5$

Table 4.1.

the clearance into microcirculation.[7] The amount and nature of proteins and mucopolysaccharides found in the ground substance affect water uptake. When skin is dried it takes up a great deal of water. This uptake can be altered by changing the concentration of skin proteins and mucopolysaccharides of the ground substance.

Topical Anti-Inflammatory Activity of Mucilage

Mucilage produces a dose-response relationship over a 1 and 5 percent concentration on inhibiting inflammation induced by topical croton oil on mouse ear swelling. A 1 percent dose inhibited inflammation 3.7 percent whereas a 5 percent dose reduced inflammation 33.7 percent. The higher response represents the beginning of the plateau (table 4.2, figure 4.2). We feel that mucilage acts as a storage container under the rind that changes from a sol to a gel when aloin is released at the base of the rind. Mucilage acts as a mechanical cover of wounds, since it probably consists of mucopolysaccharide chains that are in equilibrium with the storage form of mucopolysaccharide in the parenchyma. Also, growth factors may be present so that mucilage improves wound healing in an endocrine and in a mechanical way.

Bioavailability of Aloe Vera

There are many small and large components in aloe. Age, sex, environment, stratum corneum, dermis, and epidermis influence the absorption and distribution of aloe compounds. If the compounds are metabolized or if the blood flow through the skin is changed, it influences the clearance of aloe components. One must recognize that the skin is a dynamic system whose components function to maintain homeostasis. Aloe compounds can alter skin blood flow and bioavailability. Skin blood flow, temperature, drainage, compounds remaining in skin, dose applied to skin, the surface area, and time of exposure determine the skin penetration of aloe vera. Other components of aloe can act as a vehicle to increase the movement of compounds through the skin.[8]

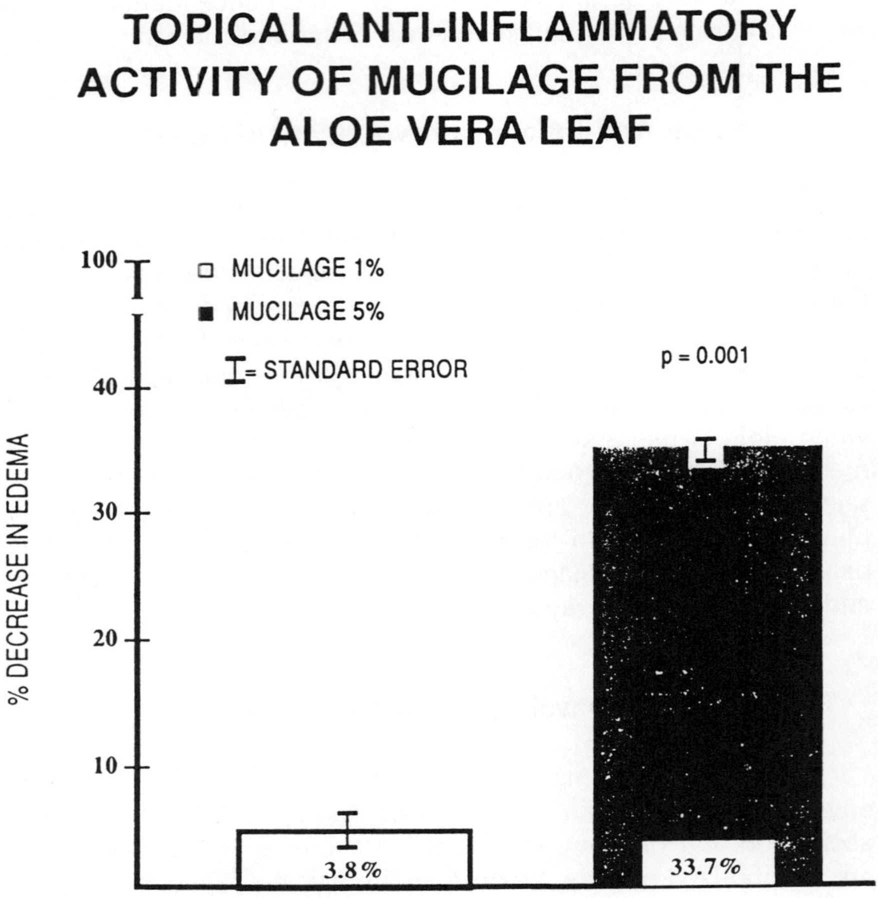

TOPICAL ANTI-INFLAMMATORY ACTIVITY OF MUCILAGE FROM THE ALOE VERA LEAF
100
40
30
20
10
% DECREASE IN EDEMA
MUCILAGE 1%
MUCILAGE 5%
= STANDARD ERROR
p = 0.001
3.8 %
33.7 %

Fig. 4.2.

TOPICAL ANTI-INFLAMMATORY ACTIVITY OF MUCILAGE FROM THE ALOE VERA LEAF

	EDEMA	
TREATMENT	EAR TISSUE WEIGHT CHANGE (MG)	%DECREASE
CROTON OIL CONTROL 25 μg/μl	7.42 ± 1.01	—
+ MUCILAGE 1%	7.14 ± 0.85	3.77
+ MUCILAGE 5%	4.92 ± 0.85 *	33.69

± = STANDARD ERROR, * $p < 0.001$

Table 4.2.

Aloe Vera Is a Vehicle for Hydrocortisone

Aloe vera hydrates and softens the skin as oils do. Yet it also covers the skin in an occlusive manner (mucilage) to prevent water loss, which is necessary for wound healing. Aloe's permeability through the skin makes it a unique biological vehicle that would allow the incorporation of both water- and oil-soluble agents. The stratum corneum acts as a barrier to steroid penetration. Aloe vera hydrates the barrier and increases the steroid penetration through the keratin layer. Aloe's large amount of fluid can aid both hydrophilic and hydrophobic compounds to move across the skin. This "dual property" of aloe vera can enhance penetration and reduce skin resistance. An agent like the steroid can be effective if the skin-aloe interface has maximum hydration, if the aloe has a low affinity for the steroid, and if the vehicle contact time with the skin is adequate. These criteria are met by aloe vera. Physicians are well aware of the pitfalls of using hydrocortisone. Aloe's novel "vehicle effect" complements the steroid's biological activity as well as increasing its physical carriage to reduce its toxic effects. Can aloe vera reduce the toxicity of any biological agent of therapeutic value? Aloe vera worked well with hydrocortisone when administered systemically in the paw-swelling assay (88.1 percent edema reduction). The croton oil ear-swelling assay showed a classic additive response between aloe and hydrocortisone (97 percent reduction in topical induced edema). There was also a 91.1 percent decrease in polymorphonuclear leukocyte infiltration. These studies clearly establish an additive vehicle effect (figures 4.3, 4.4, and 4.5).[9]

Aloe Vera Is a Vehicle for Estrogen

Estrogen-induced growth of the uterus is mediated in part by polypeptide growth factors that act to stimulate proliferation. Two growth factors, insulin-like growth factor 1 and epidermal growth factor (EGF) are associated with the induction of uterine growth by estrogens.[10] EGF acts as a mediator for estrogen on mouse uterine growth. Antibodies to EGF inhibits uterine growth 70 percent by estrogen. DNA synthesis was also recorded in the endothelial cells of uterine blood vessels. Also, progesterone potentiates the effect of

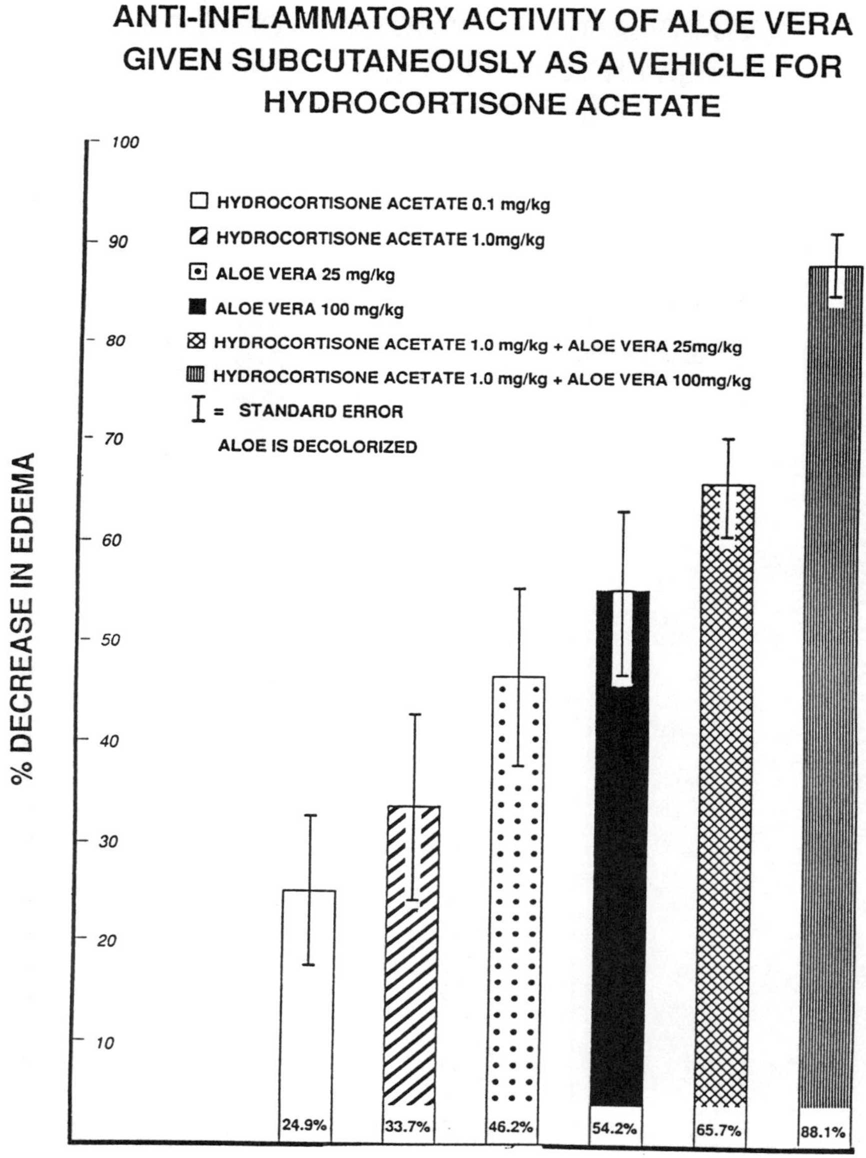
ANTI-INFLAMMATORY ACTIVITY OF ALOE VERA GIVEN SUBCUTANEOUSLY AS A VEHICLE FOR HYDROCORTISONE ACETATE
% DECREASE IN EDEMA
100
90
80
70
60
50
40
30
20
10
HYDROCORTISONE ACETATE 0.1 mg/kg
HYDROCORTISONE ACETATE 1.0mg/kg
ALOE VERA 25 mg/kg
ALOE VERA 100 mg/kg
HYDROCORTISONE ACETATE 1.0 mg/kg + ALOE VERA 25mg/kg
HYDROCORTISONE ACETATE 1.0 mg/kg + ALOE VERA 100mg/kg
= STANDARD ERROR
ALOE IS DECOLORIZED
24.9%
33.7%
46.2%
54.2%
65.7%
88.1%

Fig. 4.3.

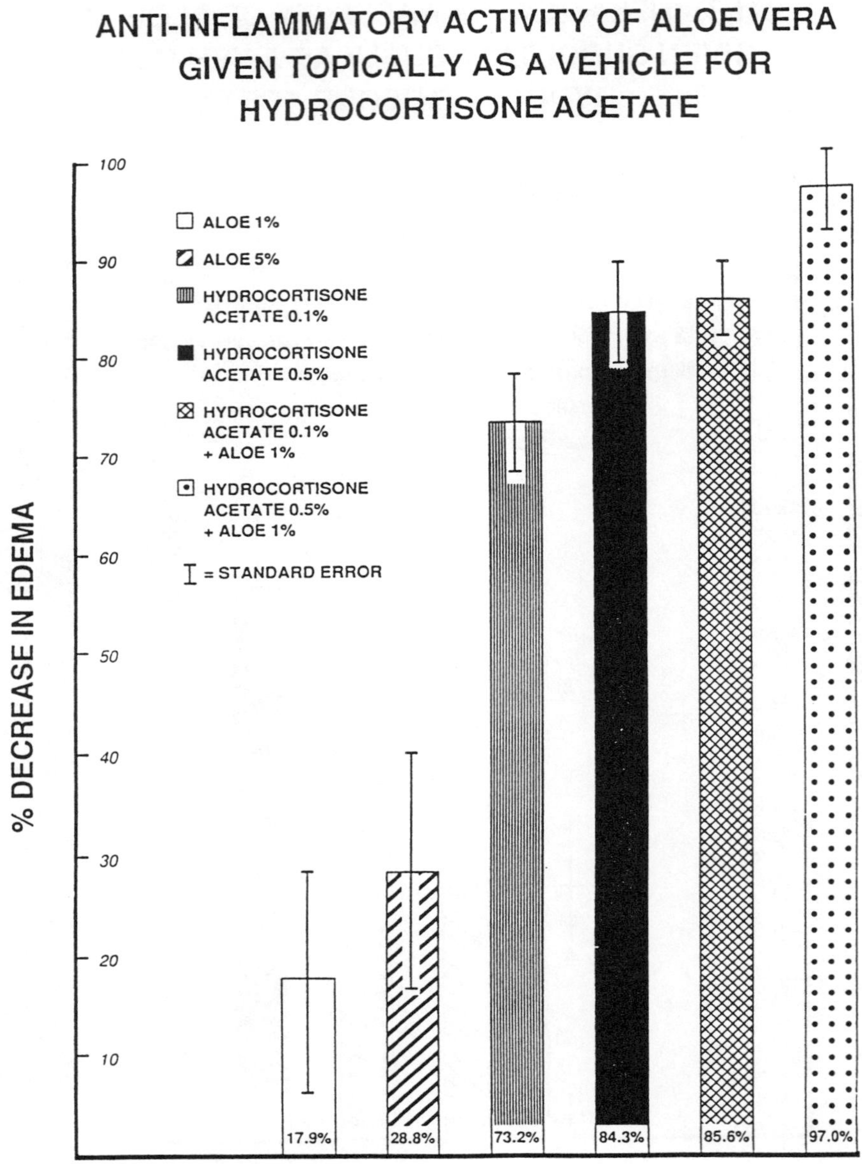
ANTI-INFLAMMATORY ACTIVITY OF ALOE VERA GIVEN TOPICALLY AS A VEHICLE FOR HYDROCORTISONE ACETATE
% DECREASE IN EDEMA
100
90
80
70
60
50
40
30
20
10
ALOE 1%
ALOE 5%
HYDROCORTISONE ACETATE 0.1%
HYDROCORTISONE ACETATE 0.5%
HYDROCORTISONE ACETATE 0.1% + ALOE 1%
HYDROCORTISONE ACETATE 0.5% + ALOE 1%
= STANDARD ERROR
17.9%
28.8%
73.2%
84.3%
85.6%
97.0%

Fig. 4.4.

THE EFFECT OF ALOE VERA AND HYDROCORTISONE ON PMN INFILTRATION INTO A MUSTARD INDUCED INFLAMMATION SITE IN RATS

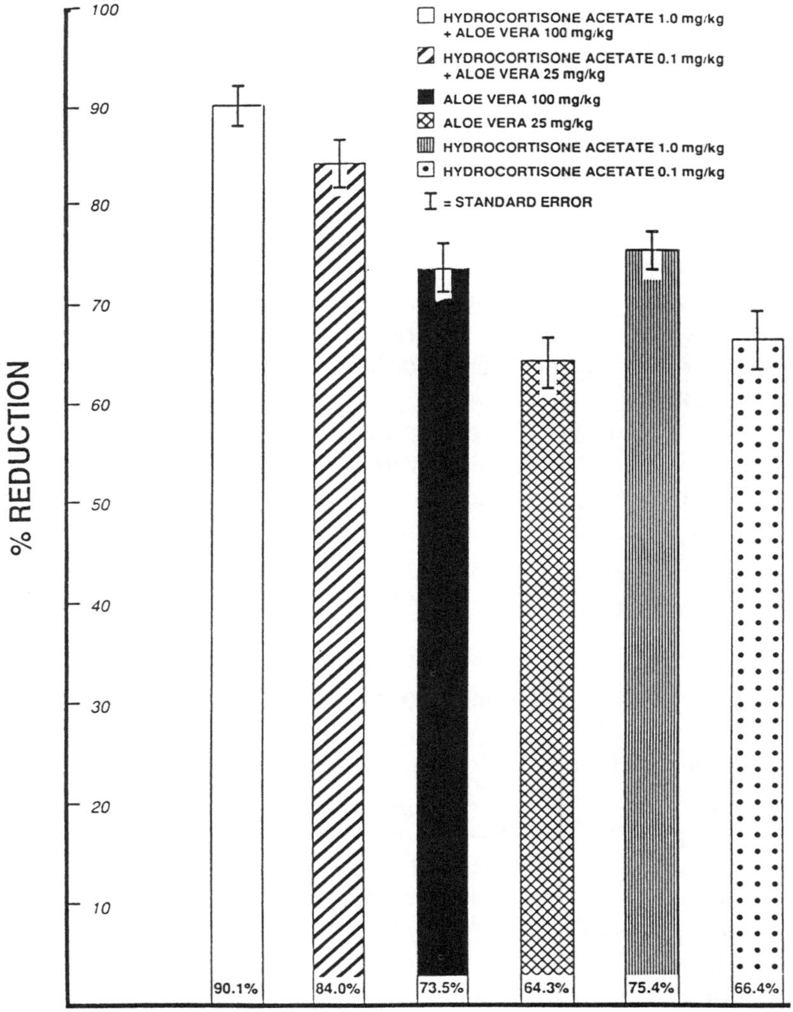

Fig. 4.5.

estrogen in insulin-like growth factor mediation of estrogen. Estrogen suppresses LH and partially FSH in the blood of overiectomized mice.[11] Possibly an ovarian factor works with estrogen to suppress blood FSH. Small amounts of estradiol (micrograms) increase total weight, dry weight, and water of the immature rat uterus in six hours.[12] The response is predictable within a narrow range of variation. In mice, the mitotic activity was recorded in the uterus and vagina.

Estrogens have a protective effect against ischemic heart disease in menopausal women.[13] They have a favorable effect on plasma lipid and high-density lipoprotein (anti-atherogenic). Estrogens have a 50 percent protective effect against the risk of coronary heart disease. Estrogens are present in willow wheat germ oil, date palm tree, clover, and alfalfa, which could be sources of protection for women.[14] E. B. Astwood[15] established an estradiol dose-response curve between 0.002 μg and 0.1 μg/day. The dilation of the rat cervix decreased from diestrus to estrous but increased during the course of gestation. This increase was due to relaxin.[16] Estradiol increased uterine nitrogen and hexosamine but decreased collagen. These items were not changed in skin.[17]

This study purposed to determine if aloe vera had estrogenic activity in ovariectomized mice. We also attempted to establish a dose-response curve for estradiol benzoate in ovariectomized mice from 0.005 to 0.1 μg. We, then, tried to determine if aloe vera would improve the estrogenic activity of estradiol in ovariectomized mice and thus act as a vehicle for reproductive hormones.

The Estrogen Assay

Adult female mice (30g; ten animals/group; HSD-ICR; Frederick, Maryland, colony) were ovariectomized, and five days later the animals were injected either with saline (controls), 100 mg/kg or 300 mg/kg of whole-plant aloe vera subcutaneously each day for seven days. On day 12, each animal was vaginally smeared to determine the stage of the estrous cycle the mice were in. The uteri were removed from each animal, blotted dry on filter paper, and weighed. The standard error for each mean was recorded. To obtain a dose-response curve for estradiol benzoate, ovariectomized mice were given corn oil (controls), 0.005,0,01, and 0.1 μg estradiol benzoate over four days. On day 5, the uteri were removed, blotted, and weighed. Also, ovariectomized mice were given saline (controls), 0.01 μg estradiol benzoate in corn oil, and 0.01 μg estradiol benzoate with aloe vera at 50 and 300 mg/kg x 4 days. On day 5, the uterus from each mouse was removed, blotted, and weighed. Aloe vera was administered subcutaneously and separate from estradiol benzoate over the four-day daily injection period.

Estrogenic Vehicle Results of Aloe Vera

Whole-leaf aloe vera subcutaneously administered daily to ovariectomized mice for seven days did not induce estrous or increase uterine weight at 100 and 300 mg/kg (table 4.3). We conclude that aloe vera does not have estrogenic activity despite the fact that sterols have estrogenic activity at higher doses than seen in aloe. It may be that other factors in aloe vera modulate this activity. T. Malini showed that sterols were estrogenic in that they increased uterine weight and produced a cornified vaginal smear.[18] However, M. I. Elghamry estimated that the estrogenic activity of sterols are 1/400 of that recorded for estradiol benzoate.[19] Plant sterols have a wide spectrum of biological activity.

The uterotropic effect of estradiol benzoate given subcutaneously for four days in ovariectomized mice was 69.2 ± 1.5 mg for estradiol benzoate at 0.005 μg dosage and 177.7 ± 7.8 mg at the higher 0.1 μg dose. The dose-response curve for estradiol benzoate on increasing uterine weight is very sensitive at small doses and has a long slope that can be repeated over and over. The variation recorded for the regression line is very small. Doses as small as one-thousandth of a microgram can be assayed on the dose-response curve (figure 4.6). Whole-leaf aloe vera increased the uterotropic effect of estradiol benzoate in ovariectomized mice administered subcutaneously over five days (figure 4.7, table 4.4). The saline-injected ovariectomized control mice had a uterine weight of 44.8 ± 0.7. This response was increased to 62.4 ± 2.6 mg (a 39.3 ± 1.6 percent increase over controls) by 0.01 μg estradiol benzoate. When the 0.01 μg estradiol benzoate was administered simultaneously with 50 mg/kg aloe vera, the uterine weights were 67.8 ± 1.3 mg (a

EFFECT OF WHOLE LEAF ALOE VERA ON VAGINAL SMEARS AND UTERINE WEIGHT OF OVARIECTOMIZED MICE.

TREATMENT MG/KG X 7	NO. OF MICE IN ESTROUS	UTERINE WT. MG.
Saline Controls	1/10	27.2 ± 2.6
100	0/9	29.0 ± 4.1*
300	0/11	29.0 ± 2.0*

*$P > 0.5$ ± = S.E.

Table 4.3.

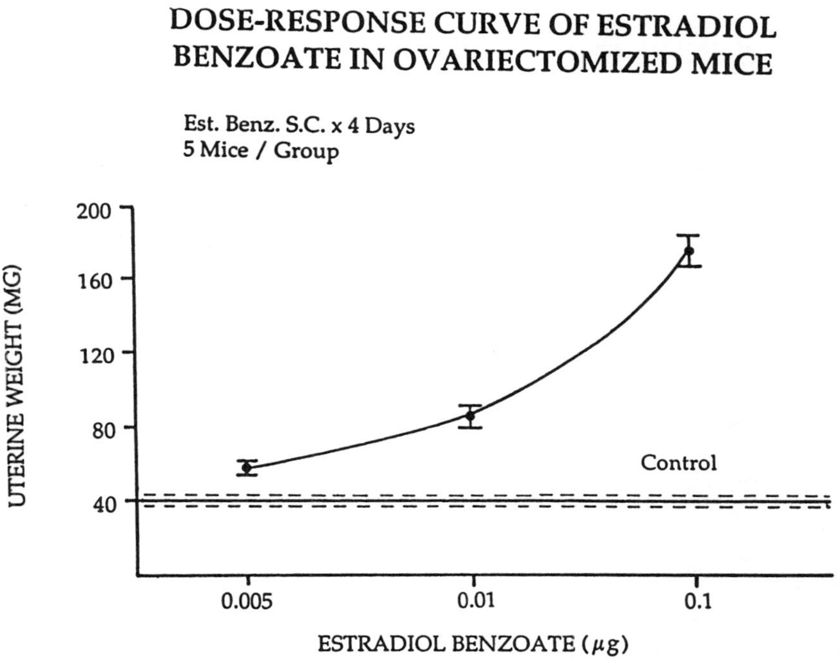
DOSE-RESPONSE CURVE OF ESTRADIOL
BENZOATE IN OVARIECTOMIZED MICE
Est. Benz. S.C. x 4 Days
5 Mice / Group
200
160
120
80
40
UTERINE WEIGHT (MG)
Control
0.005
0.01
0.1
ESTRADIOL BENZOATE (μg)

Fig. 4.6.

WHOLE LEAF ALOE VERA INCREASED THE UTEROTROPIC EFFECT OF ESTRADIOL BENZOATE IN OVARIECTOMIZED MICE ADMINISTERED SUBCUTANEOUSLY OVER 5 DAYS

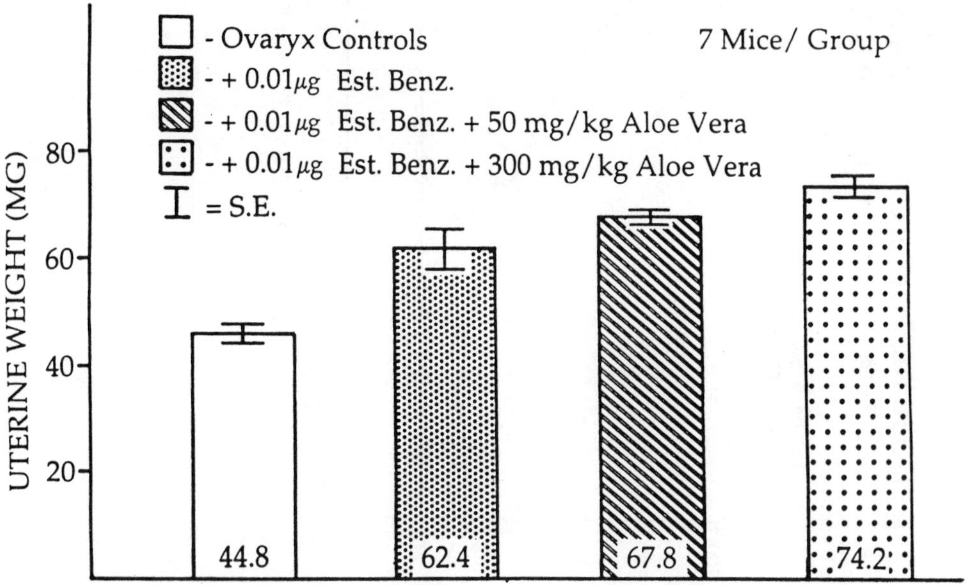

Fig. 4.7.

WHOLE LEAF ALOE VERA INCREASED THE UTEROTROPIC EFFECT OF ESTRADIOL BENZOATE IN OVARIECTOMIZED MICE ADMINISTERED SUBCUTANEOUSLY OVER 5 DAYS

Treatment	Uterine Weight Mg.	Uterine Weight % Inc.
Ovaryx (Saline) Controls	44.8 ± 0.7	-
+ 0.01μg Est. Benz.	62.4 ± 2.6	39.3 ± 1.6
+ 0.01μg Est. Benz. + 50 mg/kg Aloe Vera	67.8 ± 1.3	51.3 ± 1.0
+ 0.01μg Est. Benz. + 300 mg/kg Aloe Vera	74.2 ± 3.7	65.6 ± 3.3

7 Animals/Group. S.Q. X 4 ± = S.E.

Table 4.4.

51.3 ± 1.0 percent increase over controls). However, when 0.01 μg estradiol benzoate was given with 300 mg/kg aloe vera, uterine weights were 74.2 ± 3.7 mg. This represents a 65.6 percent increase in uterine weight over controls. In fact, aloe vera virtually doubled the uterotropic effect seen with estradiol benzoate alone. It must be remembered that aloe vera has no estrogenic activity at these doses but acts as a very good vehicle to increase the estrogenic response. Possibly aloe vera can act as a vehicle for protein hormones as well. Can aloe vera enhance the growth response (anabolic activity) of growth hormone in hypophysectomized animals? Since aloe is a vehicle, can it decrease the toxicity of valuable drugs by enabling us to reduce the dose?

Aloe Vera as a Synergistic Biological Vehicle for Testosterone Proprionate

Exogenous male hormone has ambivalent effects on the testes. Low doses indirectly inhibit spermatogenesis in normal animals by suppressing pituitary gonadotropin, whereas large doses maintain spermatogenesis in the hypophysectomized rat. The systemic effects of testosterone were reflected in the heavier ventral prostates and seminal vesicles. Androgen induces morphological changes in androgen-dependent cells. Nuclear changes and a reduced epithelium cell height observed after gonadectomy were reversed by testis extract. R. M. Melampy described after castration, a decrease in nuclear diameter and cell height which was normalized in nuclear diameter and cell height by testosterone replacement.[20] The nuclear pore complexes and tight junctions were quantified in the seminal vesicle epithelial cells of castrate- and castrate-androgen-treated male rats. Nuclear pore density was increased by male hormone. Castration causes cell atrophy, pyknotic nuclei, reduced ribonuclear protein, and nucleolar size. Male hormone treatment increases cell height and nuclear diameter.[21] Steroids act at the level of gene transcription in target cells increasing RNA synthesis. In castrate rats treated with testosterone proprionate, the amount of three polyamines increased seminal vesicle and ventral prostate.[22] They have a controlling role in the synthesis of nucleic acids and proteins. We can assume that polyamines are related to cell and organ growth. Treatment of mice with testosterone proprionate increased testicular and seminal vesicle weight as well as sertoli cell activity, but androgen has a direct inhibitory effect on steroidogenesis in active Leydig cells. Anti-androgens can block the action of testosterone on the prostate and seminal vesicle. This has clinical application for prostate hyperplasia, acne, and hirsutism. Also, a sincere effort is being made to develop agents that will inhibit fertility in the male.[23]

Methods of Administration and Androgen Preparations

Testosterone proprionate is clinically used in hypogonadism. It was demonstrated that the free compound was less effective than the ester. Esterification tends to retard absorption, which promotes a more efficient utilization of the hormone. The effect is a slow delivery of steroid hormone that lengthens duration of action. Slow absorption lengthens duration of action. An increase in the length of the chain attached to the D ring up to a certain point increases the duration and potency of action. If the chain is too long (stearate), the activity declines. Proprionate esters have enjoyed the widest use as a preparation. Testosterone proprionate is marketed dissolved in oil. However, oil has shortcomings in that it is allerogenic. It causes local inflammation on intramuscular or subcutaneous injection. The oil absorption is delayed long after the hormone is released. The hormone is eliminated in two to five days. Vehicles for testosterone have for the most part been unsuitable.[24] We therefore are considering aloe vera as a vehicle for testosterone proprionate. Aloe vera was very suitable for estradiol benzoate. Aloe has no estrogenic activity but increased the effect on uterine weight of estradiol benzoate.

Biological Methods for Measuring Androgen

If male hormone is applied directly to the sensitive tissue, the amount necessary to produce a response is about one-hundredth the amount needed by injection. We developed a method in which we applied 10 μ1 of about 5 μg androsterone directly to the comb of one-day-old white Leghorn cockerels for ten days. We obtained a fine dose-response curve, which could be used to assay extracts of urine from growth-retarded boys treated with chorionic gonadotropin. The White Leghorn one-day-old chick is the most sensitive biological end point yet developed. The experimental error for the assay is about 10 percent.

The methods involving mammals have been many and varied. They are less sensitive than the chick assays. Traditionally, the seminal vesicle and ventral prostate in the castrate rat treated with androgen over seven days gave good results. In this work, we have used the 15 gm male mouse that was castrated. The castrated immature mouse was allowed to stand for three days. It was then treated with testosterone proprionate for four days and the seminal vesicle was blotted and weighed on day 5. No attempt was made to measure the levator ani muscle, which holds the rectum. Growth of the levator ani muscle by androgen was considered an anabolic response, as opposed to the sex response increase in a seminal vesicle.

Castration in mammals causes severe changes in secondary sex characters as well as behavior. The changes are more severe if the castration is done before puberty. The penis, seminal vesicles, prostate, and Cowper's gland fail to develop. In man, similar changes occur and the voice remains high, with infantile hair development. Administration of androgen to normal animals decreases testis size, degenerates germinal epithelium, and interferes with spermatogenesis. The suppressed pituitary secretes inadequate amounts of gonadotropin to maintain functional integrity of the testis. In rats, 2 μg testosterone proprionate per day decreased testes weight 41 percent. The damaging influence of androgens on the rat testis is due to the pituitary.

This study attempted to determine if aloe vera could act as a biological "synergistic" vehicle for testosterone proprionate. The androgen dose for the immature castrate mouse of 25 μg x 4 was based on a dosage developed in immature castrate rats. Whole-leaf aloe vera was given at 150 mg/kg x 4. Aloe vera has no estrogenic or androgenic activity of its own. But since aloe enhanced the activity of estrogen, we set out to determine if it would enhance in a synergistic way the androgenic activity, as measured by the seminal vesicle weight, of testosterone proprionate–treated immature castrate mice.

The Androgen Assay

Immature castrate mice (15g; 10 animals/group; HSD-ICR Maryland Colony) were given daily subcutaneous injections (25 μg × 4) of testosterone proprionate in corn oil. Aloe vera (whole-leaf) was given subcutaneously each day simultaneously with the androgen at 150 mg/kg × 4. Control castrate mice received aqueous or corn oil injections. Also, aloe vera at 150 mg/kg × 4 was given alone, serving as an aloe vera control. The dose of testosterone was based on a dose-response curve done in immature castrate rats. The mean and standard errors of seminal vesicles were used to determine significance. An attempt was made to determine if the combined treatment was greater than the added response: A+B=C.

Aloe Vera Synergizes with Testosterone Proprionate

We constructed a testosterone proprionate dose-response curve using the immature castrate rat over seven days (figure 4.8). The reason we used the immature castrate rat is because the literature has stated over the years that the rat is the best model to use.[25] The seminal vesicle weight ranged from 132 mg to over 200 mgs over the testosterone dose range (control = 23 mg). The ventral prostate and the anabolic indices, the levator ani muscle, were less sensitive. From this data we designed a study with immature castrate mice, because mice are somewhat more sensitive to aloe and possibly to testosterone proprionate. Castrate mice received daily 25 μg testosterone proprionate in corn oil for four days. The percent increase of seminal vesicle weight rose from 18.0 ± 1.6 (oil control) to 312.3 ± 12.0 (A). When 150 mg/kg of whole-leaf aloe was given simultaneously with the 25 μg testosterone proprionate,, a 461.02 ± 28.5 percent (C) increase in seminal vesicle weight was recorded. Aloe vera, alone, given at 150 mg/Kg × 4 gave a 8.1 ± 0.9 percent increase in seminal vesicle weight (B). Please know that the combined treatment of aloe + testosterone proprionate is greater than A+B= C. Therefore, aloe vera, which has no androgenic activity, provided a synergistic relationship with testosterone proprionate (table 4.5, figure 4.9). Could aloe vera be a vehicle or modulator for most therapeutic agents? Based upon the present androgen results, it appears that aloe vera is a better vehicle for testosterone than for estradiol.

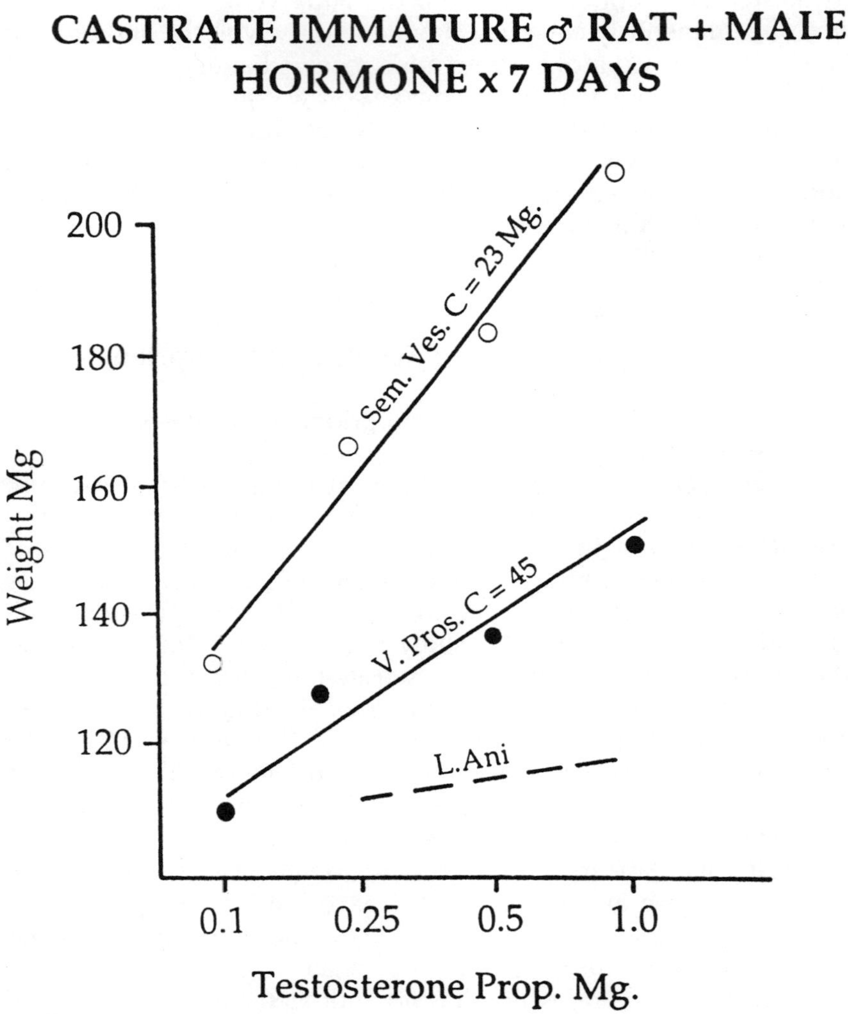
CASTRATE IMMATURE ♂ RAT + MALE HORMONE x 7 DAYS
200
180
160
140
120
Weight Mg
Sem. Ves. C = 23 Mg.
V. Pros. C = 45
L.Ani
0.1
0.25
0.5
1.0
Testosterone Prop. Mg.

Fig. 4.8.

THE SYNERGISTIC EFFECT of WHOLE LEAF ALOE VERA on TEST. PROP. STIMULATION of SEMINAL VESICLES of IMMATURE CASTRATE MALE MICE

	Seminal Vesicle	
	Weight Mg.	%Increase
Aq. Control	6.7 ± 0.6	—
Oil Control	7.9 ± 0.7	18.0 ± 1.6
Test. Prop 25μg x 4	20.9 ± 0.8	312.3 ± 12.0 (A)
Test. Prop. 25μgx 4 + Aloe 150mg/kg x 4	30.7 ± 1.9	461.0 ± 28.5 (C)
Aloe 150mg/kg x 4	7.2 ± 0.8	8.1 ± 0.9 (B)

10 Mice/Group. The combined treatment is > than A+B=C : Synergism P<0.01

Table 4.5.

WHOLE LEAF ALOE VERA SYNERGISM on TEST. PROP. STIMULATION of SEMINAL VESICLES of IMMATURE CASTRATE MALE MICE

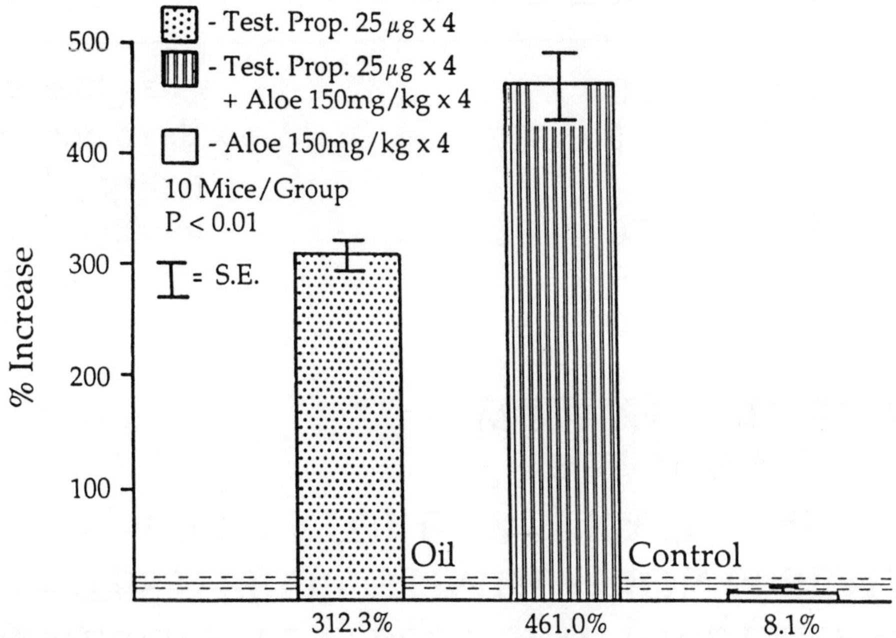

Fig. 4.9.

Gonadotropin Antagonism

A. Effect of Whole-Leaf Aloe Vera on Pituitary Gonadotropin in Unilateral Overiectomized Mice

Interleukin, a cytokine secreted by macrophages and monocytes, exhibits immune properties and plays a role in the release of gonadotropin in ovariectomized animals.[26] Interleukin inhibits LH secretion in ovariectomized male and female rats. It blocks the progesterone-induced LH surge in the ovariectomized rat primed with estradiol benzoate. Inhibin inhibits pituitary FSH and it is suggested that this effect is not entirely mediated by changes in gonadotropin-releasing hormone receptors. Inhibin starts playing a physiological role in modulating FSH secretion between eighteen and twenty days after birth.[27] Other results suggest that interleukin works at the level of the brain and gonads,[28] but not the pituitary, to inhibit reproductive function. It stimulates ACTH secretion and inhibits sexual steroid production by cultured Leydig cells and interferes with luteinization of granulosa cells in culture.[29]

Since aloe vera stimulates macrophages to produce interleukin (a polypeptide cytokine), this work was designed to see if high doses of aloe vera would block gonadotropin secretion in the unilateral ovariectomized animal. C. Rivier and W. Vale[30] reported that interleukin placed into the lateral ventricles of castrate male rats inhibited LH. Possibly the suppression of LH release involves receptive elements located with the blood-brain barrier. Stimulation of macrophages by mannose polysaccharide elevates interleukins from twelve hours up to five days.[31]

The Gonadotropin Inhibition Assay

Adult female mice (30 gm; 15 mice/group; HSD-ICR) were unilaterally ovariectomized, and the right ovary was removed and weighed. Mice were daily subcutaneously injected for seven days with whole-leaf aloe vera at 100 to 300 mg/kg. Control animals received saline injections. On day 7 the left ovary was removed and weighed. The amount of hypertrophy was measured as percent increase in weight as related to unilateral ovariectomized controls.

Standard errors of the means as well as significances were determined.

Aloe Vera Antagonizes Pituitary Gonadotropin

The increase in relative ovarian weight over seven days in unilateral ovariectomized mice receiving saline daily was 23.0 mg. Aloe vera at 100 mg/kg × 7 reduced the weight change to 18.2 mg. However, when mice were given 300 mg/kg aloe vera, the ovaries lost 1.5 mg. These data suggest that the high dose of aloe vera blocked pituitary gonadotropin, as evidenced by the fact that ovarian hypertrophy did not occur. In fact, the ovaries lost 1.5 mg. One could speculate that the high dose of aloe blocked the releasing hormone or the tropic hormone through interleukin, since aloe vera stimulates the release of interleukin from macrophages. It may be that low doses of aloe given to normal mice increase ovarian weight, in which case one must consider the possibility that aloe vera modulates the hypothalamic-pituitary control over the ovaries (table 4.6, figures 4.10 and 4.11).

B. Effect of Whole-Leaf Aloe Vera on the Uteri of Immature Mice Treated with Human Chorionic Gonadotropin

The human trophoblast secretes chorionic gonadotropin (HCG) near implantation of the blastocyst. Within a week, high levels of chorionic gonadotropin can be picked up by sensitive assay. Unlike the anterior pituitary, the trophoblastic cells are not subject to negative feedback. The subunits of HCG resemble LH, and the amino acid content as well as the sequence are identical. There is a high content of mannose and glucosamine in HCG.[32] It exerts an FSH and LH action—mainly LH. HCG stimulates the ovary to ovulate. HCG and LH can fit into the same receptor.[33] Its role in controlling steroid synthesis in pregnancy is not clear. HCG rises rapidly and reaches a peak at two months of pregnancy. It then declines toward the end of the third trimester. It may prepare the mammary gland for lactation, but the lactogen probably plays the greater role in this regard.

HCG–inhibiting substances found in the urine of children have prevented the uterotropic influence of chorionic gonadotropin in immature mice.[34] The inhibition has been studied during the menstrual

EFFECT OF WHOLE LEAF ALOE VERA GIVEN SUBCUTANEOUSLY OVER 7 DAYS ON PITUITARY GONADOTROPIN IN UNILATERAL OVARIECTOMIZED MICE.

ALOE TREATMENT MG/KG X 7	RELATIVE OVARIAN WEIGHT*		
	DAY 1	DAY 7	CHANGE
Saline Control	50.6 ±6.8	73.6 ±3.8	+23.0
100	42.7 ±3.2	60.9 ±3.6	+18.2
300	55.3 ±5.1	53.9 ** ±3.4	-1.5

15 Mice/Group *Mg/100 GM. B.W.T. **P<0.001

Table 4.6.

CHANGE IN RELATIVE OVARIAN WEIGHT BY WHOLE LEAF ALOE GIVEN SUBCUTANEOUSLY FOR 7 DAYS TO UNILATERAL OVARYX. MICE

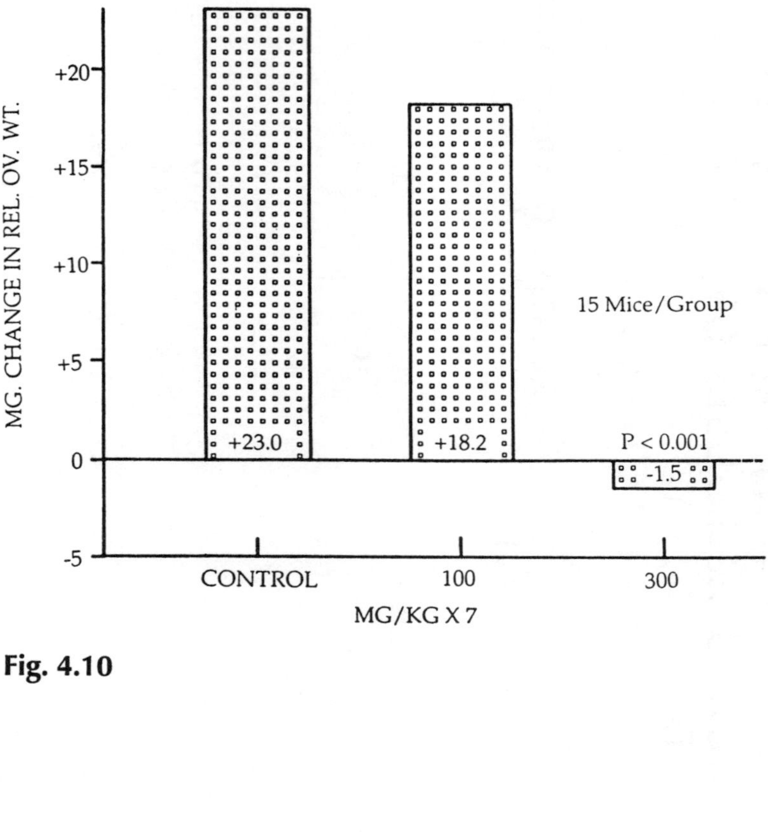

Fig. 4.10

EFFECT OF WHOLE LEAF ALOE (300 MG/KG X 7) ON UNILATERAL OVARYX. MICE

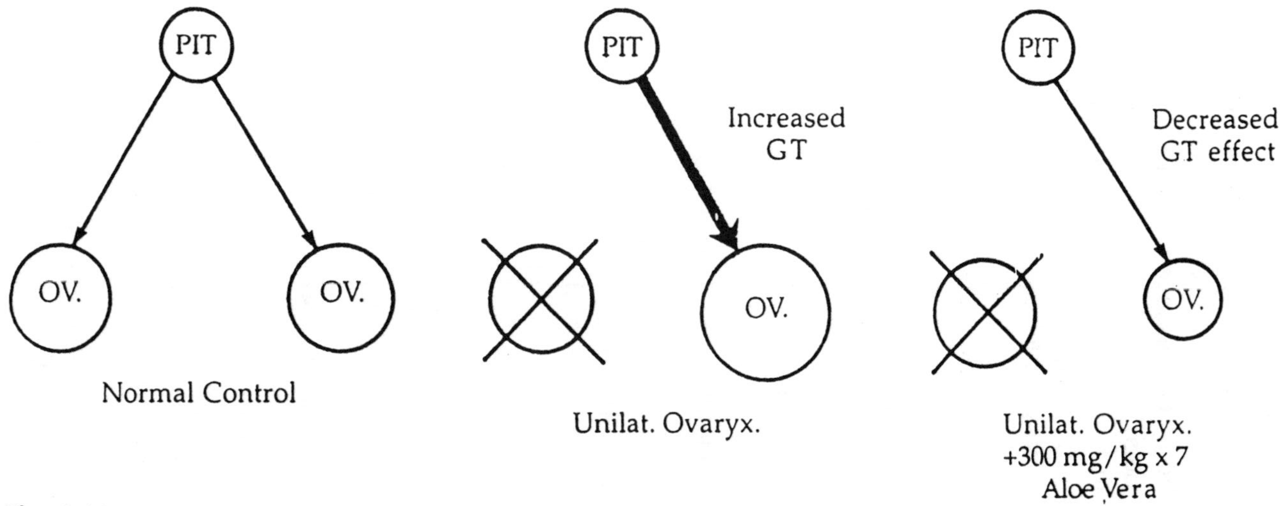

Fig. 4.11.

cycle.[35] Estrogen treatment suppresses the inhibitor and the gonadotropin. When HCG was implanted into the median eminence of the hypothalamus or pituitary, it decreased the secretion of gonadotropin.[36] HCG has a similar biological and immunological activity as LH. The recent discovery that LH/HCG has receptors in the uterus has brought about some confusion. HCG has been able to modulate metestrus uterine progesterone content.[37] It may be that HCG produces a relaxing effect on the uterus. HCG stimulates the growth of preovulatory follicle. It can induce luteinization of granulosa and theca cells.

This study attempts to determine if aloe vera would increase or decrease the response of HCG on uterine weight in immature mice. The total dose of 0.30 i.u. of HCG produces roughly a 30 percent increase in uterine weight. The aloe dose is not a maximum dose but a moderate-to-small dosage.

Chorionic Gonadotropin Inhibition Assay

Immature female mice (HSD-ICR, Frederick, Maryland, colony; 12 gm; 15 animals/group) were given subcutaneously a total dose of HCG of 0.30 i.u.: three injections of 0.05 i.u. on day 1, two injections on day 2, and one injection on day 3. Animals were also given subcutaneously a total dose of whole-leaf aloe vera of 30 mg/kg.: three injections of 5 mg/kg on day 1, two injections on day 2, and one injection on day 3. A combination group received aloe and HCG injections simultaneously. The control group received daily injections of saline. On day 4, the animals were sacrificed and their uteri were removed, blotted, and weighed. The standard errors of the means were calculated, and the significance was determined.

Aloe Vera Antagonizes Chorionic Gonadotropin

Mice treated with 0.30 i.u. of HCG had uteri that weighed 73.5 $\pm$ 3.8 mg. Combining 30 mg/kg aloe with the HCG treatment decreased the uterine weight to 63.2 $\pm$ 2.7 mg ($P<0.05$). Animals given 30 mg/Kg of aloe alone had uteri that weighed 23.5 $\pm$ 1.1 mg, which were not significantly different from saline control uteri (22.8 $\pm$ 1.2 mg) ($P<0.5$) (table 4.7, figure 4.12). Aloe vera had virtually little or no effect on HCG influence on the ovarian weight. HCG stimulates

EFFECT of WHOLE LEAF ALOE VERA on the UTERI of HUMAN CHORIONIC GONADOTROPIN TREATED IMMATURE MICE

	UTERINE WEIGHT (MG)
Control	22.8 ± 1.2
Aloe 5mg / KG X 6	23.5 ± 1.1
HCG 0.05 I.U. x 6	73.5 ± 3.8
Combination	63.2 ± 2.7*

15 Animals / Group   ± = S.E.   *$P < 0.05$

Table 4.7.

EFFECT of WHOLE LEAF ALOE VERA on the UTERI of HUMAN CHORIONIC GONADOTROPIN TREATED IMMATURE MICE

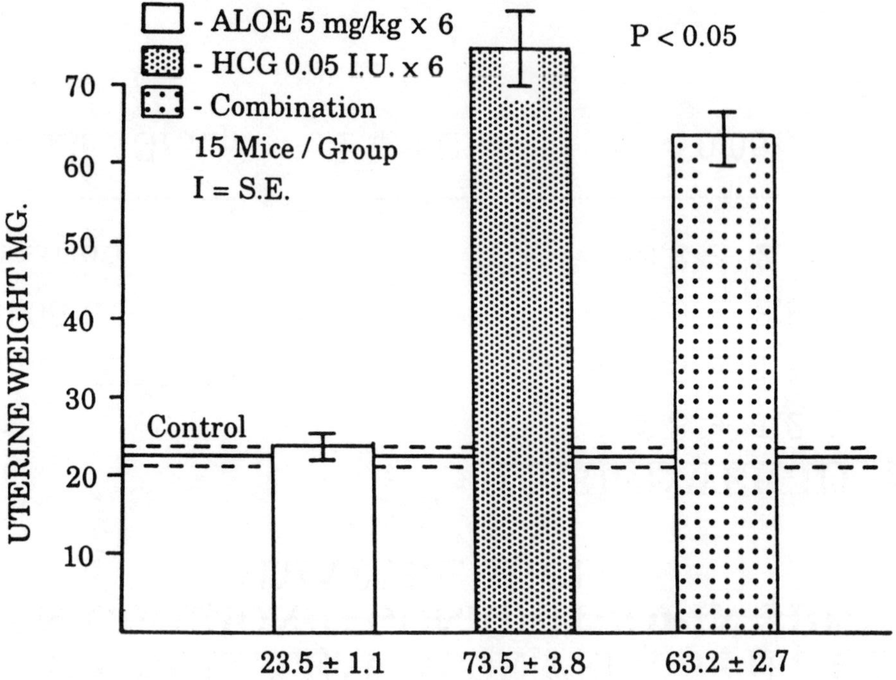

Fig. 4.12.

the ovary to increase uterine weight. Aloe vera's antagonism was recorded on the uterine weight but not on ovarian weight. We should recall that aloe vera at high doses had no estrogenic activity in ovariectomized mice, as measured by the vaginal smear and uterotropic responses. However, aloe vera improved the estradiol benzoate response at 0.01 μg by doubling the uterotropic response of the estrogen. Since aloe has no estrogenic effect by itself, this response is more than an additive effect. In a similar way, aloe gave a synergistic response with testosterone proprionate. In fact, aloe vera gave a better vehicle response with androgens than with estrogens. Since the aloe vera response was not at the ovarian level but at the uterine level (inhibitory), one must consider the possibility that aloe vera antagonizes the HCG at the controversial uterine receptor because aloe vera normally enhances the estrogenic response.

Summary

Aloe vera increases the penetration of skin by water hydration, occlusiveness, and increase of compound solubility. Aloe vera increases the anti-inflammatory activity but blocks the steroid wound-inhibiting response. Mucilage acts to keep moisture in wounds. We observed no estrogenic or androgenic activity in aloe despite the fact that it contains sterols. Aloe vera doubled the uterotropic effect seen with estradiol and had a synergistic effect with testosterone proprionate. Whole-leaf aloe vera antagonized pituitary gonadotropin, suggesting a release of interleukin, which inhibits gonadotropin. This effect of aloe on gonadotropin may be a modulation effect through interleukin. Aloe also antagonizes chorionic gonadotropin at the uterine level, but not at the ovarian level. The stimulatory and inhibitory influence of aloe vera, again, verifies the modulation and vehicle effect.

References

1. R. H. Davis, W. L. Parker, and D. P. Murdoch, "Aloe Vera as a Biological Active Vehicle for Hydrocortisone Acetate," *Journal of the American Podiatric Medical Association* 81 (1991): 1.

2. R. H. Davis, J. J. DiDonato, G. M. Hartman, and R. C. Haas,: "Anti-Inflammatory and Wound Healing Activity of a Growth Substance in Aloe Vera," *Journal of the American Podiatric Medical Association* 84 (1994): 77.
3. R. H. Davis, M. G. Leitner, J. M. Russo, and M. E. Byrne, "Wound Healing: Oral and Topical Activity of Aloe Vera," *Journal of the American Podiatric Medical Association* 79 (1989): 559.; R. H. Davis, W. L. Parker, and D. P. Murdoch, "Aloe Vera: A Biological Vehicle for Hydrocortisone," *Journal of the Pennsylvania Academy of Science* 63 (1991): 209.
4. G. Rialdi, *Cytotoxicity Assays Skin Care Instant Reports* 8 (1991): 168.
5. G. Snedecor, W. Cochran, *Statistical Methods,* 6th ed. (Ames: Iowa State University Press, 1974).
6. H. R. Elden, *Biophysical Properties of the Skin,* vol. 1 (New York: John Wiley, 1971); B. Anderson, P. Hoffman, and K. Meyer. "The O-serine Linkage in Peptides of Chondroitin 4 and 6 Sulfate," *Journal of Biological Chemistry* 240 (1965): 156.; T. Helting and L. Roden, "Biosynthesis of Chondroitin Sulfate: II Glucuronosyl Transfer in the Formation of the Carbohydrate–Protein Linkage Region," *Journal of Biological Chemistry* 244 (1969): 2799.; J. H. Fessler, "Water and Mucopolysaccharide Content as Structural Components of Connective Tissue," *Nature* 179 (1957): 426.
7. H. Baker, A. M. Kligman, "A Simple in Vivo Method for Studying the Permeability of the Human Stratum Corneum," *Journal of Investigative Dermatology* 48 (1967): 273.
8. B. Shroot, and H. Schaefer, "Skin Pharmacokinetics," *Pharmacology and the Skin* 1 (1987): 121.
9. Davis, Parker, and Murdoch, "Aloe Vera, as a Biological Active Vehicle," 1; Davis, Parker, and Murdoch, "Aloe Vera: A Biological Vehicle," 209.
10. K. G. Nelson, T. Takahashi, N. L. Bossert, D. K. Walmer, and J. A. McLachlan, "Epidermal Growth Factor Replaces Estrogen in the Stimulation of Female Genital-Tract Growth and Differentiation," *Procedures of the National Academy of Science* 88 (1991): 21; G. Norstedt, A. Levinovitz, and H. Eriksson, "Regulation of Uterine-like Growth Factor I mRNA and Insulin-like Growth Factor II mRNA by Estrogen in the Rat," *Acta Endocrinologica (Copenhagen)* 120 (1969): 466.
11. F. H. Bronson, "Suppression of Serum Follicle–Stimulating Hormone by Follicular Fluid in the Maximally Estrogenized Ovariectomized Mouse," *Endocrinology* 103 (1978): 1894.
12. E. B. Astwood, "A Six Hour Assay for the Quantitative Determination of Estrogen," *Anatomical Records* 70 (1938): 25.
13. L. G. Martin, G. M. Brenner, K. L. Jarolim, M. W. Banschback, D. L. Coon, and A. K. Wolfe, "Effect of Sex Steroids on Myocardial Anoxic Resistance," *Proceeding of the Society of Experimental Biology Medicine,* 202 (1993): 288.
14. M. X. Zarrow, E. A. Lazo-Wasem, R. L. Shoger, "Estrogenic Activity in a Commercial Animal Ration," *Science* 118 (1953): 650.
15. A. S. Astwood, "A Six Hour Assay," 25.
16. M. X. Zarrow, J. Yochim, "Dilation of the Uterine Cervix of the Rat and Accompanying Changes during the Estrous Cycle, Pregnancy and following Treatment with Estradiol, Progesterone and Relaxin," *Endocrinology* 69 (1961): 292.
17. C. F. Morgan, "A Study of Estrogenic Action in the Collagen, Hexosamine and Nitrogen Content of Skin, Uterus and Vagina," *American Journal of Anatomy* 73 (1963), 12.
18. T. Malini and G. Vanilhakumari, "Comparative Study of the Effect of B. Sitosterol, Estradiol and Progesterone on Selected Biochemical Parameters of the Uterus of Ovariectomized Rats," *Journal of Enthnopharmacology* 36 (1992): 51.

19. M. I. Elghamry, I. M. Shihata, "Biological Activity of Phytoestrogens," *Plant Medicine* 14 (1966): 352.
20. L. F. Cavazos, and R. M. Melampy, "Cytological Effects of Testosterone Proprionate on Epithelium of Rat Seminal Vesicles," *Endocrinology* 54 (1954): 640.
21. H. E. Ortiz, J. C. Cavicchia, "Androgen-Induced Changes in Nuclear Pore Number and in Tight Junctions in Rat Seminal Vesicle Epithelium," *Anatomical Records* 226 (1990): 129.
22. H. E Fjosne, M. A. Ostensen, H. Haarstad, and A. Sunde, *Prostate* 17 (1990): 1.
23. P. J. Shaughnessy and J. W. Sheffield, "Effect of Testosterone on Testicular Steroidogenesis in the Hypogonadol Mouse," *Journal of Steroid Biochemistry* 35 (1990): 729.; R. Neri, "Pharmacology and Pharmacokinetics of Flutamide," supplement to *Urology* 34 (1989): 18.; B. W. Snyder, R. C. Winneker, and F. H. Batzold, "Endocrine Profile of Win 49596 in the Rat: A Novel Androgen Receptor Antagonist," *Journal of Steroid Biochemistry* 33 (1989): 1127.
24. R. I. Dorfman and R. A. Shipley, *Androgens* (London: John Wiley, 1956).
25. Ibid.
26. C. A. Dinarello, "Biology of Interleukin," *Federation of the American Society of Experimental Biology* 2 (1988): 108.; M. L. Polan, A. Kuo, J. Loukides, and K. Bottomly, "Cultured Human Lethal Peripheral Monocytes Secrete Increased Levels of Interleukin-1," *Journal of Clinical Endocrinology Metabolism* 70 (1990): 480.; C. Rivier, and W. Vale, "In the Rat Interleukin-1a Acts at the Level of the Brain and the Gonads to Interfere with Gonadotropin and Sex Steroid Secretion," *Endocrinology* 124 (1989): 2105.; I. R. Tizard, R. H. Carpenter, B. H. McAnalley, and M. C. Kemp, "The Biological Activities of Mannans and Related Complex Carbohydrates," *Molecular Biotherapy* 1 (1989): 290.; F. You-Ji, E. Shalts, L. Xia, J. Rivier, C. Rivier, W. Vale, and M. Ferin., "An Inhibitory Effect of Interleukin-1a on Basal Gonadotropin Release in the Ovariectomized Rhesus Monkey: Reversal by a Corticotropin-Releasing Factor Antagonist," *Endocrinology* 128 (1991): 2077.
27. C. Rivier, R. Schwall, A. Mason, L. Burton, J. Vaughan, and W. Vale, "Effect of Recombinant Inhibin on Luteinizing Hormone and Follicle–Stimulating Hormone Secretion in the Rat," *Endocrinology* 128 (1991): 1548.
28. Rivier and Vale, "In the Rat Interleukin-1a Acts at the Level of the Brain," 2105.
29. E. W. Bernton, J. E. Beach, J. W. Holaday, R. C. Smallridge, and H. G. Fein, "Release of Multiple Hormone by an Action of interleukin-1 on Pituitary Cell," *Science* 238 (1987): 519.
30. Rivier and Vale, "In the Rat Interleukin-1a Acts at the Level of the Brain," 2205; Rivier, Schwall, Mason, Burton, Vaughan, and Vale, "Effect of Recombinant Inhibin," 1548.
31. Tizard, Carpenter, McAnalley, and Kemp, "Biological Activities," 290.
32. R. C. Martin, *Textbook of Endocrine Physiology* (Baltimore: Williams and Wilkins, 1976).
33. M. Herono, M. Igarashi, and S. Matsumoto, "The Direct Effect of HCG upon Pituitary Gonadotropin Secretions," *Endocrinology* 90 (1972): 1214.
34. L. J. Soffer, M. Fogel, and A. Z. Rudavsky, "Gonadotropin-Inhibiting Substances," *Israel Journal of Medical Science* 1 (1975): 1267; M. Reiss, J. J. Pearse, R. H. Davis, et al., "Inhibition of the Biological Action of Gonadotropin, Thyrotropin and Corticotropin by Small Amounts of Serum and Cerebral Spinal Fluid," *Journal of Endocrinology* 29 (1964): 83.

35. L. J. Soffer, and M. Fogel, "Effect of Urinary Gonadotropin-Inhibiting Substance upon the Action of Human Chorionic Gonadotropin and Human Post Menopausal Urinary Gonadotropin," *Journal of Clinical Endocrinology* 23 (1963): 870.
36. Herono, Igarishi, and Matsumato, "The Direct Effect of HCG," 1214.
37. P. Bonnamy, A. Benham, and P. Leymarie, "Human Chorionic Gonadotropin Affects Tissue Levels of Progesterone and Cyclic Adenosine 3,5—Monophosphate in the Metestrus Rat Utereus in-Vitro," *Biology of Reproduction* 40 (1989): 511; J. S. Richards, and K. Bogovich, "Effect of Human Chorionic Gonadotropin and Progesterone on Follicular Development in the Immature Rat," *Endocrinology* 111 (1982): 1429.

5

The Gowda Experiment

Dr. D. C. Gowda

Dr. D. C. Gowda of the University of Mysore in India (with his associates B. Neelisiddaiah and V. Anjaneyalu) published in *Carbohydrate Research* "Structural Studies of Polysaccharides from Aloe Vera."[1] The mucilagenous jelly from Aloe plicatilis Miller was considered to be a linear (1–4) linked glucomannan having a glucose-to-mannose ratio of 1:2.8. Others suggested the jelly to have equal amounts in the polysaccharide of D-glucose and D-mannose with about 2.4 percent uronic acid. Nevertheless, the structure of the polysaccharide was not investigated. Therefore, Dr. Gowda made a detailed study of the chemical nature of the mucilagenous jelly of aloe vera.

Dr. Gowda extracted the jelly from the leaves of aloe vera with 50 percent aqueous ethanol, followed by precipitation with ethanol giving a polysaccharide mixture, which, after dissolution with HCL, dialysis, and precipitation with ethanol, produced a coarse white fibrous powder. The yield was 0.7 percent based on the weight of the wet jelly. The material was composed of glucose and mannose in a molar ratio of 1:6, with traces of galacturonic acid, arabinose, xylose, and galactose. The precipitation was further purified by repeated precipitation with aqueous ethanol until there was no change in the glucose-to-mannose ratio. Methylation studies indicated that the glucose and the mannose are (1→4) linked in the polysaccharide. The jelly of aloe plicatilis was considered to be a single linear glucomannan, whereas aloe vera was considered to have four linear glucomannans.

The Magic Bullet in Aloe Vera

The traditional approach to natural substances like aloe vera is to extract aloe in search of the active component. Aloe vera has some two hundred active components, so a search for one active substance, a "magic bullet" would be difficult. However, one can isolate fractions that are active in a certain biological direction and when possible identify the active agent. We have shown that amino acids, vitamins, growth factors, aspirin-like substances, sterols, and immune mechanisms have biological activity. Some components are stimulators, and others are inhibitors.[2] Some components in both areas synergize so that the total activity in each system is greater than the sum of the active components. Some ingredients antagonize each other to produce a masking effect. The balance between the inhibition and stimulation in aloe helps us to understand the secrets and miracles found in the aloe plant. The powerful anti-inflammatory activity of sterols in aloe is buffered by the wound-healing influence of growth factors. The end result is that aloe vera has a multiplicity of therapeutic influences with little or no toxicity.

Biological Modulation

All living systems have the ability to receive stimuli and select an appropriate response. The selection process is referred to as a modulation. The modulation in plants may involve enzymatic and chemical reactions as well as nuclear activity and growth factors. The inhibitory and stimulatory systems within aloe vera allow it to act as a modulator of inflammation and wound healing. Most likely, the modulation of aloe represents the interaction between many components, as opposed to the action of any single entity. When a living tissue is confronted with injury or trauma, the local cells and vasculature must recognize the nature of the stimulus and take the appropriate course of action to maintain homeostasis. This balance involves compounds, mediators, and immune mechanisms. R. P. LaBadie found that aloe vera gel contains at least two classes of substances with immunomodulatory activity.[3] One component stimulates antibody information, whereas another inhibits antibody production. This relationship represents biological modulation when applied to inflammation or wound healing. The assessment of single ingredients in aloe vera for their cellular and humoral immune function has received much attention. Claims and theories have been put forth for ascorbate as an immune modulator. Ascorbate is an immune stimulator, and we have shown that it inhibits inflammation and adjuvant-induced arthritis (inhibitor).[4] Modulation of neutrophil motility has been recorded for vitamin C. Phagocytosis and anti-oxidant modulation are being considered.

A Natural Approach to Treating Wounds and Inflammation, Even in the Diabetic

Aloe vera reduced inflammation and improved wound healing in both the normal and diabetic states, in a dose-response fashion.[5] Diabetes mellitus affects 10 million Americans and represents the sixth leading cause of death in the United States. Diabetes exhibits poor wound healing due to poor collagen formation and reduced wound tensile strength. The diabetic fibroblast suffers from premature aging. The diminished inflammatory response for normal phagocytosis of cellular debris is related to an altered metabolic, immune, and cardiovascular posture. Over a dose range of 1 to 100 mg/kg decolorized aloe vera improved wound healing in a dose-response manner in diabetes. Mustard-induced edema was inhibited 60 and 80 percent, respectively, by 10 and 100 mg/kg aloe vera in diabetes. Aloe vera was analgesic in both diabetic and nondiabetic patients. These findings suggest that aloe works effectively in an abnormal physiological state. Combined methanol-water (1:1) and water extracts of fresh aloe leaves were dialyzed to give crude polysaccharide fractions, which exhibited actions to lower plasma sugar levels on I.P. injections in normal mice. These two fractions are designated as arborans A and B.[6] Be on the lookout for fractions that can elevate blood sugar because a modulation of blood sugar by aloe seems evident.

The Aloe Vera Extract and the Biological Assay

The extraction mixture was prepared by adding 400 g of lyophilized aloe vera (decolorized) to 3,200 mls of 50 percent ethanol (1:8

ratio). Unlike in the Gowda procedure,[7] we did not further add ethanol or dialyze to obtain a precipitate, because this would alter the original ethanol percentage. The ethanol-aloe mixture was ultracentrifuged at 3,000 RPMs for ten minutes. The supernatant was separated from the precipitate and both fractions were then frozen to −80° Centigrade. Once thoroughly frozen, both fractions were dried to a powder using a Labconco 4.5 liter freeze-dryer. The supernatant freeze-dried powder, at 1 mg, was equivalent to 1.03 mg of original aloe vera freeze-dried powder. One milligram of the precipitate powder was equivalent to 36 mg of original aloe vera powder.

Adult ICR mice were anesthetized with ether and shaven on both sides of the back. A sterile 6 mm Baker biopsy punch was used to induce a wound on each side of the vertebral column (10–12 wounds/group). Anterior-posterior wound diameter measurements were made using a vernier caliper on days 0 and 4. Mice were given daily subcutaneous injections with 150 mg/kg aqueous unextracted aloe vera over the experimental period. The aloe vera supernatant and precipitate powders were also injected at 150 mg/kg using the same regimen. Control mice received daily injections of saline on a 10 ml/kg basis. Standard errors for each mean value were calculated.[8] The student's "t" test was used to determine significant differences (the p value) between means.

The topical anti-inflammatory activity of the supernatant and precipitate extracts were measured using the croton oil–induced ear-swelling assay.[9] Adult male mice were given 10 μl of 25 μg/μ1 croton oil topically on the inner surface of the right ear using a Hamilton microsyringe. Ear weight differences, as determined by using a 6 mm Baker punch, between the right and left (untreated) ears represented the amount of edema. Aqueous solutions were prepared by adding freeze-dried aloe vera, supernatant, and precipitate in distilled water to give 5 percent solutions in terms of the original aloe vera. Aloe vera, supernatant, and precipitate, at concentration of 5 percent, were applied in volumes of 10 μl per animal, thirty minutes after the croton oil application. The wound-healing activity was compared to the previously obtained anti-inflammatory activity data from a 50 percent ethanol extract of aloe vera.[10]

Assuming that the total biological activity in the original aloe vera is 100 percent calculation of percent anti-inflammatory activity in the 50 percent supernatant and the wound-healing activity in the

50 percent precipitate was determined. This approach might reflect any antagonism of activity present.

The Results and Discussion

The wound-healing activity of a 50 percent ethanol extract of aloe vera was evaluated in mice given 150 mg/kg/day, subcutaneously, over four days (figure 5.1). Animals treated with unextracted aloe vera had a reduction in wound diameter of 29.4 ± 4.4 percent. An average reduction of 47.1 ± 5.7 percent was recorded for mice receiving the 50 percent ethanol precipitate of aloe vera. There was no reduction in wound healing in the mice receiving the supernatant as compared to the untreated control. The wound-healing response obtained by the original aloe vera and the 50 percent ethanol precipitate was not significantly different ($P>0.5$). Since no improvement in wound healing was observed in the 50 percent ethanol supernatant–treated mice, most or all of the wound-healing activity appears to reside in the aloe vera precipitated with 50 percent ethanol.

Biological Activity in Aloe Vera

A comparison of the wound-healing and the anti-inflammatory activities from a 50 percent ethanol extract of aloe vera showed that most of the anti-inflammatory activity (78 percent) was present in the supernatant, as compared to 32 percent recorded in the precipitate (table 5.1 and figurer 5.2). The original aloe had the greatest amount of anti-edema activity.[11] On the other hand, little or no wound-healing activity was recorded for the supernatant (0 percent). Based on mean values, theoretically, the precipitate could have as much as 160 percent wound-healing activity in reference to the unextracted aloe. Possibly the supernatant could be masking some of the ability of the precipitate to heal wounds (figure 5.3).

Components in Aloe Vera and Modulation

The many components in aloe vera that contribute to the total biological activity make it difficult, if not impossible, to identify a

WOUND HEALING ACTIVITY OF A 50% ETHANOL EXTRACT OF ALOE VERA IN MICE GIVEN 150 MG/KG/DAY S.C. OVER 4 DAYS

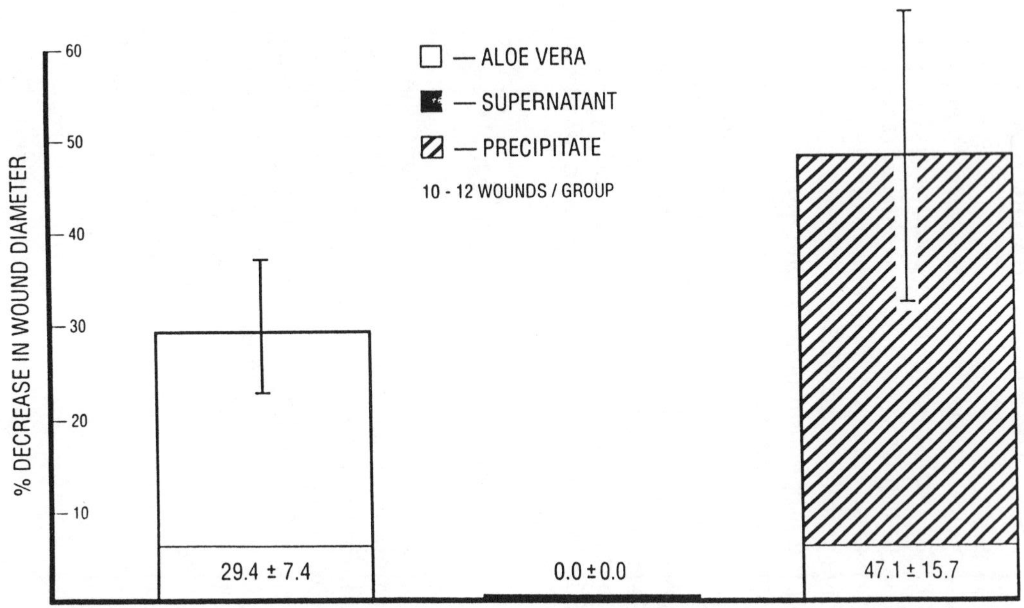

Fig. 5.1.

THE ISOLATION OF THE WOUND HEALING AND ANTI-INFLAMMATORY ACTIVITIES FROM A 50% ETHANOL EXTRACT OF ALOE VERA

	% DECREASE	
	WOUND DIAMETER	EDEMA
ALOE VERA	29.4 ± 7.4 (100)	37.4 ± 4.5 (100)
SUPERNATANT	0.0 ± 0.0 (0)	29.2 ± 2.5 (78)
PRECIPITATE	47.1 ±15.7 (160)	12.1 ± 1 (32)

( )=% STIMULATORY (WOUND HEALING) AND INHIBITORY (ANTI-INFLAMMATORY) ACTIVITY IN ALOE VERA.

Table 5.1.

THE ISOLATION OF THE WOUND HEALING AND ANTI-INFLAMMATORY ACTIVITIES FROM A 50% ETHANOL EXTRACT OF ALOE VERA

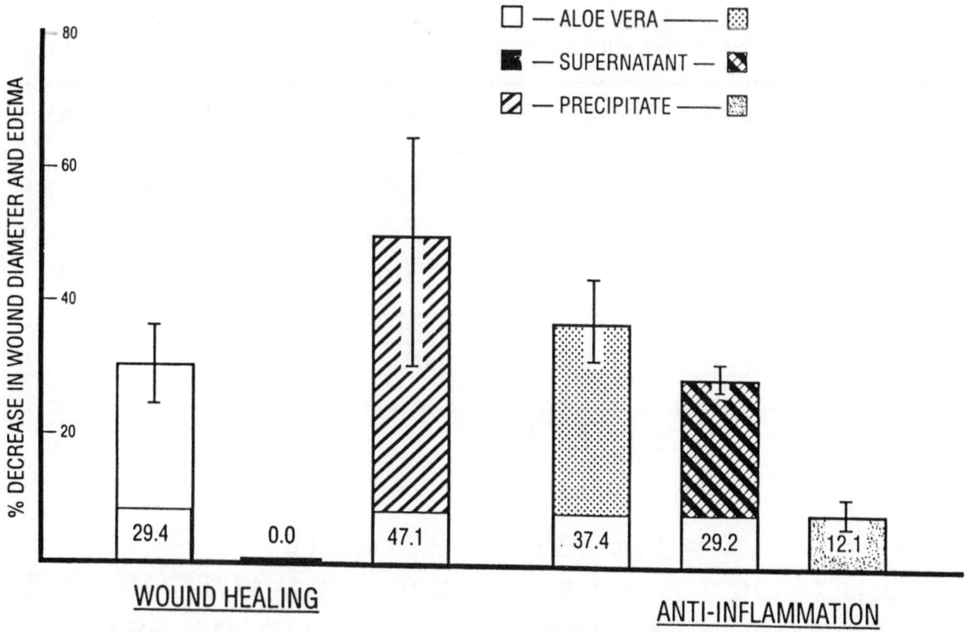

Fig. 5.2.

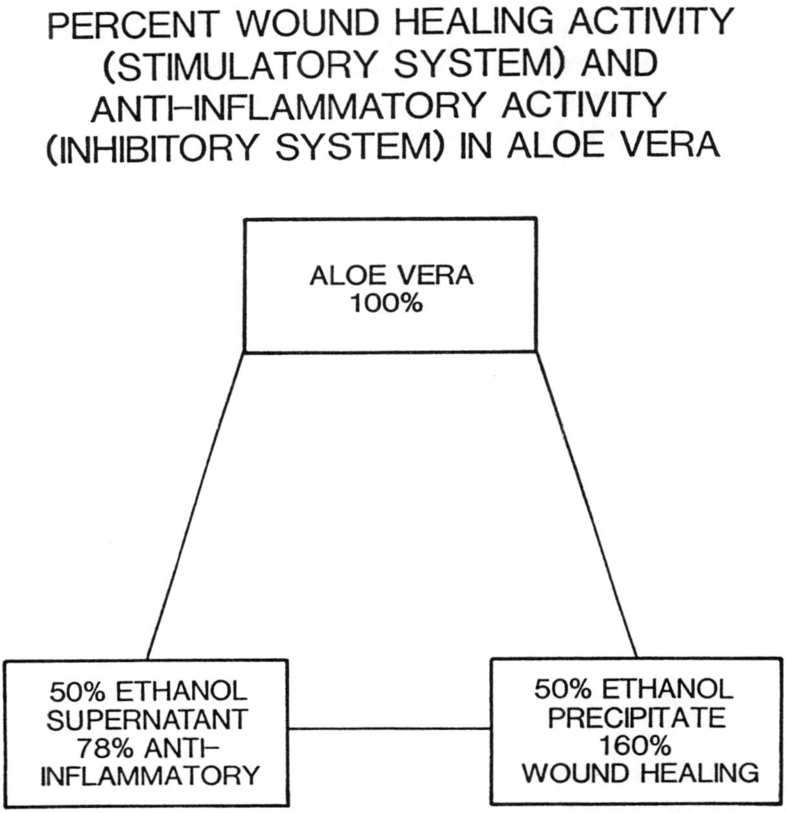
PERCENT WOUND HEALING ACTIVITY
(STIMULATORY SYSTEM) AND
ANTI-INFLAMMATORY ACTIVITY
(INHIBITORY SYSTEM) IN ALOE VERA
ALOE VERA
100%
50% ETHANOL
SUPERNATANT
78% ANTI-
INFLAMMATORY
50% ETHANOL
PRECIPITATE
160%
WOUND HEALING

Fig. 5.3.

single active ingredient. In fact, one tablespoon of aloe vera contains over two hundred different chemicals that have biological activity.[12] We have not accounted for all the active components and activity in aloe vera. To suggest that one ingredient is responsible for wound-healing and anti-inflammatory activity seems presumptive. We have shown certain amino acids, vitamins, RNA, and immune mechanisms to be anti-inflammatory, and so we have grouped these and other ingredients together to form the inhibitory system.[13] I.E. Danhof suggests that the glycoproteins (enzymes) form a major part of this system.[14] The wound-healing or stimulatory system consists of mucopolysaccharide growth factors and other components found in the precipitate. Many active ingredients synergize such that the final sum total of the activity in each system is greater than the sum of the components.[15] Some ingredients antagonize each other so that a masking effect is present. A possible antagonism by the anti-inflammatory or inhibitory system on the wound-healing components appears possible because the 50 percent ethanol precipitate of aloe vera could have 160 percent more wound-healing activity than the original aloe when the anti-inflammatory influence in the supernatant is removed. If a modulation exists between the two systems, synergy, and antagonism within and between the two systems help us to understand the mechanisms contained in the plant gel.

The Aloe Plant

The carbohydrate (polysaccharide) found in the precipitate of a 50 percent ethanol extract of aloe and the glycoprotein (enzymes) in the supernatant are made in the outer rind layers of cells of the aloe leaf. The excess carbohydrate that is needed by the plant for energy is transported to the inner parenchyma and stored as gel fillet. The gel fillet contains 99.5 percent water and 0.5 percent solids, as compared to 12.4 percent solid found in the outer rind. This represents a twenty-four-fold differential in solids relative to fillet. We should mention that the amount of solid formed from the 50 percent ethanol in the precipitate was about thirty-five times that recorded for the supernatant. This represents most of the biological activity of the aloe leaf. Even though a main component of the ethanol precipitate is mucopolysaccharide, which contributes to growth and wound repairs, it does not represent the largest total in biological activity. Thus one should not throw out the supernatant material—both systems are important as biological modulators. Both systems play a major role in the function of the cardiovascular, endocrine, and immune systems.

If the rind is removed from the gel fillet, a slimy mucilage is left behind on the tray. When the mucilage is allowed to dry on an overhead transparency, a "fern reaction"–like complex carbohydrate can be seen. This means that the mucilage contains polysaccharide, which can be extracted. At one time we thought that the mucilage acted as a vehicle to transport synthetized substances throughout the leaf. We now know that the mucilage acts as a container for the inner gel fillet. It combines with aloe and aloin to form a seal so that the gel will not leak out. The combination of mucilage, aloin, and aloe makes a powerful adhesive or glue.

Process of Wound Healing and Aloe Vera

An initial inflammation causes the release of mediators (prostaglandins and bradykinins), which produce a vasodilation and an increased vascular permeability.[16] PMNs and monocytes migrate into the clot, which helps unite the wound edges.[17] The wound then becomes filled with granulation tissue, which is composed of capillaries, fibroblasts, macrophages, and mast cells (proliferation). Collagen fibrils become evident within the wound area, causing an increase in wound strength. Adequate oxygen is needed for this phase of wound healing. In the remodeling phase, fibroblasts form ground substance, collagen, glycoprotein, and proteoglycans. This is a complex process in which the strength and form of the wound tissue are returned to the normal homeostatic state. Aloe vera has anti-inflammatory components such as amino acids,[18] vitamin C,[19] aspirin-like compounds,[20] and mannose,[21] which can normalize the acute vascular response. We have shown that aloe vera can block the PMN response[22] but does not reduce connective tissue formation. In fact, I. E. Danhof[23] and W. Winters[24] have shown that aloe vera stimulates fibroblasts to increase in number in a dose-response fashion. These findings would tend to indicate that aloe increases the remodeling and tensile strength of wounds by causing the fibroblasts to produce collagen. Growth factors in aloe vera must be present for the fibroblast stimulation.[25]

The epidermis thickens at its cut edges due to mitosis of cells in the basal layer. Epithelial cells from the edges of the wound proliferate and migrate along the cut edges of the dermis beneath the surface scab, so that epithelial cells fuse at the midline, producing a continuous thin epithelial layer. Fibroblasts from the lower dermis fill in the wound area as it forms ground substance. If a wound is dry, the scab is deep and epithelial cells migrate downward before moving horizontally through the dermis.[26] Epidermal regeneration is then slowed, producing less new dermis. If the wound is covered, so that the wound is kept wet, basal cells migrate over the surface from the edge to the exudate. The cut edges of the epidermis are sealed over by dividing cells and migrating epidermal cells. The proliferation and migration of cells under occlusion in a wet wound require the presence of oxygen. Oxygen is required for the epidermal regeneration. Aloe vera may act in an occlusive manner to keep the wound moist and at the same time allow oxygen to penetrate the wound for regeneration.[27] Aloe vera prevents water loss from the wound to increase mitosis, proliferation, and migration of epidermal cells. Possibly aloe vera may stimulate the epidermal growth process by adding gibberellin, auxin, or mannose phosphate to the wound. Clearly, fibroblast proliferation and function may be improved by aloe, suggesting that it contains fibroblast growth factor or that it stimulates macrophages.[28]

Carrageenan-Inflamed Synovial Pouch

We studied the seven-day-old air synovial pouch to determine if it can be used as an experimental model that mimics the inflamed joint cavity of rheumatoid arthritis induced by injecting carrageenan into the air pouch. This model we felt could be used to measure the stimulatory system (repair) and the inhibitory system (inflammation) in aloe vera simultaneously. The seven-day-old air synovial pouch was used to determine if it can be employed as a model that reflects inflammation and repair by injecting carrageenan into the pouch. The vascularity of the pouch wall and the number of mast cells in pouch fluid were used to evaluate the anti-inflammatory activity of aloe vera in a simulated synovial cavity. The weight of the sample of pouch wall and the fibroblasts were used to measure the growth aspect of aloe vera.

The Air Pouch Assay

The air pouch synovium model was employed by us to study anti-inflammatory activity of aloe vera as it relates to crippling joint diseases like rheumatoid and adjuvant arthritis. Adult mice ICR mice (30 gm.; 18–20/group) were anesthetized with ether and the entire dorsal surface was shaved using an animal clipper. Using a twenty-five-gauge × 1½" needle, 30 ml of air was subcutaneously injected to form an air pouch. The pouch was sealed by pinching the skin gently on removing the needle. The animals were divided into three groups: saline controls, represented by the non-irritated mice who received 1 ml saline directly into the pouch; the 1 percent carrageenan mice, represented by the inflamed mice who received the 1 ml of 1 percent carrageenan alone into the pouch; the 1 percent carrageenan mice whose pouch received 10 percent aloe vera. This latter group is called the aloe-treated mice. Mice were individually numbered using an ear punch. All pouches were maintained for seven days and were constantly checked for leakage. On the seventh day 1 percent carrageenan was administered into the pouch, which served as irritant controls. Aloe-treated mice received the 1 percent irritant, and two hours later 1 ml of 10 percent freeze-dried decolorized aloe vera was administered into the air pouch. Saline controls received 1 ml of 0.9 percent saline at the same time the aloe was given. All injections into the pouch were 1 ml volumes using a 27-gauge needle.[29]

An inflammation response by 1 percent carrageenan was recorded twenty-four hours after the administration. Mast cells migrated from the synovium under the mouse skin muscle band into the synovial fluid inside the ear cavity. A drop of synovial fluid was placed on an albuminized slide, fixed in alcohol overnight stained with Wright's Quick Stain. The number of cells per twenty fields was counted under oil immersion. The degree of vascularity was recorded for each animal and rated 0 to 3. The zero response represented no vascular response, whereas a 3 represented a maximum vascular response. Photographs were taken of the wall vascularity of animals from each group. A piece of skin was removed from the dorsal wall of the air pouch of each animal by means of a 6 mm Baker biopsy punch. The sample of the skin of the pouch wall was weighed to the nearest 0.01 mg on a Mettler balance. The mast cell count and the vascularity are indications of acute inflammation. The increased weight of the pouch wall represents a growth response and repair by an increase in the number of fibroblasts produced by 10 percent aloe vera in the synovial-like membrane. The anti-inflammatory activity of aloe prevented the occurrence of chronic inflammation, as recorded by the acute anti-inflammatory vascular and mast cell response. A section of the synovial wall was placed in a 10 percent formalin and stained with hematoxylin-eosin. Mean values were calculated for each endpoint as well as the corresponding standard errors of the mean. The student's "t" test was used to determine the significant differences between means.[30]

The Carrageenan-Inflamed Synovial Pouch Response to Aloe Vera Confirms Our Biological Results from the Gowda Experiment

Hans Selye adapted an air pouch method to evaluate inflammation.[31] The histology of the irritant-induced inflamed wall as well as the cells and biochemistry of the fluid could be used to test synthetic and natural anti-inflammatory agents. We have shown that croton oil–induced inflammation could be reduced in a dose-response fashion by tryptophan by evaluating the vascularity of the air pouch wall.[32] The injection of air under the skin forms an air pouch whose lining cells closely resemble synovial cells in rodents.[33] Intra-articular injections in rats have been used to study synovial cell response to injury, but the damage is non-specific. The air pouch permits easy study of injury in synovial-like tissue. According to the pouch age, it progressively develops phagocytic-like lining cells and organized vasculature that acts as a mechanical barrier to the products of the inflammatory response.[34] The six-day-old pouch seems to be an ideal test model to study the anti-inflammatory activity of aloe vera as it mimics the human synovium. This model is easy and gives us reproducible results (figure 5.4).

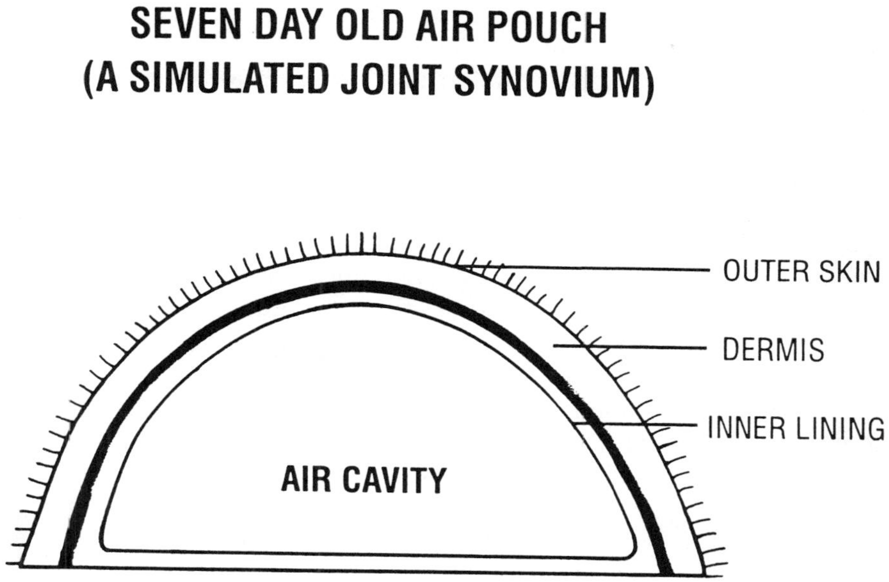
SEVEN DAY OLD AIR POUCH
(A SIMULATED JOINT SYNOVIUM)
OUTER SKIN
DERMIS
INNER LINING
AIR CAVITY

Fig. 5.4.

Mast Cells

Table 5.2 and figure 5.5 shows the effects of aloe vera on the number of mast cells in fluid aspirated from air pouch cavities treated with 1 percent carrageenan. No mast cells were found in aspirated fluid from saline control mice. The number of mast cells was increased to 13.4 ± 0.8 per 20 fields in animals treated with carrageenan ($P<0.001$). Administration of 10 percent aloe vera reduced the mast cell response 52.2 percent ($P<0.001$). Mast cells are found in connective tissue that increase in inflammation and migrate into tissue fluid. Mast cells were seen in the inner lining of the air pouch that were increased by the carrageenan-induced inflammation. The best response was recorded twenty-four hours after the carrageenan injection.[35] However, the histamine content in pouch fluid and tissue was noted 30 minutes after the irritant injection. The role of mast cells in connective tissue during the inflammation is not clearly understood. The connective tissue mast cells seen in our study are larger, with many uniform granules, as well as having a higher histamine content.[36] There is an increase in mast cells in the synovial lining of patients with rheumatoid arthritis and rat adjuvant arthritis.[37] The majority of mast cells in tissue seemed to be near blood vessels, suggesting, possibly, that they play a role in the carrageenan-induced inflammation. In any event, 10 percent aloe vera reduces the acute inflammation when injected into the inflamed pouch, as well as decreasing the mast cell numbers in pouch fluid.

Vascular Response and the Pouch Wall

Table 5.3 and figure 5.6 show the effects of aloe vera on a 1 percent carrageenan–irritated simulated joint synovial model. A biopsy punch weight of the air pouch wall revealed no significant increase in weight in 1 percent carrageenan–treated mice over saline control animals ($P>0.5$). However, administration of 10 percent aloe into the carrageenan-treated mice increased the wall punch biopsy weight from 21.4 ± 0.9 to 27.3 ± 1.9 mg ($P<0.01$). This represents a 27.6 percent increase in biopsy weight by 10 percent aloe vera. Inflammation causes a redness and vasodilation of the air pouch wall. Carrageenan (1 percent) increased the vascular rating of the air pouch

EFFECT OF ALOE VERA ON THE NUMBER OF MAST CELLS IN FLUID ASPIRATED FROM AIR POUCH CAVITIES TREATED WITH 1% CARRAGEENAN

	NO. OF MAST CELLS*
SALINE CONTROL	0.0 ± 0.0
1% CARRAGEENAN	13.4 ± 0.8
+ 10% ALOE VERA	6.4 ± 0.7**

* NO. OF MAST CELLS / 20 FIELDS; ** $p < 0.001$; 5 MICE/GROUP

Table 5.2.

EFFECT OF ALOE VERA ON THE NUMBER OF MAST CELLS IN FLUID ASPIRATED FROM AIR POUCH CAVITIES TREATED WITH 1% CARRAGEENAN

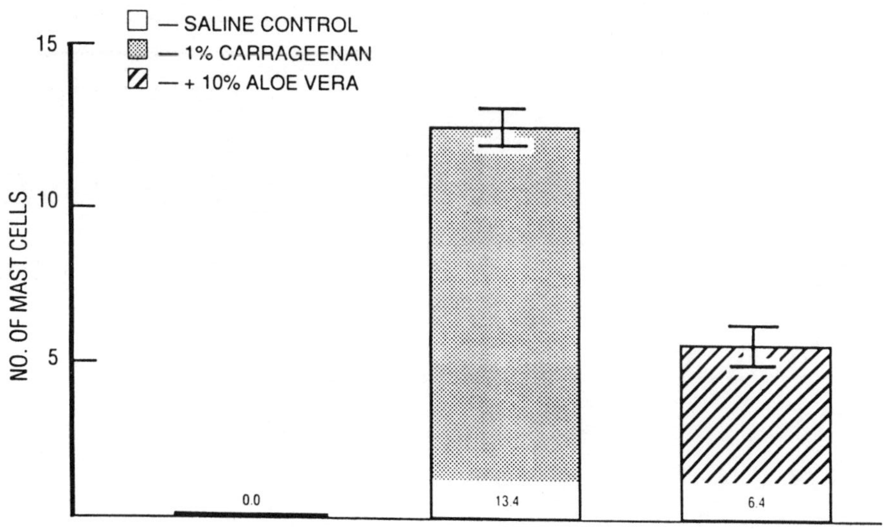

Fig. 5.5.

EFFECT OF ALOE VERA ON A 1% CARRAGEENAN IRRITATED SIMULATED JOINT SYNOVIAL MODEL

	AIR POUCH WALL	
	BIOPSY PUNCH (MG)	VASCULAR RATING (0-3)
SALINE CONTROL	21.2 ± 0.9	0.0 ± 0.0
1% CARRAGEENAN	21.4 ± 0.9	2.6 ± 0.1
+ 10% ALOE VERA	$27.3 \pm 1.9^{*}$	$1.3 \pm 0.2^{**}$

18-20 MICE/GROUP; * < 0.01, ** $p < 0.001$

Table 5.3.

EFFECT OF ALOE VERA ON A 1% CARRAGEENAN IRRITATED SIMULATED JOINT SYNOVIAL MODEL

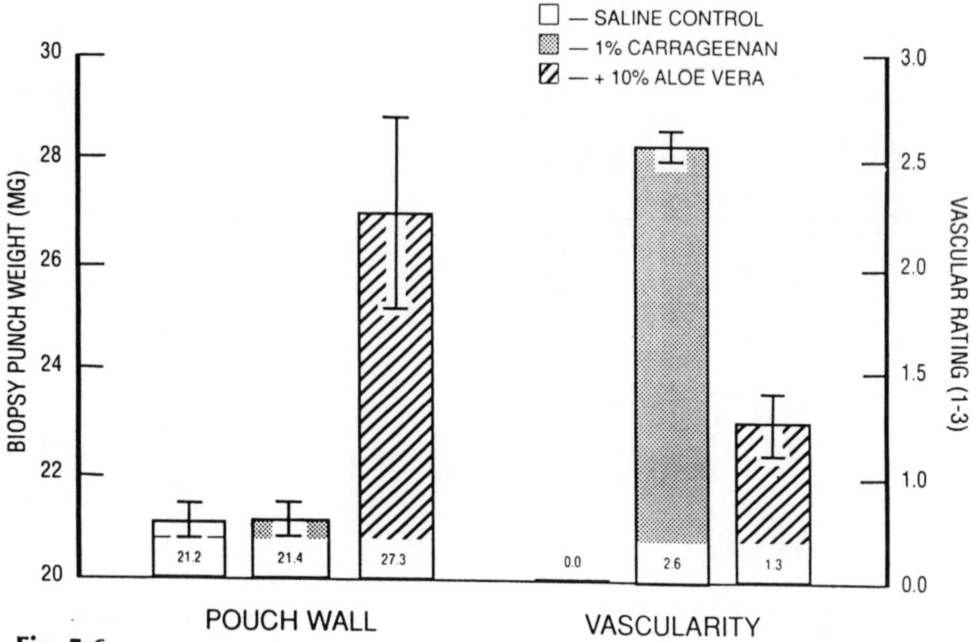

Fig. 5.6.

wall from 0.0 ± 0.0 to 2.6 ± 0.1 ($P<0.001$). This response is very similar to the mast cell response, and both represent acute inflammation. Administration of 10 percent aloe vera into the air pouch treated with 1 percent carrageenan inhibited the pouch wall redness and vasodilation 50 percent ($P<0.001$). Pictures were taken of the inflammatory vasodilation of 1 percent carrageenan and the acute anti-inflammatory response of 10 percent aloe vera. Since the acute anti-inflammatory response of 10 percent aloe vera occurred in the first 0 to 6 hours, the increase in air pouch punch biopsy weight by aloe represents a healing and repair response.

Since aloe vera stimulates fibroblast growth and repair by wound healing, the increase in pouch wall weight does not represent a chronic inflammatory effect.[38] We have shown that aloe vera has no anti-fibrosis activity in chronic inflammation. In fact, doses up to 400 mg/kg did not block chronic inflammation.[39] Aloe vera has no chronic anti-inflammatory activity but rather stimulates fibroblast growth and function for wound healing and repair. The 27.6 percent increase in biopsy weight by 10 percent aloe vera represents an increase in fibroblast numbers (growth response) of the inner synovial lining as observed histologically. This is a growth-repair effect of aloe vera and not a chronic inflammatory response. The wound healing/repair and the acute anti-inflammatory activity of aloe vera were recorded simultaneously in this air pouch test model. Aloe vera inhibited acute inflammation, as evidenced by the inhibition of mast cells and vasodilation of pouch vessels. Aloe vera stimulated fibroblast growth-repair of the air pouch wall, as seen by the increase in biopsy weight, as well as the increase in fibroblast numbers in the synovial inner lining. This is not a chronic inflammatory response. The synovial air pouch can be used as an in vivo model to simultaneously study the acute anti-inflammatory and wound healing (fibroblast stimulation) activities of aloe vera. This experimental synovial model should provide data for future application of aloe vera.

Immunomodulatory Compounds in Aloe Vera

LaBadie and his group found there was modulatory activity with regard to human complement and PMNs.[40] One fraction could inhibit the production of free oxygen radicals by activated PMNs. This activity could not be attributed to non-specific effects like toxicity, stimulant binding, or scavenger activity. The results of LaBadie's work indicate that the aqueous extract of aloe vera gel has at least two classes of substances with immuno-modulatory activity. He points out that aloe vera has healing effects in experimentally induced disorders in laboratory animals such as bacterial infections, carrageenan-induced edema, and adjuvant arthritis. Similar results have been recorded in our laboratory.

Summary

We have shown that a 50 percent ethanol extract precipitate of aloe vera improved wound healing 47.1 percent as compared to the 29.4 percent recorded for the unextracted aloe vera. Little or no wound-healing activity was found in the supernatant. Based on mean values, the precipitate could have as much as 160 percent wound-healing activity in reference to the original unextracted aloe vera. Possibly the supernatant with its anti-inflammatory activity could be "masking" some of the wound-healing activity of the precipitate. Aloe vera has an inhibitory system (anti-inflammatory activity) and a stimulatory system (wound-healing activity), which may act as a modulator of wound healing and inflammation. Administration under the skin forms an air pouch with an inner lining that can be inflamed by carrageenan to mimic human synovitis. The air cavity became lined with an increased number of mast cells, which go into the cavity fluid. The vascularity of the pouch wall was increased by carrageenan-induced inflammation. Both these end points of inflammation were inhibited by the administration of 10 percent aloe vera directly into the air pouch. The fibroblast stimulation activity of aloe vera recorded in wound healing was observed in this study. The air pouch wall biopsy weight was significantly increased ($p<0.01$) by aloe vera. Also, histological examination of the synovium revealed that aloe vera stimulated the fibroblast numbers. Since aloe vera has little or no toxicity even at very high does, we interpret the fibroblast response in the air pouch not as chronic inflammation, but rather a growth-repair response. This simultaneous inhibition of inflammation and the growth repair response by aloe vera verifies the data we recorded from our biological Gowda experiment.

References

1. D. C. Gowda, B. Neelisiddaiah, and V. Anjaneyalu, "Structural Studies of Polysaccharides from Aloe Vera," *Carbohydrate Research* 72 (1979): 201.
2. R. H. Davis, "Inhibitory and Stimulatory Systems in Aloe Vera," *Aloe Today,* Winter 1992.
3. L. A. Hart, P. H. Enckevort, H. Van Dijk, R. Zaat, R. T. D. DeSilva, and R. P. LaBadie, "Two Functionally and Chemically Distinct Immunomodulatory Compounds in the Gel of Aloe Vera," *J. Ethnopharmacology* 23 (1988): 61.
4. R. H. Davis, P. S. Agnew, and E. Shapiro, "Effect of Aloe, Vitamin C and RNA on Adjuvant Arthritis," *Pennsylvania Academy of Science* 58 (1984): 114; D. C. Hanley, W. A. Solamon, B. Saffran, R. H. Davis, "The Evaluation of Natural Substances in Treatment of Adjuvant Arthritis," *Journal of the American Podiatric Association* 72 (1982): 275.
5. R. H. Davis, M. G. Leitner, J. M. Russo, "Aloe Vera Improves Wound Healing and Reduces Inflammation in Diabetes," *Pennsylvania Academy of Science* 61 (1987): 84.
6. H. Hikino, M. Takahaski, L. Murakami, C. Konno, "Isolation and Hypoglcemic Activity of Arborans A and B, Glycans of Aloe Arborescens Var. Natalensis Leaves," *International Journal of Crude Drug Research* 24 (1986): 183.
7. Gowdy, Neelisaddaiah, and Anjaneyalu, "Structural Studies," 201.
8. G. W. Snedecor, and W. G. Cochran, *Statistical Methods,* 6th ed. (Ames: Iowa State University Press, 1974).
9. R. H. Davis, J. Kabbani, and J. Maro, "Aloe Vera and Inflammation," *Pennsylvania Academy of Science* 60 (1986): 67.
10. R. H. Davis, W. L. Parker, R. T. Samson, and D. P. Murdoch, "The Isolation of an Active Inhibitory System from an Extract of Aloe Vera," *Journal of the American Podiatric Medical Association* 81 (1991): 258.
11. Ibid.
12. B. C. Coats, and R. E. Holland, *Creatures in Our Care: The Veterinary Uses of Aloe Vera,* (Dallas, TS: , n.p. 1990).
13. Davis, Kabbani, and Maro, "Aloe Vera and Inflammation," 67.
14. I. E. Danhof, *Remarkable Aloe,* Grand Prairie, TX, self-published, Omnimedicus Press, 1987).
15. B. C. Coats, *The Silent Healer: A Modern Study of Aloe Vera* (Garland, TX: self-published, 1979).
16. R. H. Davis, W. L. Parker, and D. P. Murdoch, "Aloe Vera as a Biologically Active Vehicle for Hydrocortisone Acetate," *Journal of the American Podiatric Medical Association* 81 (1991): 1.
17. P. Dineen, G. Hildick-Smith, *The Surgical Wound* (Philadelphia Lea and Febiger, 1981); H. I. Maibach, and D. T. Rovee, *Epidermal Wound Healing* (Chicago: Yearbook Medical Publishers, 1972); J. R. Perez-Polo, J. DeVellis, and B. Haber, *Growth and Trophic Factors,* (New York: Alan R. Liss, 1983).
18. M. B. Forst, and R. H. Davis, "Effect of Tryptophane, Anthranilic Acid and Ribonucleic Acid on Adjuvant Arthritis," *Journal of the American Podiatric Medical Association* 69 (1979): 643.

19. R. H. Davis, K. Y. Rosenthal, L. R. Cesario, and G. R. Rouw, "Vitamin C. Influence on Localized Adjuvant Arthritis," *Journal of the American Podiatric Medical Association* 80 (1990): 14.
20. Coats, *The Silent Healer.*
21. D. O. Willenborg, C. R. Parish, W. B. Cowden, "Phosphosugars Are Potent Inhibitors of Central Nervous System Inflammation," *Federation of the American Society of Experimental Biology,* 3 (1989): 1968.
22. Davis, Kabbani, and Maro, "Aloe Vera and Inflammation," 67; R. H. Davis, and N. P. Maro, "Aloe Vera and Gibberellin Anti-Inflammatory Activity in Diabetics," Journal of the American Podiatric Medical Association, 79 (1989): 24.
23. Danhof, *Remarkable Aloe.*
24. W. Winters, R. Benavides, W. J. Clouse, "Effect of Aloe Extracts on Human Normal and Tumor Cells in Vitro," *Economic Botany* 35 (1981): 89.
25. Perez-Polo, DeVellis, and Haber, *Growth and Trophic Factors*; Davis and Maro, "Aloe Vera and Gibberellin," 24.
26. Davis, Parker, and Murdoch, "Aloe Vera as a Biologically Active Vehicle,"; J. T. Scales, "Wound Healing and the Dressing," *British Journal of Industrial Medicine,* 20 (1963): 82.
27. Davis, Parker, and Murdoch, "Aloe Vera as a Biologically Active Vehicle,"; J. C. Forrester, "The Tape Closed Wound—a Bioengineering Analysis," *Journal of Scientific Research* 9 (1969): 537.
28. Danhof, *Remarkable Aloe.*
29. J. C. W. Edward, A. D. Sedgwick, and D. A. Willoughby, "The Formation of a Structure with Features of Synovial Lining by Subcutaneous Injection of Air, An in Vivo Tissue Culture System," *Journal of Pathology* 134 (1981): 147.
30. Snedecor and Cochran, *Statistical Method.*
31. Selye, Hans, *The Stress of Life* (New York: McGraw: Hill, 1956), 151–61.
32. R. H. Davis, H. S. Pitkow, and K. A. Shovlin, "Anti-Inflammatory Effect of Tryptophan in a Selye Pouch," *Journal of the American Podiatric Association* 71 (1981): 690.
33. Edwards, Sedgwick, and Willoughby, "The Formation of a Structure," 1947.
34. A. D. Sedgwick, Y. M. Sin, A. R. Mackay, A. Alduaij, and D. A. Willoughby, "Studies into the Mode of Action of Non-Steroidal Anti-Inflammatory Drugs Using a Model of Facsimile Synovium," *Journal of Pharmacologic Pharmacology* 36 (1983): 171.
35. Y. M. Sin, A. D. Sedgwick, E. P. Chea, and D. A. Willoughby, "Mast Cells in Newly Formed Lining Tissue during Acute Inflammation: A Six Day Air Pouch Model in the Mouse," *Annals of the Rheumatic Disease* 45 (1986): 873.
36. Ibid.
37. A. J. Crisp, "Mast Cells in Rheumatoid Arthritis," *Journal of the Royal Society of Medicine* 77 (1984): 450; k. Hiroshata and I. Kobayashi,: "Fine Structure of the Synovial Tissue in Rheumatoid Arthritis," *Kobe Journal of Medical Science* 10 (1964): 195.kk
38. Danhof, *Remarkable Aloe.*
39. R. H. Davis, "A Natural Influence on Adjuvant Induced Arthritis in Rats," *Pennsylvania Academy of Science* 56 (1982): 112.
40. Hart, Van Enckevort, Van Dijk, Zaat, DeSilva, and LaBadie, "Two Functionally and Chemically Distinct Immunomodulatory Compounds," 61.

6

Improved Wound Healing by Aloe Vera

Aloe Acts Like a "Crazy Glue"

If an animal should puncture the leaf, one observes that the leaf is able to seal the wound and prevent the gel fillet from leaking to the outside. Every aloe farmer who removes the leaf at harvest observes that at the point of severance of the leaf, the leaf seals and contracts to prevent aloe gel from escaping. We measured the cross-sectional contraction of the leaf at various distances from the tip. The closer the cuts across the leaf were to the base of the leaf, the greater the contraction. This response was due to a greater cross-sectional area as one moves from the tip to base. The amount of mucilage per unit volume of aloe gel increases to cause a greater sealing of the leaf wound. We punctured the leaf at specific points along the leaf and found the sealant time was very accurate. How does this sealant action take place? The mucilage in the presence of aloe gel hardens and acts as a "Crazy Glue" to seal the leaf hole so that the gel does not leak out. When mucilage is mixed with aloe and applied to the surfaces of two wooden sticks, the force (tensile strength) required to pull the sticks apart was 1228.2 ± 30.3 grams ($N = 9$). We felt that if we could transfer this phenomena to the human incisional wound, we would have a major discovery in wound healing and an important therapeutic use for aloe vera.[1] Our research on the movement of water through the skin using gel fillet suggests that aloe vera gel fillet in high doses can remove water from the skin. However, if mucilage is mixed with aloe, we feel this will not occur because of the occlusive properties (covering) of mucilage. Mucilage redirects the water into the skin in the presence of aloe. The transformation of the mucilage from a liquid (sol) to a gel we call a sol-gel transformation. Our electron microscope observations, as well as the "fern reaction," suggest that mucilage is a long chain polysaccharide. The burial custom in the first century was to cover the body with aloe that weighed half the body weight. For example, they covered Jesus' body with 100 pounds of aloe and wrapped it with linen strips. We can estimate that he weighed about 200 pounds. The aloe (plus mucilage) and linen sealed and preserved the body. It kept the air out. They first wrapped the fingers, then the arms, and then the whole body until it looked like a mummy (John 19). This was one of the great secrets of those early days.

Aloe and mucilage form a colloidal system in which the particles are of such a size that they do not settle to form a precipitate but hang in the liquid phase. The constant agitation of the particles suggests they have energy that counteracts gravity. The colloidal particles have electric charges, which go against gravity, and an envelope of water around them aids the colloidal process. The change from a sol (liquid) to a gel (solid) can be brought about by a change in temperature, pH, concentration, agitation, and pressure. It is the gel form that acts as a "Crazy Glue" capable of sealing the hole in the leaf so that gel fillet does not leak out. The particles are polysaccharide, and the surrounding liquid consists of water with dissolved materials.[2] The wind moves the aloe leaf and imparts energy to the solid particles (the gel) to convert it to a liquid sol so that the leaf can move the aloe from the leaf tip to the center of the aloe plant. In this way, aloe vera production is increased.

Connective Tissue Is Important to Wound Healing

The connective tissue serves an important function of connecting tissues together. Connective tissues form basement membranes, blood vessels, body cavity linings, and intra-organ frameworks. Connective tissue cells produce materials that support other tissues. The chief component of connective tissue is collagen. Collagen is a tough fibrous protein that connects tissues together. It plays the major role in giving wounds tensile strength.[3] The fibroblast makes the collagen by forming three peptide chains. The process requires proline, lysine, ascorbic acid, and oxygen. A deficiency of any one of these factors prevents collagen synthesis. In the early phases of wound healing there is a reduction in collagen, but during remodeling the mechanical strength of the wound increases due to a greater maturation of wound collagen. Collagen gives wounds its tensile strength. The ground substance contains water, electrolytes, glycoproteins, and proteoglycans. Connective tissue contains varying amounts of ground substance between the cells and collagen fibers. The proteoglycans are large protein polysaccharides, also, synthesized by fibroblasts. These large complex molecules are glycosaminoglycans—long chains of modified sugars. They hold water to give connective tissue much flexibility. Connective tissue has the capability of repair, as in wound healing by making and remodeling collagen and proteoglycans.[4]

Collagen is composed of proline, glycine, and lysine. Proteoglycans are made up of sugars. In many ways, the biochemistry of connective tissue reminds us of the composition of aloe vera. Glucosamine is an important precursor of proteoglycans, and it makes up about 50 percent of hyaluronic acid and chondroitin sulfate. Since glucosamine stimulates the production of collagen and proteoglycans, it would enhance cartilage repair in osteoarthritis. Since aloe vera stimulates the fibroblast to increase wound tensile strength, it may stimulate glucosamine to form collagen and proteoglycans.[5] Aloe vera increases wound tensile strength and collagen formation, but zinc and vitamin C must be present. Our experience with aloe vera suggests that it might be used to repair joint cartilage, damaged tendons, and wounds that do not heal. Supplementing aloe vera with glucosamine would be an interesting treatment to stimulate connective tissue repair.

Mechanical Properties of Skin

Skin contains cells, a fibrous network of collagen, elastin, and ground substance. This mixture determines the mechanical properties of skin. Skin exhibits tension and extensibility. Skin tension determines the mechanical response to an incised wound. It also plays a critical part in wound contraction. Tension varies with age and is related to the content and direction of elastic fibers of the dermis. The breaking strength of the skin increases fourfold with increasing age. The thickness of skin also increases with age and parallels the collagen content. Extensibility declines with age. In general, the mechanical properties of skin correlate with the meshwork of collagen fibers. Our experience tells us that the breaking strength of skin depends upon the rate at which the force is applied. During the stretching of skin, the interstitial fluid is displaced. These properties change with age, skin thickness, and composition.[6]

Tensile Strength Measurement

The tensile strength of wounds is measured as the force or load applied per unit of cross-section area.[7] The breaking strength is the force required to break a wound. Skin thickness increases with age, and thus breaking strength can increase with age. The tensile strength is not a function of the length of the incision, but breaking strength is. In measuring tensile strength, the application of force, skin thickness, and incision length must be controlled. The method of measuring tensile strength usually includes the measurement of force required to pull apart a wound in an intact animal or excised wound tissue. A receptacle attached to one edge of the wound can be filled with water until the wound breaks. The receptacle and fluid are weighed as an expression of wound tensile strength. In our tensile strength studies in diabetic animals, we used clips fixed to each side of the skin wound. One was fixed and the other led over a pulley to a container to which we added water until the wound was disrupted. This apparatus gave us a good measure of tensile strength. Some instruments (computerized) cost up to $30,000.[8] We have devised a plastic syringe (cost is $5.00) with mm markings on the plunger that go up to 220 mm of air pressure. The peritoneal cavity is filled with air until the wound is disrupted and the volume of air is recorded. This method is very sensitive and accurate for measuring tensile strength to wounds. It is our feeling that measurement of force to disrupt a wound in living animals is more meaningful than similar measurements made of excised tissue. Since collagen is a fibrous protein and the hexosamine-containing component is amorphous, one can assume that collagen contributes most to the total tensile strength of wounds. The tensile strength of wounds is closely related to cross-linking of the already-formed collagen fibers. There is virtually no correlation between hexosamine content of wounds and tensile strength.

Factors Affecting Wound Tensile Strength (Figure 6.1)

Severe anemia interferes with wound healing. A sharp reduction in wound tensile strength was recorded in rabbits when hemoglobin was reduced to 35 percent by bleeding. One of the functions of blood is to carry oxygen to tissues. Increasing local tissue oxygen concentration improves the rate of wound healing. Maximum wound healing was obtained at about 30 percent oxygen, but at 12 percent wound healing was impaired. Low oxygen tension occurs in the early stage of wound healing, and gradually increases as healing progresses. Oxygen is critical and limits the healing rate. Wounds healed more quickly at an environment temperature of 30° C than at the normal room temperature of 18–20° C. Warm environments favored healing, whereas cold temperatures were detrimental to wound healing. Local application of adrenocortical steroids inhibited the formation of granulation tissue. In fact, cortisone retards the production of all mesenchymal cellular elements of repair. Stress stimulates ACTH and causes an increased secretion of adrenal corticoids, which depress connective tissue elements of wound healing. Collagen synthesis and mucopolysaccharide synthesis are inhibited by cortisone and chronic stress. Histamine plays an important role in the early stages of wound healing. Depletion of skin histamine retarded wound healing and lowered tensile strength. However, injected histamine did not appear to influence healing. Attempts to inhibit histamine formation showed no effect on wound healing. The results at this time make it difficult to determine the influence of histamine on wound tensile strength.[9]

Nutritional Influence on Wound Healing

Water Content of Wounds

R. J. Adamsons measured the water content of incised wounds in guinea pigs and found that the greatest increase in water occurred during the first twenty-four hours. Increases in water content of a wound were due to metabolic water. The water content of the wound had no positive relationship to the tensile strength (figure 6.2).[10]

FACTORS AFFECTING WOUND TENSILE STRENGTH

ANEMIA AND BLOOD LOSS ⇩

OXYGEN TENSION ⇧

CORTICOIDS ⇩

STRESS ⇩

HISTAMINE?

Fig. 6.1.

Whole-plant aloe vera (50 mg/kg × 4) was able to increase the percentage of water in wound connective tissue over controls (figure 6.3). A high water content is normal for healing wounds because it represents a new specialized tissue that differs biologically and chemically from unwounded tissue.

Protein Depletion

Depletion of protein contributes to poor wound healing.[11] It prolongs the inflammatory, or lag phase. There is a decrease in fibroblast numbers, proteoglycans, and collagen synthesis. Methionine can be converted to cystine, which can reverse the effects of protein depletion. The formation of disulfide bonds appears to be critical for the proper alignment and attachment of the peptide chains needed to form tropocollagen. Sulfur containing amino acids may be important to the wound-healing process. Histidine-deficient animals have a reduced wound-breaking strength. Protein depletion can be correlated with a decrease in wound tensile strength. J. M. Daly[12] fed rats a protein deficient diet for six weeks. The results showed that wound tensile strength was reduced from 222 mm Hg (controls) to 166 mm Hg (six weeks protein depletion diet) (Table 6.1). Feeding of dextrose was of no value but 5 percent amino acids could restore the tensile strength toward normal. No significant impairment of wound healing is associated with essential fatty acid deficiency.

Vitamin C and Wound Healing

The primary defect in ascorbic acid deficiency was the failure of fibroblasts to produce collagen. Vitamin C is essential for the process of hydroxylation of proline, which is used for the actual construction of the collagen molecule. Collagen's helix coil is stabilized by hydroxyproline and hydroxylysine.[13] During collagen synthesis, collagen lysis and synthesis occur at the same time. When vitamin C is absent, collagen lysis predominates. Lack of ascorbic acid leads to scurvy and wound degeneration. Administration of vitamin C improves wound healing. However, if vitamin C is deficient, an improper sequence of amino acids is produced. The procollagen chains

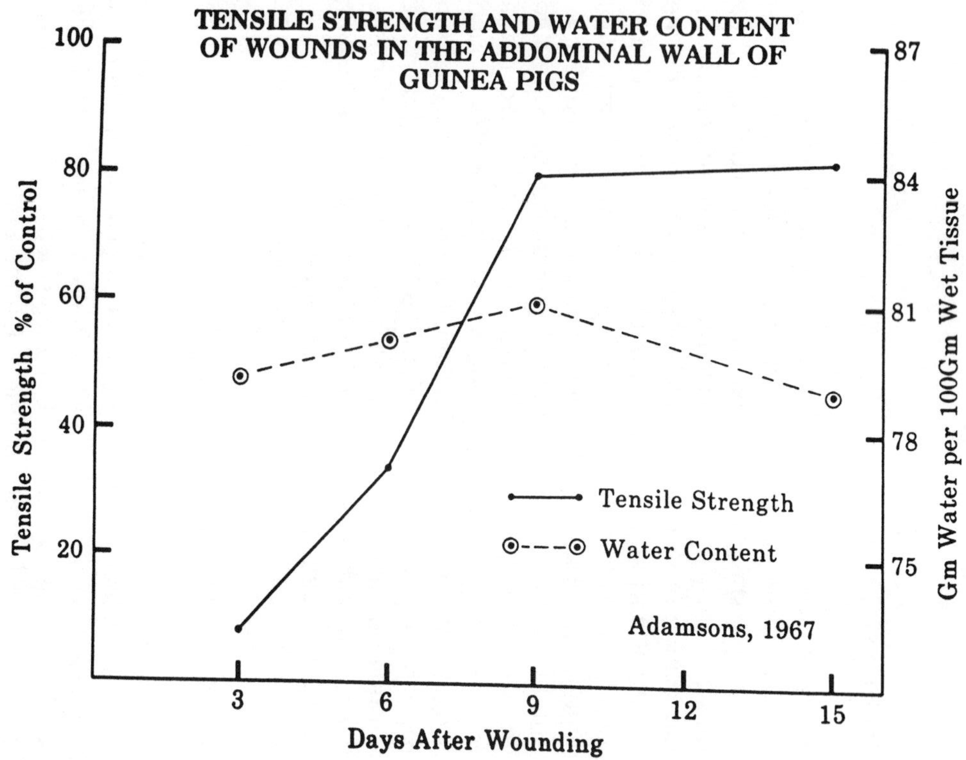
TENSILE STRENGTH AND WATER CONTENT OF WOUNDS IN THE ABDOMINAL WALL OF GUINEA PIGS
Tensile Strength % of Control
100
80
60
40
20
Gm Water per 100Gm Wet Tissue
87
84
81
78
75
Tensile Strength
Water Content
Adamsons, 1967
3
6
9
12
15
Days After Wounding

Fig. 6.2.

EFFECT OF WHOLE PLANT ALOE VERA ON THE PERCENT WATER IN WOUND CONNECTIVE TISSUE

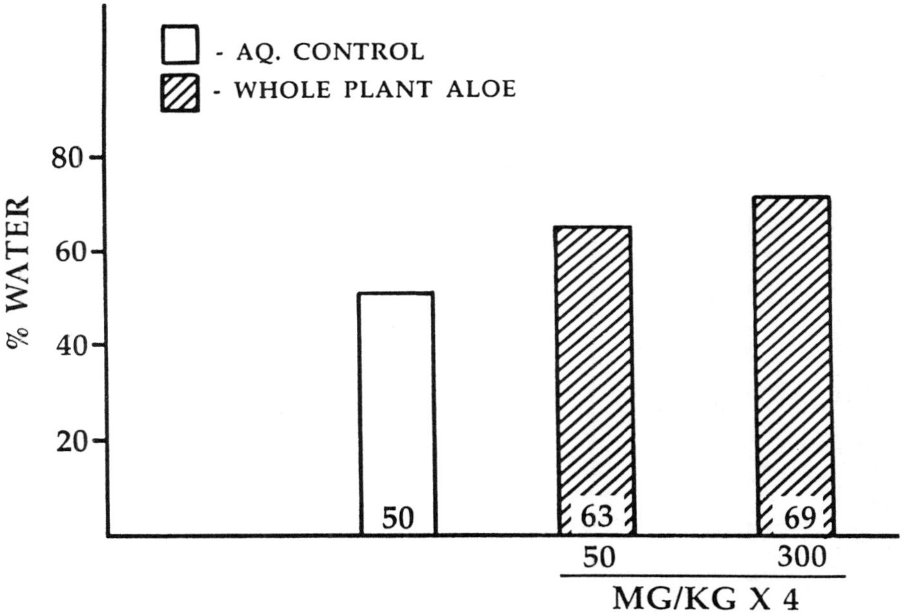

Fig. 6.3.

PROTEIN DEPLETION INFLUENCE ON WOUND HEALING TENSILE STRENGTH IN RATS

DURATION OF PROTEIN DEPLETION (WKS)	TENSILE STRENGTH MMHg
CONTROL	222
2	178
6	166

DALY, 1972

Table 6.1.

are not secreted from the cell, satisfactory polymerization does not occur, and the clinical picture of scurvy results. Adamson shows the wound tensile strength and hydroxyproline concentrations in wounds of scorbutic and vitamin C–treated guinea pigs (figure 6.4). As the percentage of hydroxyproline in wounds increased, the tensile strength increased proportionately. This proves that vitamin C is needed for collagen synthesis, tensile strength, and hydroxyproline formation. Vitamin A may also be a necessary cofactor for collagen synthesis and cross-linkage.

Zinc Deficiency

Zinc deficiency has an adverse effect on wound healing by inhibiting epithelialization, tensile strength, and collagen.[14] Zinc is a cofactor in various enzyme systems responsible for cellular proliferation, such as reverse transcriptase and DNA polymerase. Multiplication of fibroblasts is needed for collagen formation but is inhibited by zinc deficiency. Zinc deficiency in normal mice decreases wound tensile strength from 1441 ± 142 to 559 ± 103. However, supplementation with zinc brought the tensile strength back to normal. In diabetes, wound tensile strength is reduced, which can be normalized by administering zinc (table 6.2). Supplemental zinc may accelerate wound healing to an above-normal rate. Magnesium may also be needed for wound healing.

Aloe vera contains vitamin C, zinc, water, growth factors, and a small amount of protein.[15] These ingredients and others contribute to a positive nutritional influence on wound healing. Aloe vera inhibits inflammation and improves open wound and incisional wound healing.

Whole-Leaf Aloe Vera–Mucilage (1:1 Ratio)

We observed a "fern reaction" with mucilage, suggesting that mucilage is a long chain polysaccharide. When water was removed from mucilage, it closely resembled a bandage. If mucilage is placed over an open wound, the wound remains moist and does not drop, as a dry wound does. Mucilage has an occlusive nature that improves

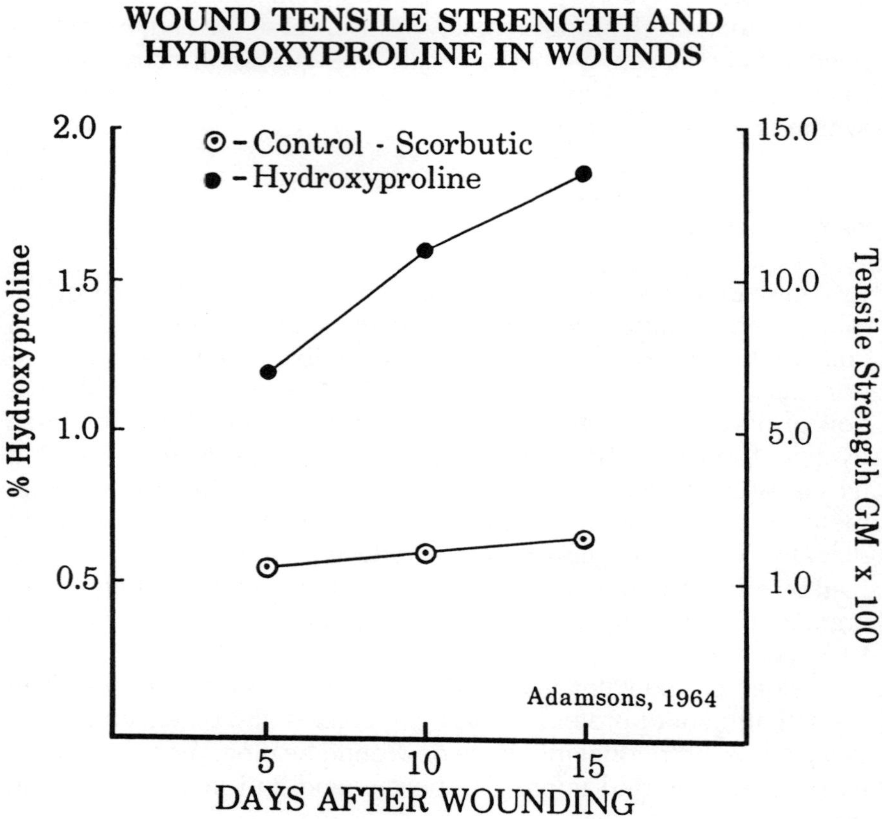

WOUND TENSILE STRENGTH AND
HYDROXYPROLINE IN WOUNDS
- Control - Scorbutic
- Hydroxyproline
% Hydroxyproline
2.0
1.5
1.0
0.5
Tensile Strength GM x 100
15.0
10.0
5.0
1.0
Adamsons, 1964
5
10
15
DAYS AFTER WOUNDING

Fig. 6.4.

WOUND TENSILE STRENGTH IN ZINC DEFICIENT AND DIABETIC MALE MICE

	Relative Tensile* Strength	P Value
Control	1441 ± 142	
Zinc Deficient	559 ± 103	<0.001
Zinc Supplemented	1653 ± 147	>0.2
Control	1619 ± 153	
Diabetic	1244 ± 139	0.05
Diabetic + Zinc Supplemented	1630 ± 160	>0.5

* Tensile Strength = GM/B.WT x 100.

Table 6.2.

wound healing by a mechanical and endocrine means. The growth factors in mucilage stimulate fibroblasts and epidermal cells for growth and repair. If we could transfer the sol-gel transformation from the leaf to the wound, it would be a major discovery in wound healing.

The sol-gel transformation of dilutions of a 1:1 mixture of freeze-dried whole-leaf aloe and mucilage indicates that diluting the gel with water reduces the gelation. Normally, aloe vera is hydroscopic—that is, it quickly picks up water. However, with the 1:1 aloe mixture, dilution to 50 percent and 100 percent with water causes a delay in the transformation from a sol to a gel (figure 6.5). It appears that a 1:1 mixture of aloe with mucilage causes the water to move away from aloe, as shown by the decrease in viscosity with time. Water is prevented from being absorbed into the aloe by the mucilage. In fact, when we compare the gain and loss of water by the gel, mucilage, and the 1:1 ratio of mucilage and aloe, we find that only the aloe gel gains water. Both the mucilage and the combination of the aloe gel and the mucilage (1:1 ratio) lost water (figure 6.6). We have reversed the movement of water away from the aloe by the occlusive nature of mucilage. This will increase the movement of water (containing growth factors) toward the skin having inflammation and wounds. We feel that mucilage represents a storage form of polysaccharide whose molecules are closer together. Possibly, the polysaccharide is a lipid form rather than the protein form seen in the internal center of the leaf. This would clearly explain the occlusive nature of mucilage, as compared to the penetrating nature of aloe vera proper.

The tensile strength of the aloe-mucilage (1:1 ratio) gel is 1228.2 ± 30 gms (N = 9). It took this amount of force to pull two sticks apart that we glued together with the aloe-mucilage (1:1 ratio). The coefficient of standard error variation was only 2.5 percent. When the temperature of the gel was increased from 23°C (72.4°F) to 54°C (129.2F), a breakage of the gel was observed (figure 6.7). Since this temperature could never be reached in the human body, the aloe-mucilage gel might be used as a bone glue. The mucopolysaccharide fibers of the aloe-mucilage gel are strong, probably bonded together by factors that provide us with a large tensile strength that will mend wounds and hold even bones together. This combination is non-toxic and is not altered by temperature. We made an observation on the

EFFECT OF DILUTION ON THE VISCOSITY OF ALOE VERA AND MUCILAGE (1:1 RATIO)

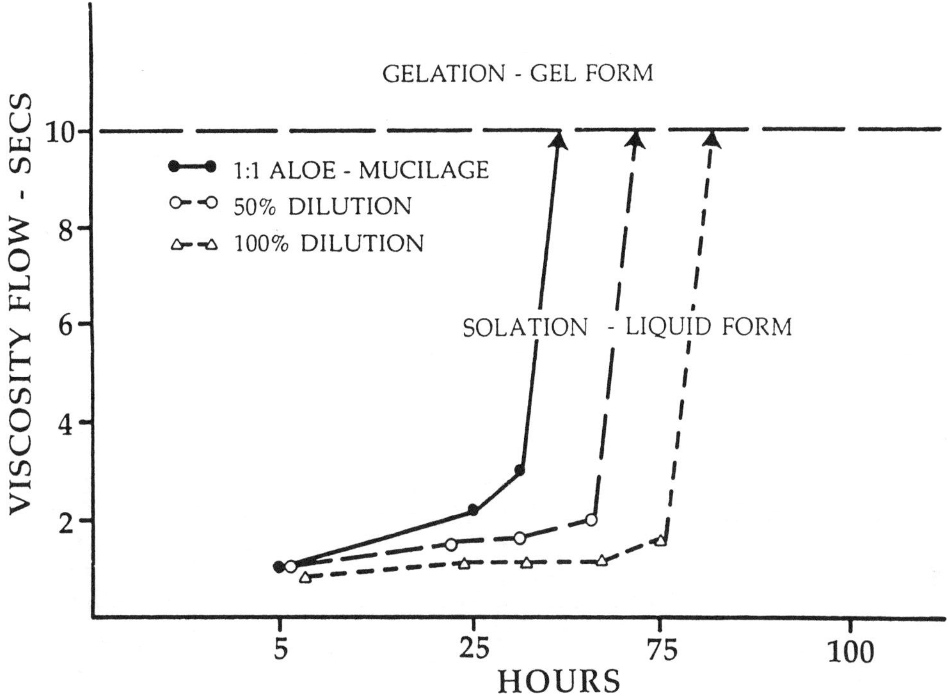

Fig. 6.5.

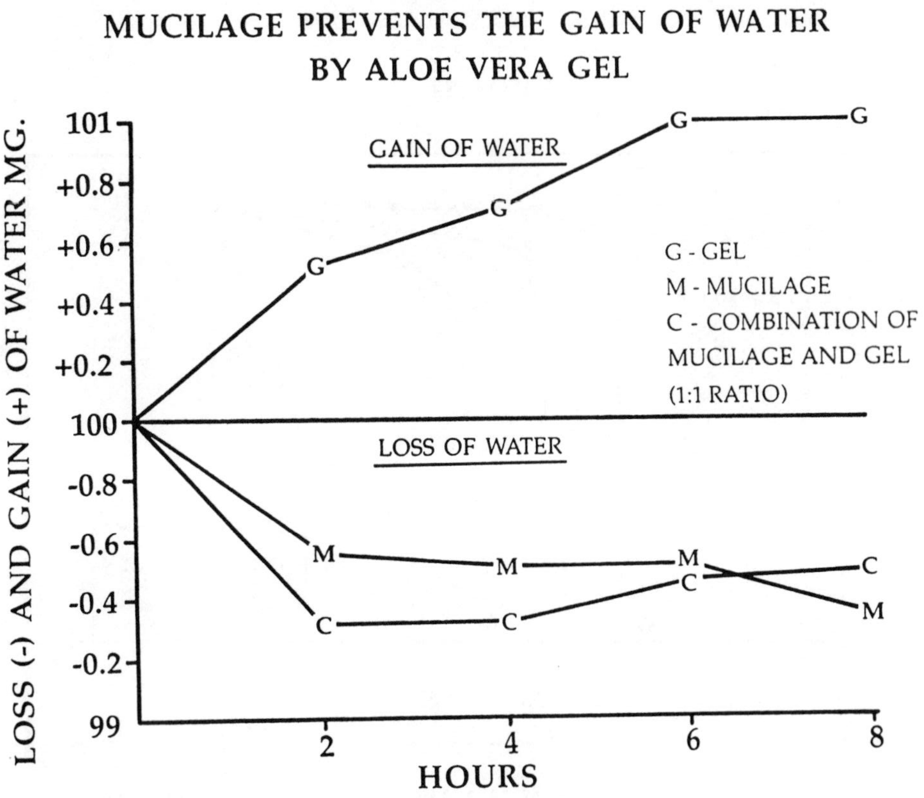
MUCILAGE PREVENTS THE GAIN OF WATER
BY ALOE VERA GEL
LOSS (-) AND GAIN (+) OF WATER MG.
101
+0.8
+0.6
+0.4
+0.2
100
-0.8
-0.6
-0.4
-0.2
99
GAIN OF WATER
LOSS OF WATER
G - GEL
M - MUCILAGE
C - COMBINATION OF
MUCILAGE AND GEL
(1:1 RATIO)
G
M
C
2
4
6
8
HOURS

Fig. 6.6.

EFFECT OF INCREASING TEMPERATURE ON THE BREAKAGE OF THE 1:1 ALOE-MUCILAGE GEL AREA

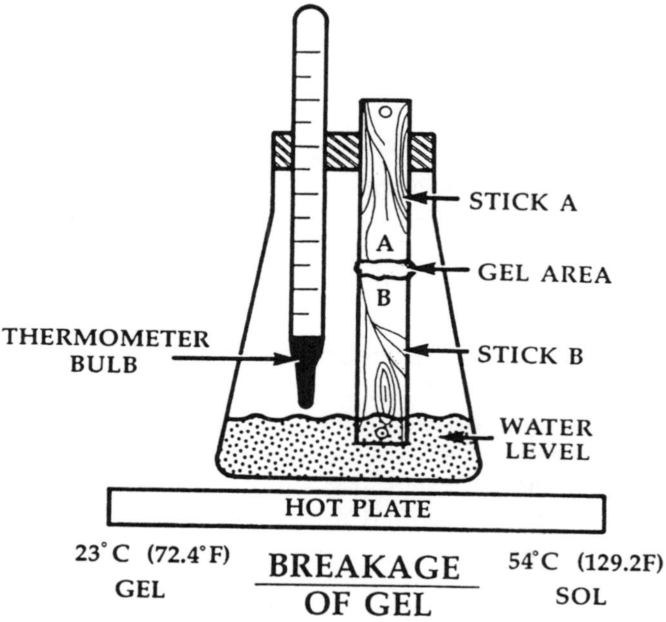

Fig. 6.7.

wound-healing effect of the 1:1 mixture of mucilage–aloe vera gel placed on an open wound for three days. The gel mixture improved wound healing fourfold when compared to untreated controls. This was due to the occlusive and endocrine properties of the 1:1 gel. More work needs to be done using this gel on open wounds (table 6.3). A comparison of whole-leaf freeze-dried aloe powder and aloe liquid on wound tensile strength at 50 mg/kg × 4 dose revealed that the percentage of increase in tensile strength was 13.1 percent for powder as compared to 22.0 for liquid aloe vera (figure 6.8). Since proteoglycans in wound connective tissue need water to expand and bind collagen to increase wound tensile strength, possibly the water in liquid aloe can help to explain the difference in response.

A Topical Wound-Healing Preparation of Whole-Plant Aloe and Mucilage (1:1 Ratio)

Figure 6.9 shows the topical effect of whole-plant aloe combined with mucilage at 1:1 ratio at 1 and 5 percent dose in petrolatum over four days with 0.5 percent aloe pulp on wound tensile strength. The 1 percent aloe and mucilage (1:1 ratio) increased the tensile strength of the wound 18 percent. However, increasing the dose of the combination to 5 percent produced a 60 percent increase in tensile strength over controls. Adding 0.5 percent aloe pulp to the 5 percent aloe and mucilage increased the wound tensile strength still further to 131 percent. A dose-response relationship is evident with a further increase in response by adding the aloe pulp. The mucilage with its growth factors and tightly woven mucopolysaccharide chains combined with aloe to form a strong gel in which the polysaccharide chains bonded together to increase tensile strength. Adding the aloe pulp caused these fibers to form a network with the 1:1 gel, which gave us the strongest preparation thus far seen with aloe vera. In fact, using this preparation to bind two pieces of wood together would increase the tensile strength such that it is difficult to pull them apart. We have transposed from the leaf the sealing effect of aloe and mucilage to an animal wound and have added the additional component of aloe pulp fibers to increase the strength of the gel network. Whether or not the aloe pulp fibers contribute biological activity is not known. We feel that the aloe pulp will enhance the bind between

AN OBSERVATION: THE WOUND HEALING EFFECT OF A 1:1 MIXTURE OF MUCILAGE-ALOE VERA GEL PLACED ON THE WOUND FOR 3 DAYS.

	% REDUCTION OF WOUND
UNTREATED CONTROL	11
MUCILAGE-ALOE GEL	46

ADULT MALE MICE

Table 6.3.

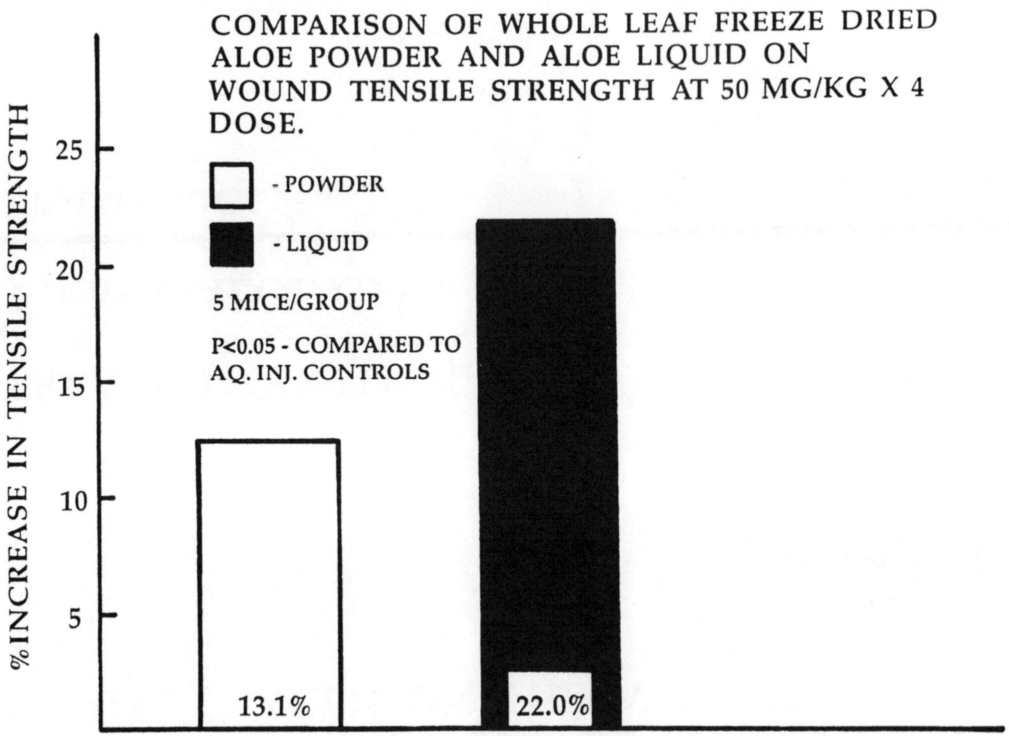

COMPARISON OF WHOLE LEAF FREEZE DRIED ALOE POWDER AND ALOE LIQUID ON WOUND TENSILE STRENGTH AT 50 MG/KG X 4 DOSE.
- POWDER
- LIQUID
5 MICE/GROUP
P<0.05 - COMPARED TO AQ. INJ. CONTROLS
%INCREASE IN TENSILE STRENGTH
25
20
15
10
5
13.1%
22.0%

Fig. 6.8.

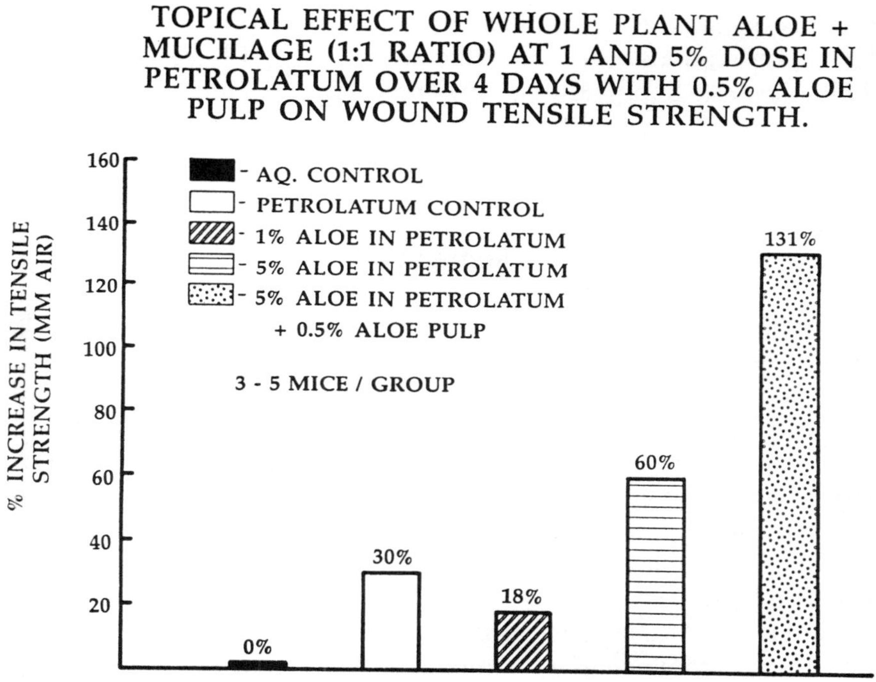
TOPICAL EFFECT OF WHOLE PLANT ALOE + MUCILAGE (1:1 RATIO) AT 1 AND 5% DOSE IN PETROLATUM OVER 4 DAYS WITH 0.5% ALOE PULP ON WOUND TENSILE STRENGTH.
% INCREASE IN TENSILE STRENGTH (MM AIR)
160
140
120
100
80
60
40
20
- AQ. CONTROL
- PETROLATUM CONTROL
- 1% ALOE IN PETROLATUM
- 5% ALOE IN PETROLATUM
- 5% ALOE IN PETROLATUM + 0.5% ALOE PULP
3 - 5 MICE / GROUP
0%
30%
18%
60%
131%

Fig. 6.9.

the mucopolysaccharide fibers of the mucilage and aloe to produce a great wound-healing preparation. This preparation could be used on wounds that don't heal (diabetic wounds), as well as a bone glue. Possibly this combination could be placed under the skin and act as a slow-release vehicle for hormones and valuable drugs that are toxic, such as digitalis. This combination would be an excellent bandage for "open wounds"; however, the wound would have to be filled with aloe paste to provide a concentration gradient for the movement of water. Aloe vera powder is hydroscopic. The presence of mucilage with aloe forces the water toward the wound.

Summary

When an aloe farmer severs the leaf, he notices that the leaf is able to seal the wound to prevent the escape of gel fillet to the outside. The mucilage in the presence of aloe gel hardens and acts like a "Crazy Glue." In wound healing, collagen is a tough protein that connects the incisional wound tissues together. It plays the major role in establishing wound tensile strength. Proteoglycans are made up of sugars and provide flexibility to connective tissue. Aloe vera stimulates fibroblasts to increase wound tensile strength. We have discussed the mechanical properties of skin and the measurement of wound tensile strength. The importance of water, protein, vitamin C, and zinc in reference to wound healing was discussed. A whole-leaf aloe vera–mucilage (1:1 ratio) significantly increased wound tensile strength such that we feel we have transferred the sealant properties of aloe from the aloe leaf to the animal wound. This was further increased by the addition of aloe pulp fibers. The combination of mucilage and aloe also forms an excellent bandage for open wounds.

References

1. R. H. Davis, "Comments on the Aloe Leaf," *Autumn* 4 (1992).
2. R. H. Davis, "The Conductor-Orchestra Concept of Aloe Vera," *Cosmetics and Toiletries Manufacturing Worldwide* 95 (1995): 21.
3. T. J. Ryan, "An Environment for Healing the Role of Occlusion," *Royal Society of Medicine,* 88 (1985): 31.

4. T. T. Irwin, "Wound Healing," *Archives Emergency Medicine* 2 (1985): 3.; I. A. Silver, *The Physiology of Wound Healing: Theory and Surgical Practice* (New York: Appleton–Century Crofts, 1980), 11–28.
5. L. R. Bucci, "Glucosamine–a New Potent Nutraceutical for Connective Tissue," *Nutritional Supplement Advisor,* (May 1992), 56.
6. T. Gibson, R. M. Kenedi, and J. E. Craik, "The Mobile Micro-Architecture of Dermal Collagen: A Bioengineering Study," *British Journal of Surgery* 52 (1965): 764.
7. W. Van Winkle, "The Tensile Strength of Wounds and Factors That Influence It," *Surgery Gynecological Obstetrics,* October 1969, 819.
8. R. H. Davis, M. G. Leitner, and J. M. Russo, "Aloe Vera Improves Wound Healing and Reduces Inflammation in Diabetes," *Pennsylvania Academy of Science,* 61 (1987): 84.; R. H. Davis, "Effect of Zinc Deficiency and Alloxan Induced Diabetes on Mouse Wound Healing," *Pennsylvania Academy Science* 41 (1983): 9.; E. D. Engel, N. E. Erlick, and R. H. Davis, "Diabetes Mellitus: Impaired Wound Healing from Zinc Deficiency," *Journal of the American Podiatric Association,* 71 (1981): 536.
9. Van Winkle, "The Tensile Strength of Wounds," 1969.
10. R. J. Adamsons, F. Musco, and I. F. Enquist, "The Water Content of Healing Incisions," *Surgery, Gynecologic Obstetrics,* April 1967, 734.
11. S. A. Localio, W. Casale, and J. W. Hinton, "Tissue Protein Depletion; a Factor in Wound Disruption," *Surgery, Gynecologial Obstetrics* 86 (1968): 107.
12. J. M. Daly, H. M. Vars, and S. B. Dudrick, "Effects of Protein Depletion on Strength of Colonic Anastomoses," *Surgery, Gynecological Obstetrics* 13 (1972): 15.
13. T. V. Taylor, S. Rimmer, B. Day, J. Butcher, and I. W. Dymock, "Ascorbic Acid Supplementation in the Treatment of Pressure-Sores," *Lancet,* September: 1974, 544.; P. L. Schwartz, "Ascorbic Acid in Wound Healing—a Review," *Journal of the American Dental Association* 56 (1970): 497; M. B. Rubin, "Vitamins and Wound Healing," *Plastic Surgical Nursing,* Spring 1984, 16.
14. Davis, "Effects of Zinc Deficiency and Alloxan Induced Diabetes," 9.; M. Chvapil, "Zinc and Other Factors of the Pharmacology of Wound Healing," in *Wound Healing and Wound Infection: Theory and Surgical Practice* (New York: Appleton Century-Crofts, 1980), 135; R. F. Liszewski, "The Effect of Zinc on Wound Healing: A Collective Review," *Journal of the American Otolaryngological Association,* 81 (1981): 104.
15. B. C. Coats, *The Silent Healer: A Modern Study of Aloe Vera* (Garland, TX: self-published, 1979).

7

Gibberellin: A Growth Factor in Aloe Vera

Gibberellin is a plant-derived growth factor present in aloe vera that plays a major role in the plant's growth and development. Gibberellin represents only one of five major types of plant growth factors that have been identified. Gibberellin was shown to be produced by rice fungus by a Japanese plant pathologist named Kurosawa working on Formosa. He and his colleagues isolated the gibberellin and showed that it was involved in growth and development of plants. Gibberellin could cause growth of sugarcane, barley, wheat, rice, and maize. Gibberellin could be absorbed on charcoal and eluted off by acetone, alcohol, or ether. It is stable to autoclaving, freezing, sunlight, and exposure to ultraviolet light.[1] Magnesium sulfate led to the formation of a growth-inhibiting filtrate. We feel that charcoal removes gibberellin from aloe vera (whole-leaf), which can be eluted off with alcohol.[2]

Microgram amounts of gibberellin increased growth of dwarf peas to the tall variety (a 500 percent increase in a few days).[3] Gibberellin increases the rate of cell elongation by stimulating new RNA and protein synthesis. This response could not be duplicated with auxin. Possibly gibberellin suppresses the action of "inhibitor" genes in the dwarf plants. Gibberellin does not show the polar movement within the plant that is characteristic of auxin. Gibberellin stimulates the shoot but inhibits the roots.

The amylase activity of germinating barley and wheat seeds was increased on a weight basis proportionally to the applied gibberellin. Gibberellin promotes the conversion of tryptophan to indole acetic acid in a way that creates a synergistic response. Most of the effects of gibberellin were not duplicated by auxin. No toxicity studies are available for gibberellin.

Gibberellin is a growth factor for plants, but no one has shown, as far as we know, its anti-inflammatory and wound-healing therapeutic potential in laboratory animals. Also, no in vitro studies have been done in this regard. Gibberellin has been shown to produce stem elongation in genetic dwarf varieties in certain plants. These same growth factors also stimulate leaf growth and cell division at the root apex.[4] Gibberelic acid (GA_3) was used in this study because it tends to be the most active of all of the chemically identified gibberellins[5] (figure 7.1). On a cellular level, gibberellins have actions that are similar to those of steroid hormones in mammals, in spite of their very different chemical and structural properties. Gibberellin increases phospholipid synthesis as well as proliferation of the rough endoplasmic system and Golgi system.[6] It is likely that the mechanism for gibberellin's wound-healing activity is related to its ability to stimulate protein synthesis as well as the DNA-RNA cellular systems.[7] Since gibberellin must be a component of the aloe gel, possibly this glycoside accounts for much of aloe's wound-healing activity. The exact mechanism of action of gibberellin at the cellular level is not yet fully understood. Unlike steroids, gibberellin has both anti-inflammatory and wound-healing activity. Gibberellin and related compounds may offer an alternative therapy for managing inflammation and wounds even under an abnormal physiological state such as diabetes.

This chapter attempts to show that gibberellin stimulates wound healing and tensile strength, that gibberellin produces the wound-healing effect in a dose-response manner, and that aloe vera and gibberellin inhibit PMN infiltration (inflammation) comparably over the same dose range in diabetes, to evaluate auxin and other related compounds on croton oil–induced ear swelling; to show that gibberellin blocks hydrocortisone acetate inhibition on wound healing similar to aloe vera; to show the effect of aloe-related growth substances on wound tensile strength; and to determine if gibberellin and aloe vera are additive in their combined effect on wound tensile strength.

Basic Wound Healing

The wound-healing process goes through three distinct phases: the inflammatory phase, the proliferative phase, and the remodeling

THE CHEMICAL STRUCTURE
OF GIBBERELLIC ACID (GA_3)

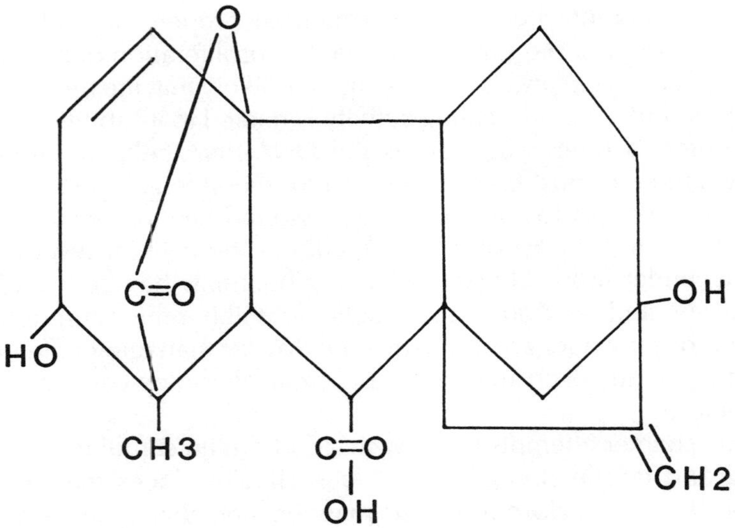

Fig. 7.1.

phase.[8] *The inflammatory phase* is the immediate response to injury with vasoconstriction and the formation of a fibrin-platelet clot. The injured tissues release histamine, which cause vascular permeability to plasma proteins. By diapedesis, the PMNs enter the wound and engulf bacteria. Macrophages secrete hydrolytic enzymes, which digest debris and clear the wound area. Plasma cells make antibodies to foreign antigens and bacteria. The fibrous tissue and exudate becomes incorporated into the clot to form a scab. *The proliferative phase* begins with the migration of epidermal cells over moist, healthy tissue. The epidermis grows under the dry wound surface. As cells migrate, they secrete a proteolytic enzyme that cuts away the base of the scab to aid movement. Macrophages are attracted to the wound area. They secrete fibroblast growth factors, which increase the number and function of fibroblasts. Fibroblasts proliferate and synthesize proteoglycans and collagen. Vitamin C is necessary for the hydroxylation of proline and lysine in collagen formation.[9] Since oxygen is needed for collagen formation, a poor vascular supply hinders collagen synthesis. Macrophages tend to encourage capillary bud formation.[10] Years ago we believed that an open wound was needed to supply oxygen until it was found that an occlusive (covered) wound had better wound healing. Oxygen was extracted from the blood vessels. An open wound dried and dropped so that the fibroblasts and epidermal cells bumped into each other. The epidermal and fibroblast growth factors could not produce their maximal effects. As a result, wound healing was inhibited. We feel that aloe vera prevents drying by its occlusive nature (mucilage) and its growth factors enhance the proliferation and migration of cells. *The remodeling phase* represents a reorientation of collagen fibers by a process of lysis and resynthesis. Molecular cross-linking and dehydration of the fibers strengthen the scar tissue. A good environment for wounds includes: an occlusive cover that keeps the wound moist but contributes valuable growth factors for cell migration and proliferation and protection against bacterial contamination, whose actual presence and toxin elaboration can inhibit wound healing. Aloe vera increased the wound healing over a dose range of 1 to 100 mg/kg in a dose-response fashion.[11] Aloe provides a good environment for wound healing. I. Danhof[12] found that tritiated thymidine uptake by skin fibroblasts was increased as the dose of aloe vera was increased. The plant growth factors in aloe vera—for example, the gibberellins and auxins—enhance the proliferation of cells as well as cellular migration, which exerts a major positive influence on wound healing. Healing may also be accelerated by the transfer of water from aloe to injured tissue. This assumes that the solid concentration of aloe is just right.

The physician's concern is to reduce the size of the wound as quickly as possible after an injury, with minimal side effects. This lessens the chance of infection. J. E. Crewe reported that aloe vera improved wound healing with tissue regeneration.[13] This response could be explained by the fact that aloe dilates capillaries to increase blood flow to the injured area. Tensile forces originate from collagen, but fiber shortening accounts for changes in granulation tissue of the wound bed. Rowe's experiments demonstrated very early that aloe vera could increase the healing of damaged areas.[14] Wound healing can be influenced by many factors. However, anything that interferes with the three phases of normal repair will have deleterious effects on the end result. Two major influences in ensuring adequate wound healing are meticulous surgical technique and systemic factors such as alcoholism, platelet-inhibiting drugs, anemia, obesity, age, and corticosteroids. Sometimes a wound can be complicated by delayed healing. This can occur when there is good wound care, occlusive dressings, good surgical technique, and adequate nutrition. A postulated mechanism as to why these efforts fail to close a wound in the normal time frame is a poor inflammatory response with a decreased signaling by macrophages through growth factors for cell proliferation.[15] Possibly aloe vera and/or gibberellin could stimulate macrophages to release traditional growth factors that could improve wound healing. Aloe vera and/or gibberellin could directly enhance wound repair.

Growth Factors Important to Wound Healing

Cells in a wound communicate with each other through substances known as growth factors.[16] Growth factors are polypeptide hormones that are stored by most cells and are secreted into local tissues. Once the growth factor contacts its target cell, it binds to a receptor on the cell surface; then a biological response can be propagated. Growth factors are responsible for the ordered, controlled functions of cells involved in healing and non-healing wounds. Macrophages (figure 7.2) are large phagocytic cells that line blood passages and are found in connective tissue. They are part of the reticulo-endothelial system. They have mitochondria and lysosome enzymes that kill bacteria. The increased metabolism of these cells in the process forms oxygen radicals. Macrophages secrete some one hundred substances, and their biological activity ranges from the induction of cell growth to cell death. They can influence every aspect of the immune and inflammatory responses. Macrophage products may affect each other's actions and the secretion of other cells.[17]

The injury of tissue has considerable effect on the form of subsequent repair.[18] Fibrin and products of lysis activate macrophages, which stimulate angiogenesis. Activated platelets release into wounds a number of growth factors such as TGF-β and PDGF. These molecules can activate fibroblasts and macrophages. Steroids inhibit inflammation and thus impair wound healing. This is due to the suppression of macrophages. Macrophages release growth factors on stimulation by fibrin, cytokines, endotoxins, hypoxia, and lactate in wounds.[19] Our focus has been on four major types of peptide hormones (growth factors) that have clinical significance: epidermal growth factors, fibroblast growth factors, platelet-derived growth factors, and transforming growth factor–β (figure 7.3).

Epidermal Growth Factor (EGF) is a fifty-three–amino acid polypeptide that is stored in the macrophages and platelet. It stimulates the proliferation and differentiation of epidermis as well as the synthesis of DNA, RNA, protein, and hyaluronic acid. EGF accelerates the rate of wound contraction. It increases the collagen content of cotton pellet–induced granulomas in rats. The increase in wound collagen was 50 percent, due to the increase in the number of fibroblasts and the rate of angiogenesis. This growth factor targets the transmembrane glycoprotein receptor located on the endothelial, fibroblast, and epithelial cell surfaces.[20]

Fibroblast Growth Factor (FGF): The basic and acidic FGFs are closely related to polypeptides that are multifunctional. The basic FGF is made in many cells, whereas the acidic FGF is synthesized in the brain and retina. FGF stimulates growth of a variety of cells derived from mesoderm and neuroectoderm. FGF is the major stimulator of angiogenesis. Heparin can modulate the bioactivity of FGF.[21]

MACROPHAGE - LARGE PHAGOCYTE (RES)

1. In Connective Tissue - Lines Blood Passages.
2. Mitochondria.
3. Lysosome Enzymes - Kills Bacteria and Removes Tumor Cells.
4. Forms Oxygen Radicals.
5. Forms Growth Factors - Stimulates Fibroblasts.
6. Participates with Lymphs - Antibody Formation.

Fig. 7.2.

GROWTH FACTORS IMPORTANT TO WOUND HEALING

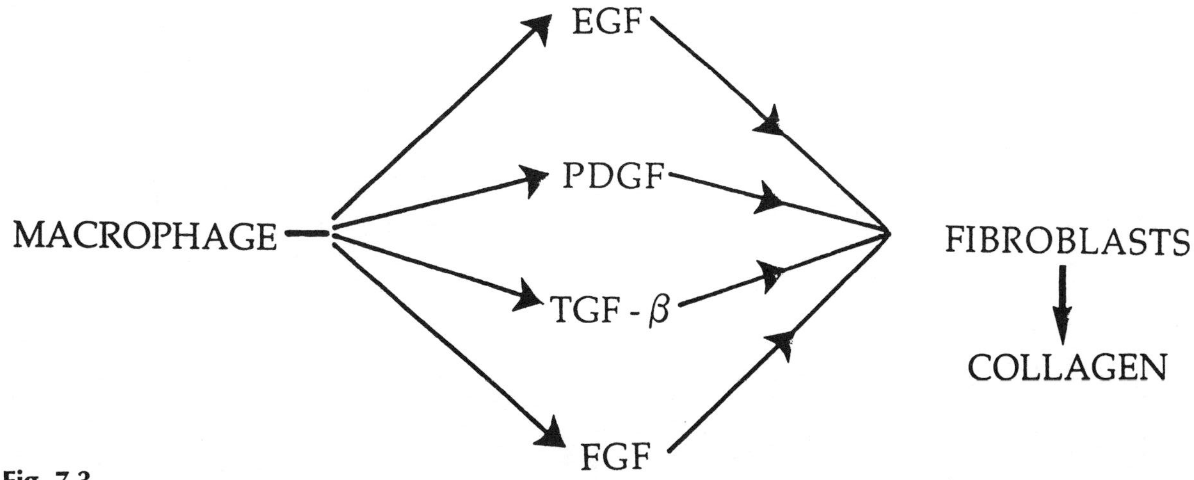

Fig. 7.3.

Platelet-Derived Growth Factor (PDGF) is a potent activator of cells of mesenchymal origin. It stimulates chemotaxis, proliferation, and gene expression in macrophages and fibroblasts. It is synthesized in megakaryocytes and carried in alpha granules of platelets. It augments wound-breaking strength 50 to 70 percent. Cellularity and granulation tissue formation were significantly increased after a single application of PDGF to incisional wounds. PDGF exaggerates the acute inflammatory phase of repair, thereby accelerating the normal cascade of tissue repair.[22]

Transforming Growth Factor–β is a polypeptide hormone that is predominantly synthesized and secreted by platelets and, to a minor extent, macrophages. Transforming growth factor–β possesses its own receptor on most cell types and shares no cross reactivity with other growth factors. It has been proven that transforming growth factor β regulates the activities of other growth factors present in a wound. Transforming growth factor–β has the ability to potentiate or retard the effects that the other growth factors have on endothelial, epithelial, and fibroblastic cell types. This action is dependent upon the gene expression of the target cell action and, possibly, the concentration of other growth factors present.[23]

Collagen research once dominated the wound-healing efforts. However, control of collagen synthesis is still a mystery. We observed that aloe vera can stimulate fibroblasts directly to form collagen and proteoglycans.[24] It is also possible for aloe vera (or gibberellin?) to stimulate or modulate the macrophage to produce growth factors that enhance collagen formation by stimulating fibroblasts. Specific clones of fibroblasts make collagen while others synthesize proteoglycans. Also, genetic factors modulate collagen synthesis. Ascorbate, oxygen, and specific amino acids are critical to collagen synthesis.[25] Wound healing is a continuous sequence of signals and responses in which epithelial and endothelial inflammatory cells, platelets, and fibroblasts interact to restore the tissues to normal function. Most investigators emphasize inflammation and coagulation to explain the burst of cell replication that is the foundation of wound healing. All wounds are not the same. Some heal largely by epithelialization. Deeper wounds bring in angiogenesis and contraction. To define wound healing, one must think of it as an interacting sequence of components.

Aloe Vera and Gibberellin Anti-Inflammatory Activity in Diabetes

Infiltration of PMNs into an inflamed wound area is an important response to injury. The PMN activity might be a chemotactic response to protein products released from injured tissues.[26] These cells first marginate to the walls of the microcirculation in the injured area, then emigrate between the endothelial cells of the vessel wall and migrate from the vessel through the ground substance to the site of injury. Phagocytes, found in acutely traumatized tissue, are responsible for release of tissue-damaging lysosomal enzymes.[27] Aloe vera reduces pain in normal animals, and there are suggestions in the literature about it possessing anti-convulsing activity. The magnesium in aloe could contribute to the sedative and anti-convulsive activity if such effects are present. Animal studies indicate that nerve conduction velocity is reduced in diabetes due to axon dwindling and degeneration. Also, the uptake of amino acids by the dorsal root is impaired.[28]

Aloe vera inhibits inflammation and adjuvant-induced arthritis. It improves wound healing and reduces edema and pain but does not reduce granuloma tissue around a foreign substance under the skin.[29] Diabetic animals were used in this study because of their poor wound-healing and anti-inflammatory capabilities. Biochemical alterations in the microvasculature of diabetics prolongs the healing response as well as altering the anti-inflammatory response. The purpose of this work is to determine if gibberellin, a plant growth hormone, could account for some of the anti-inflammatory activity in aloe vera.

Polymorphonuclear Leukocyte Infiltration Assay

Adult male ICR mice (20 to 30 g, eight animals/group) were injected intraperitonally with 200 mg/kg streptozotocin to induce diabetes. The streptozotocin (powder basis) was mixed into a solution with 0.9 percent saline. The control animals received no injections. Five days later, two animals from each group, with the exception of the control groups, were randomly chosen to test for diabetes. Blood sugars were determined to certify that the animals were diabetic.

Under ether anesthesia, all mice were shaven on one side. A marking pencil was used to outline an area the size of a nickel. Each animal was injected subcutaneously within this area with 0.2 cc of 2 percent gelatin (0.4 percent NaCl, 1 percent ethanol) solution to form a bleb. This was immediately followed by a second subcutaneous injection of 2, 20, and 100 mg/kg colorized aloe vera or gibberellic acid. The aloe vera and gibberellin were injected into an area outside the designated circle. A non-diabetic and a diabetic control group each received saline injections in place of the gelatin irritant, as well as the aloe vera or gibberellin. A third non-diabetic control group received the gelatin injection and saline in place of the aloe vera or gibberellin.

The animals were killed three hours following the second injection. Incisions were made along the indicated circumscribed area so that subdermal tissue could be removed and stained. Polymorphonuclear leukocyte infiltration in the circumscribed inflamed area was determined by staining the subdermal tissue with Wright Stain. Three separate sections of each excised tissue were randomly chosen for viewing.

Results and Discussion

Gibberellin may be an active anti-inflammatory ingredient in aloe vera. Two percent gelatin caused a 30 percent increase in polymorphonuclear leukocyte infiltration in inflammation. This response was reduced by aloe vera in a dose-response fashion to 68 percent and as much as 60.1 percent with the maximum dose of gibberellin in diabetic animals. These responses were significant at $p < 0.001$ (tables 7.1 and 7.2). By substituting gibberellin, a growth hormone glycoside, for aloe vera, virtually identical results were obtained. Gelatin-treated diabetic mice receiving 2 mg/kg of gibberellin had a polymorphonuclear leukocyte count of 28.8 ± 0.8 ($p > 0.05$) neutrophils, showing no significant effect at this dosage relative to the diabetic 2 percent gelatin control group that received no gibberellin injection. The experimental animals receiving 20 mg/kg of gibberellin showed a significant decrease in polymorphonuclear leukocyte infiltration. The neutrophil cell count was 21.2 ± 0.8 ($p < 0.001$), which is a 25.1 percent reduction in neutrophil infiltration, while

EFFECT OF ALOE VERA ON PMN INFILTRATION IN DIABETIC MICE

TREATMENT	PMN COUNT NO./HPF	% REDUCTION
Saline Control	17.4 ± 0.6	–
Saline Diabetic	10.8 ± 0.5	–
2% Gelatin	28.4 ± 0.8	–
+ Aloe Vera 2 mg/kg	28.2 ± 0.7	0.7
+ Aloe Vera 20 mg/kg	17.0 ± 0.6	40.1
+ Aloe Vera 100 mg/kg	9.1 ± 0.5	68.0

8 Animals/group (24 counts)

Table 7.1.

EFFECT OF GIBBERELLIN ON PMN INFILTRATION IN DIABETIC MICE

TREATMENT	PMN COUNT NO./HPF	% REDUCTION
Saline Control	18.1 ± 0.7	–
Saline Diabetic	9.5 ± 0.6	–
2% Gelatin	28.3 ± 0.5	–
+ Gibberellin 2 mg/kg	28.8 ± 0.8	0.0
+ Gibberellin 20 mg/kg	21.2 ± 0.8	25.1
+ Gibberellin 100 mg/kg	11.3 ± 0.7	60.1

8 Animals/group (24 counts)

Table 7.2.

aloe vera showed a similar count of 17.0±0.6 ($p < 0.001$) at the same dosage. At 100 mg/kg, aloe vera reduced the polymorphonuclear leukocyte cell count 68 percent below the 2 percent gelatin control, showing a mean value of 9.1±0.5 ($p < 0.001$) neutrophils/high power field. At this same dose, gibberellin reduced the count 60.1percent with a mean count of 11.3 ± 0.7 ($p < 0.001$). These data show that aloe vera and gibberellin are parallel in activity and possibly could suggest that the activity of each has a similar origin.

The chemical determinant for growth and differentiation depends on plant growth hormones called auxins. These are essential for growth. Gibberellin (GA_3) tends to be the most active of all the chemically identified gibberellins.[30] This plant hormone tends to be universally distributed in tall plants. Gibberellin mediates plant tissue growth because it enhances cell enlargement. The ability for gibberellin to increase cell elongation depends on the RNA and protein synthesis.[31] Since aloe vera and gibberellin have similar dose-response curves in inhibiting the infiltration of PMNs into an area of inflammation, it may be that gibberellin is a major anti-inflammatory contributor in aloe vera. We know that sterols, amino acids, and vitamin C contribute to the anti-inflammatory activity. The attraction of PMNs to the inflamed area is caused by leukotrienes. Possibly aloe and gibberellin block leukotrienes.[32] As far as I know, these results showed for the first time that gibberellin produced a biological benefit in animals.

Gibberellin Stimulates Open Wound Healing

Since gibberellin enhances RNA and protein synthesis in plants and has anti-inflammatory activity in animals,[33] we attempted to determine if gibberellin would improve open wound healing when daily subcutaneously injected over a seven-day period, 2, 10, and 100 mg/kg. Would gibberellin stimulate wound healing in a dose-response fashion similar to aloe vera? Is the mechanism for gibberellin's wound-healing activity related to its ability to stimulate protein synthesis as well as the DNA-RNA cellular systems? A wound-healing response by gibberellin has never been demonstrated in animals.

The Open Wound Assay

Adult male ICR mice (30g, 15 animals/group) were anesthetized with ether and shaven on both sides of the back. A sterile 6 mm Baker biopsy punch was used to induce a wound on each side of the vertebral column. Anterior-posterior wound diameter measurements were made using a vernier caliper on days 0, 4, and 7. Three treatment groups received daily subcutaneous injections of a gibberellic acid (GA_3) solution at dosages of 2, 10, and 00 mg/kg, respectively. Control mice received daily injections of saline on a 10 ml/kg basis.

Results and Discussion

Control animals receiving saline demonstrated an average decrease in wound diameter of 3.48 mm (60.0 percent). The group receiving 2 mg/kg gibberellic acid had a mean decrease of 3.65 mm (65.3 percent). This response was not significantly different from the control ($p > 0.05$). Animals injected daily with 10 mg/kg of gibberellic acid responded with an average decrease in wound diameter of 3.85 mm (71.6 percent). This represents a significant response at $p < 0.05$. The third treatment group receiving gibberellic acid at 100 mg/kg produced a mean decrease of 4.65 mm. This represents a mean decrease of 81.7 percent, which is significant at $p < 0.001$ (table 7.3 and figure 7.4). The analysis of variance (ANOVA) between and within all study groups yielded a Fisher, or "F," ratio of 16.48. This value is significant at $p < 0.001$.

Wound Tensile Strength

This study attempts to compare the effect of gibberellin with growth-related substances on wound tensile strength. Another experiment was designed to show the wound tensile strength activity of gibberellin in aloe vera as a vehicle. A question that requires an answer is whether or not gibberellin will block hydrocortisone acetate inhibition on wound healing as aloe vera does. Possibly gibberellin in aloe vera acts as a buffer against powerful sterols that have anti-inflammatory activity but inhibit wound healing. Anti-inflammatory

THE EFFECT OF GIBBERELLIN ON WOUND HEALING IN MICE

TREATMENT	% DECREASE IN WOUND DIAMETER	p VALUE
SALINE CONTROL	60.0 ± 8.3	———
GIBBERELLIN 2 mg/kg	65.3 ± 11.3	> 0.05
GIBBERELLIN 10 mg/kg	71.6 ± 12.1	< 0.05
GIBBERELLIN 100 mg/kg	81.7 ± 7.0	< 0.001

ANOVA $p < 0.001$ 15 MICE / GROUP ± = S.E.

Table 7.3.

THE EFFECT OF GIBBERELLIN ON WOUND HEALING IN MICE

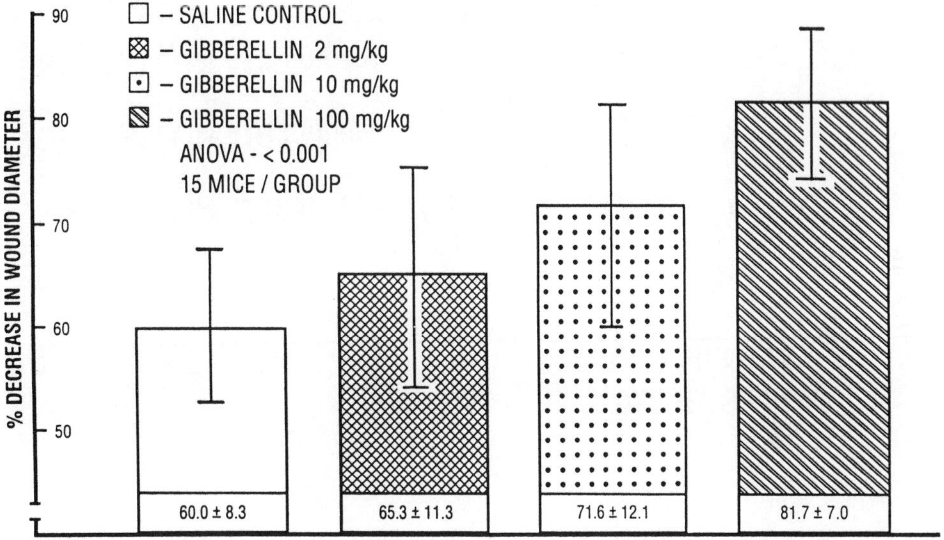

Fig. 7.4.

agents in aloe vera can block the initial inflammation in the wound-healing process and inhibit the wound repair. Growth factors such as gibberellin in aloe vera can block this wound inhibition so that aloe has both anti-inflammatory activity and wound-healing activity at the same time.

Wound Tensile Strength Assay

Adult male Sprague Dawley mice (30g, 7–13 animals/group, HSD-ICR, Frederick, Maryland, colony) had a one-inch surgical incision placed on their shaven back under ether anesthesia. Each wound was closed with a 9 mm wound clip at quarter-inch spacings, for a total of three fastens per wound. Mice were injected with aloe vera growth-related substances to show their effect on wound tensile strength subcutaneously administered at 100 mg/kg $\times$ 4. These growth-related substances found in aloe include: gibberellin (A_3), whole-leaf aloe, glucosamine phosphate, mannose-6-phosphate, indole–3–acetic acid, and chondroitin phosphate. Some of these substances are related to growth in connective tissue. Six hours after the day 4 injection, the tensile strength of wounds was measured by injecting air into the peritoneal cavity. The amount of air injected into the peritoneal cavity that caused the wound to burst apart was recorded. This volume of air was considered as a measurement of wound tensile strength. In another study, mice were daily subcutaneously injected for four days starting on the day of surgery with 50 mg/kg of whole-leaf aloe vera or with 50 mg/kg gibberellin or with the combination (50 mg/kg aloe + 50 mg/kg gibberellin). This study was designed to determine if aloe vera had an additive vehicle effect on wound tensile strength with gibberellin. A third experiment was performed to determine if gibberellin blocks the hydrocortisone acetate inhibition on wound tensile strength. Hydrocortisone-treated mice were subcutaneously injected with either 0.01 or 1.0 mg/kg for four days. In addition, mice were subcutaneously injected with 100mg/kg of gibberellin. On day 4, six hours after the last injection, the wound tensile strength was measured by injecting air into the abdominal cavity until the wound on the back burst.

Gibberellin Enhances Wound Tensile Strength

Gibberellin A_3 increased wound tensile strength when given subcutaneously at 100 mg/kg $\times$ 4 better than whole-leaf aloe vera at the same dosage. The glucosamine, mannose-6-phosphate and indole-3-acetic acid had values of 32.3, 30.3, and 26.0 percent, respectively. Chondroitin phosphate increased wound tensile strength 19.4 percent (table 7.4 and figure 7.5). L. Bucci reports that glucosamine phosphate is an important precursor of connective tissue and has documented its use in surgical wound healing.[34] Nevertheless, it was less active than aloe and gibberellin. Chondroitin sulfate is a major structural component of hyaluronic acid and gave us the smallest wound tensile strength response. Mannose phosphate is an important sugar in the active polysaccharide chain of "the aloe vera molecule."[35] Mannose-6-phosphate has significant anti-inflammatory activity and "open wound" healing activity. However, it increased wound tensile strength 30.3 percent, suggesting that it does fit into the fibroblast receptor to stimulate proteoglycans and collagen to increase connective tissue. Auxin (indole–3–acetic acid) had a similar response on wound tensile strength as mannose-6-phosphate and glucosamine phosphate. Indole–3–acetic acid gave a 37 percent topical anti-inflammatory response at the 5 percent dose in the croton oil–induced ear swelling assay. We can conclude that gibberellin and aloe vera increase wound tensile strength relative to other growth or connective tissue substances in the following sequence: gibberellin > aloe > glucosamine phosphate > mannose-6-phosphate > indole–3–acetic acid > chondroitin phosphate. Possibly, aloe vera and gibberellin stimulate these substances to increase wound healing.

Aloe Vera Has an Additive "Vehicle Effect" with Gibberellin on Wound Tensile Strength

The wound tensile strength of whole-leaf aloe vera subcutaneously administered as a vehicle for gibberellin showed a clear-cut additive response (table 7.5 and figure 7.6). Mice treated with 50 mg/kg aloe vera increased wound tensile strength 14.8 $\pm$ 0.6 percent. A 36.1 $\pm$ 1.5 percent increase was recorded for gibberellin at the

EFFECT OF ALOE - RELATED GROWTH SUBSTANCES ON WOUND TENSILE STRENGTH SUBCUTANEOUSLY ADMINISTERED AT 100 MG/KG X 4

	% Increase Over Controls
Gibberellin A_3	104.8
Whole Leaf Aloe	78.3
Glucosamine Phosphate	32.3
Mannose - 6 - Phosphate	30.3
Indole - 3 - Acetic Acid	26.0
Chondroitin Phosphate	19.4

7 MICE/GROUP

Table 7.4.

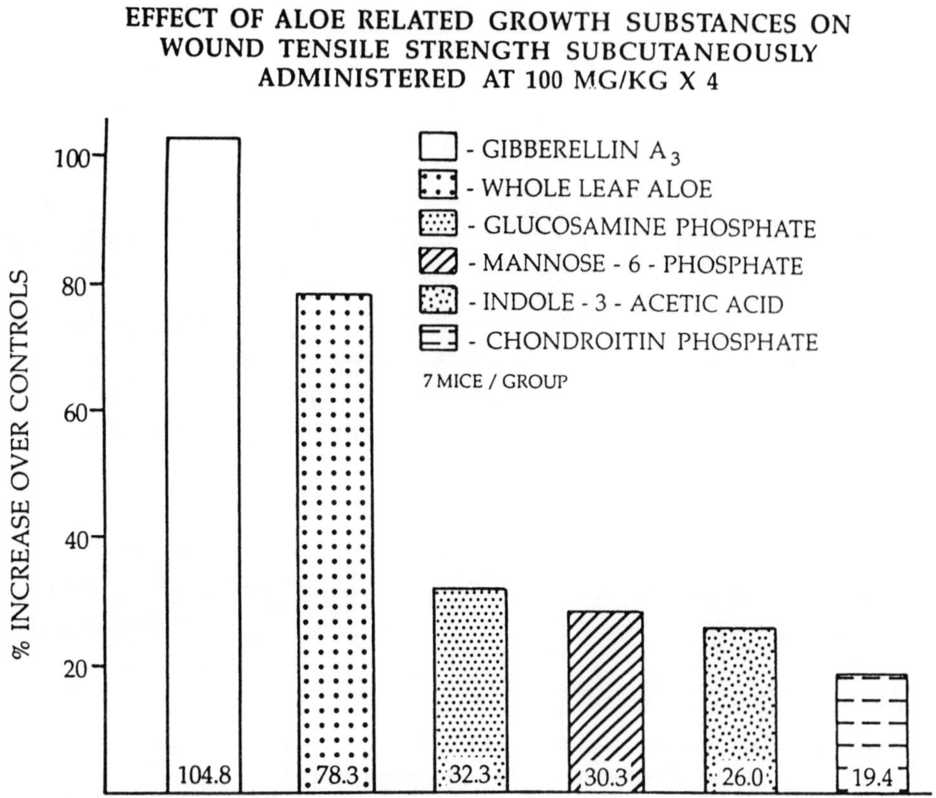
EFFECT OF ALOE RELATED GROWTH SUBSTANCES ON
WOUND TENSILE STRENGTH SUBCUTANEOUSLY
ADMINISTERED AT 100 MG/KG X 4
% INCREASE OVER CONTROLS
100
80
60
40
20
- GIBBERELLIN A 3
- WHOLE LEAF ALOE
- GLUCOSAMINE PHOSPHATE
- MANNOSE - 6 - PHOSPHATE
- INDOLE - 3 - ACETIC ACID
- CHONDROITIN PHOSPHATE
7 MICE / GROUP
104.8
78.3
32.3
30.3
26.0
19.4

Fig. 7.5.

WOUND TENSILE STRENGTH OF ALOE (WHOLE LEAF) VERA SUBCUTANEOUSLY ADMINISTERED AS A VEHICLE FOR GIBBERELLIN: AN ADDITIVE EFFECT.

Treatment mg/kg X 4	Wound Tensile Strength % Increase
Aloe - 50	14.8 ± 0.6^{A}
Gibberellin - 50	36.1 ± 1.5^{B}
Combination - 50 + 50	49.7 ± 2.2^{C}

A + B = C ($P > 0.5$)   10 - 13 Mice /Group. $\pm$ = S.E.

Table 7.5.

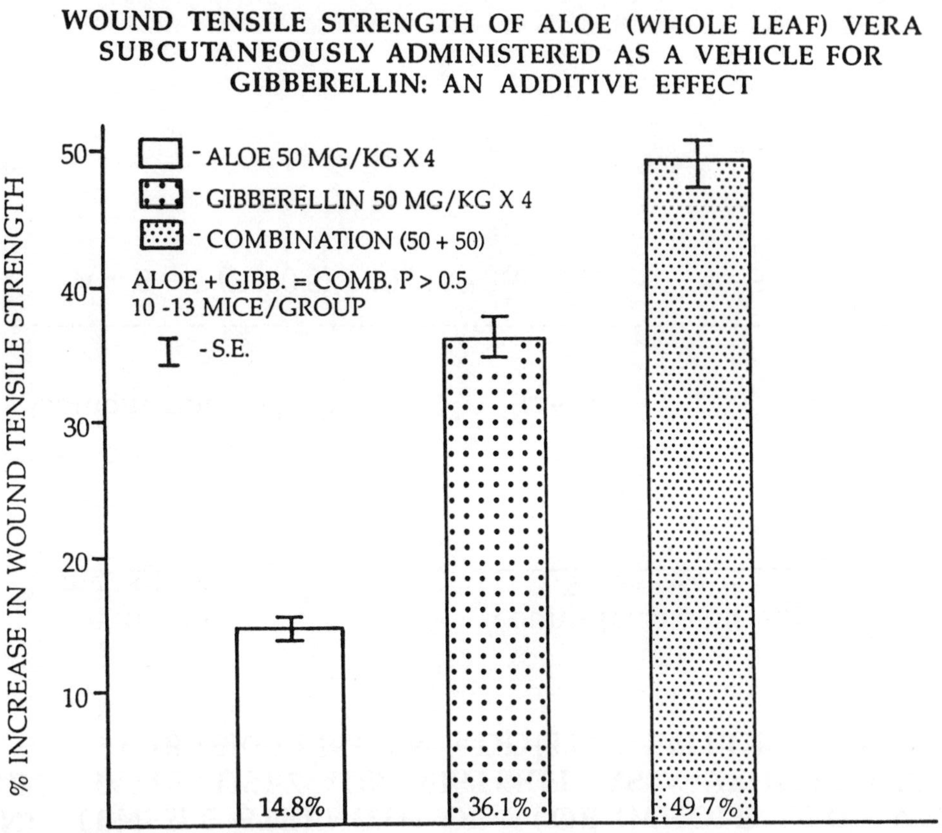
WOUND TENSILE STRENGTH OF ALOE (WHOLE LEAF) VERA SUBCUTANEOUSLY ADMINISTERED AS A VEHICLE FOR GIBBERELLIN: AN ADDITIVE EFFECT
% INCREASE IN WOUND TENSILE STRENGTH
50
40
30
20
10
- ALOE 50 MG/KG X 4
- GIBBERELLIN 50 MG/KG X 4
- COMBINATION (50 + 50)
ALOE + GIBB. = COMB. P > 0.5
10 -13 MICE/GROUP
- S.E.
14.8%
36.1%
49.7%

Fig. 7.6.

same dose. When the mice were given the combination of aloe and gibberellin at 50 mg/kg each, a 49.7 percent increase in wound tensile strength was noted. Thus aloe (A) + gibberellin (B) = the combination (C) $P > 0.5$. This additive response means that the biological activities of each component could be added together when given together. Aloe vera, therefore, is a good vehicle for gibberellin. We should note that in this study a different batch of gibberellin was used relative to the comparative study. It probably was less active, but it showed a good additive response with aloe vera.

Gibberellin Blocks Hydrocortisone Acetate Inhibition on Wound Healing Similar to Aloe Vera

Hydrocortisone reduces wound healing by blocking macrophage function.[36] These cells provide secretions and fibroblast stimulation that improve wound healing. Macrophages stimulates collagen formation, fibroblast proliferation, and tissue repair. If hydrocortisone inhibits macrophages, it will inhibit the wound-healing processes. Macrophages need cholesterol for maximum function. Since hydrocortisone lowers cholesterol, it would inhibit macrophages and fibroblasts so that wound repair is inhibited. While aloe vera has no chronic anti-inflammatory influence, it does have the ability to block the detrimental effect of the steroid on wound healing. Aloe vera stimulates the macrophage and fibroblast, which are inhibited by hydrocortisone. Does gibberellin act like aloe vera in blocking the wound-healing inhibition of hydrocortisone?

Gibberellin blocks the hydrocortisone acetate inhibition of wound tensile strength as much as aloe vera does (table 7.6 and figure 7.7). Mice treated with 0.01 mg/kg hydrocortisone did not inhibit wound healing and in combination with 100 mg/kg gibberellin produced 11.0 ± 0.4 percent increase in wound tensile strength. Wound tensile strength was blocked -45.7 ± 3.7 percent by 1.0 mg/kg hydrocortisone, which was reversed to an increase in wound tensile strength of $+78.2 \pm 2.7$ percent. The pattern of the gibberellin response is similar to aloe vera. Is gibberellin responsible for the wound-healing and anti-inflammatory activity of aloe vera? These data would tend to suggest that gibberellin is a very important factor in aloe vera in this regard.[37]

GIBBERELLIN BLOCKS THE HYDROCORTISONE ACETATE INHIBITION ON WOUND HEALING AND TENSILE STRENGTH

TREATMENT MG/KG	% CHANGE IN WOUND TENSILE STRENGTH (- or +)
0.01 HAC	0.0
+ 100 Gibb.	+ 11.0 ± 0.4
1.0 HAC	- 45.7 ± 3.7
+ 100 Gibb.	+ 78.2 ± 2.7

7 Mice/Group. Gibb. blocks HAC. $P<0.001$

Table 7.6.

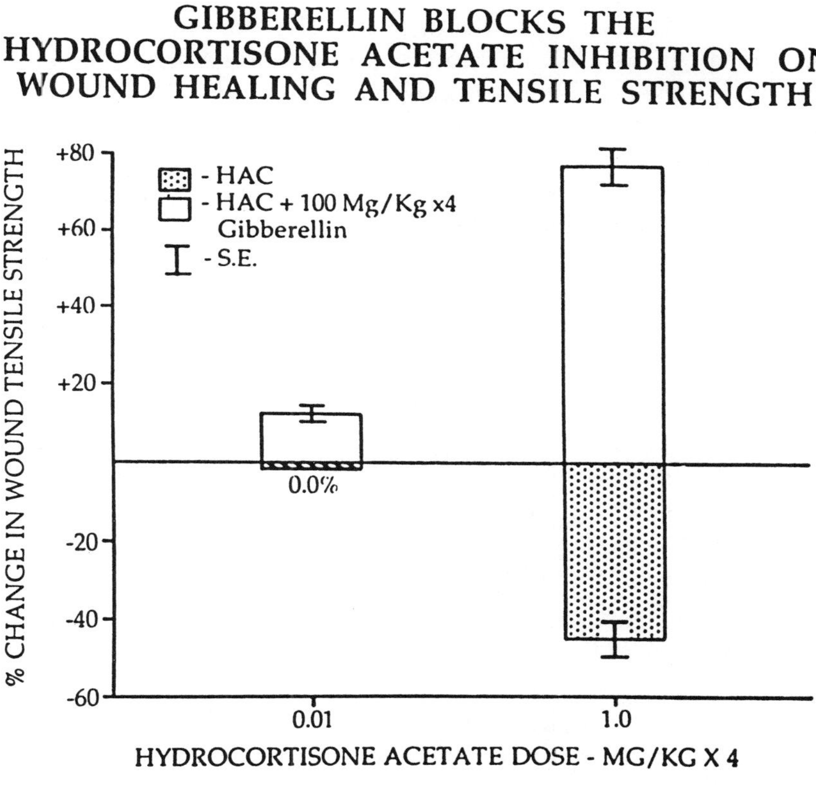
GIBBERELLIN BLOCKS THE
HYDROCORTISONE ACETATE INHIBITION ON
WOUND HEALING AND TENSILE STRENGTH
% CHANGE IN WOUND TENSILE STRENGTH
+80
+60
+40
+20
-20
-40
-60
- HAC
- HAC + 100 Mg/Kg x4
Gibberellin
- S.E.
0.0%
0.01
1.0
HYDROCORTISONE ACETATE DOSE - MG/KG X 4

Fig. 7.7.

Summary

Gibberellin increases the rate of cell elongation by stimulating RNA and protein synthesis in plants, but little or no work has been shown about its anti-inflammatory and wound-healing potential in laboratory animals. A consideration was given to basic wound healing and the growth factors important to wound healing. Gibberellin and aloe blocked the infiltration of PMNs into an inflamed area in a similar dose-response fashion in diabetic animals that have poor wound-healing and anti-inflammatory capabilities. This possibly could suggest that gibberellin was the active anti-inflammatory agent in aloe vera. Gibberellin stimulates open wound healing over a dose range of 2 to 100 mg/kg. Gibberellin also enhances wound tensile strength and, when put in aloe vera, has an additive "vehicle effect." Gibberellin blocks the hydrocortisone acetate inhibition on wound healing as much as aloe vera does.

References

1. B. Stone and T. Yamaki, "The History and Physiological Action of the Gibberellins," *Annual Reviews of Plant Physiology* 8 (1957): 181.
2. J. MacMillan, *Analysis of Plant Hormones and Metabolism of Gibberellins* (Oxford: Oxford University Press, 1984).
3. J. E. Graebe, "Gibberellin Biosynthesis and Control," *Annual Reviews of Plant Physiology* 38 (1987): 419.
4. Ibid.
5. A. Crozier, C. Kno, R. C. Durley, et al., "The Biological Activities of 26 Gibberellins in Nine Plant Bioassays," *Canadian Journal of Botany* 48 (1970): 867.
6. J. Darnell, H. Lodish, and D. Baltimore, *Molecular Cell Biology* New York: (Scientific American Books, 1986).
7. R. Maksymovich, C. Elsner, and A. B. Maksymovich, "Inter-Node Elongation in Xanthium Plants Treated with Gibberellic Acid Presented in Terms of Relative Elemental Rates," *American Journal of Botany* 71 (1984): 239; A. V. Grimestone, H. Harris, and R. T. Johnson, "Prospects in Cell Biology," *Journal of Cell Science.* 4 (1986): 115.
8. A. Johnson, "Towards Rapid Tissue Healing," *Nursing Times*, November 1984, 39; H. I. Mailbach, and D. T. Rovee, *Epidermal Wound Healing* (Chicago: Year Book Medical Publishers, 1972).
9. P. L. Schwartz, "Ascorbic Acid in Wound Healing—a Review," *Journal of the American Dietetic Association* 56 (1970): 497.
10. S. J. Liebovich and R. Ross, "The Role of Macrophage in Wound Repair," *American Journal of Pathology* 78 (1975): 71; C. F. Nathan, "Secretory Products of Macrophages," *American Society of Clinical Investigation* 79 (1987): 319.

11. R. H. Davis, "Biological Activity of Aloe Vera," *SOFW Journal* 119 (1993): 646.
12. I. Danhof, *Aloe through the Ages,* vol. 1 (Grand Prairie, TX: Omnimedicus Press, 1987).
13. J. E. Crewe, "The External Use of Aloe," *Minnesota Journal of Medicine* 20 (1937): 538.
14. T. D. Rowe, "Effect of Fresh Aloe Vera in the Treatment of Third Degree Roentgen Reactions on White Rats," *Journal of the American Pharmacology Association* 29 (1940): 348.
15. S. J. Skokan and R. H. Davis, "Principles of Wound Healing and Growth Factor Considerations," *Journal of the American Podiatric Medical Association* 83 (1993): 223.
16. T. K. Hunt, "Basic Principles of Wound Healing, *Advances in Understanding Trauma and Burn Injury* 30 (1990): 122.
17. Leibovich and Ross, "The Role of Macrophage," 71; Nathan, "Secretory Products," 319.
18. Hunt, "Basic Principles," 122.
19. T. K. Hunt, D. R. Knighton, K. K. Thakral, et al., "Studies on Inflammation and Wound Healing. Angiogenesis and Collagen Synthesis Stimulated in Vivo by Resident and Activated Wound Macrophages," *Surgery* 96 (1984): 48.
20. G. L. Brown, L. J. Curtsinger, M. White, et al., "Acceleration of Tensile Strength of Incisions Treated with EGF and TGF-B," *Annals of Surgery* 208 (1988): 788; G. L. Brown, L. B. Nanney, J. Griffen, "Enhancement of Wound Healing by Topical Treatment with Epidermal Growth Factor," *New England Journal of Medicine* 321 (1989): 76.
21. J. B. West, *Physiological Basis of Medical Practice,* 12th ed. (Baltimore: Williams and Wilkins, 1990), 842; D. Gospodarowicz, G. Neufeld, and L. Schweigerer, "Fibroblast Growth Factor: Structural and Biological Properties," *Journal of Cellular Physiology Supplement* 5 (1987): 15; A. Baird, P. Mormede, and P. Bohlen, "Immunoreactive Fibroblast Growth Factor of Peritoneal Exudate Suggests Its Identity with Macrophage Derived Growth Factor," *Biochemical Biophysiological Research Communications* 126 (1985): 358.
22. G. F. Pierce, T. A. Mustoe, and B. W. Altock, "Role of Platelet Derived Growth Factor in Wound Healing," *Journal of Cellular Biochemistry* 45 (1991): 319.
23. M. D. Sporn, A. B. Roberts, L. M. Wakefield, et al., "Transforming Growth Factor–β: Biological Function and Chemical Structure," *Science* 233 (1986): 532.
24. R. H. Davis, J. J. DiDonato, G. M. Hartman, and R. C. Haas, "Anti-Inflammatory and Wound Healing Activity of a Growth Substance in Aloe Vera," *Journal of the American Podiatric Medical Association* 84 (1994): 77.
25. J. C. Houck, S. G. Barnes, and C. Chang, "Products of Collagenolysis: An Important Mediator of Cell Infiltration during Inflammation," *Immunopathology of Inflammation,* 1971, 39–51.
26. Ibid.
27. G. Weissmann, P. Dukor, and G. Sessa, "Studies on Lysosomes: Mechanisms of Enzyme Release From Endocytic Cells and a Model for Latency in Vitro," *Immunopathology of Inflammation,* 1971, 107–17.
28. B. C. Coats, *The Silent Healer: A Modern Study of Aloe Vera* (Garland, TX: self-published, 1979); T. Miyoshi, and I. Goto, "Serial in Vivo Determination of Nerve Conduction Velocity in Rat Tails," *Electroenceph. Clin. Neurophysiol.* 35 (1973): 125–31; R. J. Green, R. King, P. K. Thomas, and D. N. Baron,

"Sodium-Potassium ATPase Activity in the Dorsal Root Ganglia of Rats with Streptozotocin-Induced Diabetes," *Diabetologia* 28 (1985): 104–7.

29. R. H. Davis, E. Shapiro, and P. S. Agnew, "Topical Effect of Aloe with RNA and Vitamin C on Adjuvant Arthritis," *Journal of the American Podiatric Medical Association* 75 (1985): 229; R. H. Davis, J. Kabbani, and N. P. Maro, "Aloe Vera and Wound Healing," *Journal of the American Podiatric Medical Association* 77: (1986): 165; R. H. Davis, J. Kabbani, and N. P. Maro, "Aloe Vera and Inflammation," *Pennsylvania Academy of Science* 60 (1986): 67.
30. A. Lang, "Structure and Metabolism," *Annual Reviews of Plant Physiology* 21 (1970): 537. 1970; J. L. Key, "Hormones and Nucleric Acid Metabolism," *Annual Reviews of Plant Physiology* 20 (1969): 449.
31. J. L. Key, N. M. Burnett, and C. Y. Lin, "RNA and Protein Biosynthesis and the Regulation of Cell Elongation by Auxin," *Annals of the New York Academy of Science* 144 (1967): 49; L. D. Nooden and K. V. Thimann, "Evidence for a Requirement for Protein Synthesis for Auxin-Induced Cell Enlargement," *Proceedings of the National Academy of Science* 50 (1963): 194.
32. Davis, "Biological Activity," 646.
33. Key, "Hormones," 449.
34. L. Bucci, "Glucosamine: A New Potent Nutraceutical for Connective Tissues," *Podiatric Products* 9 (1992): 56.
35. Davis, Di Donato, Hartman, and Haas, "Anti-Inflammatory and Wound Healing Activity," 77.
36. A. G. Gelman, T. W. Rall, and A. S. Nies, et al., *Goodman and Gelman's The Pharmacological Basis of Therapeutics*, 8th ed. (New York: Pergamon Press, 1990); J. E. Balow and A. S. Rosenthal, "Glucocorticoid Suppression of Macrophage Migration Inhibitory Factor," *Journal of Experimental Medicine* 137 (1973): 1031; R. F. Diegelmann, K. I. Cohen, and A. M. Kaplan, "The Role of Macrophages in Wound Repair: A Review," *Plastic Reconstructive Surgery* 68 (1981): 107; A. C. Guyton,: *Textbook of Medical Physiology*, 8th ed. (Philadelphia: W. B. Saunders, 1991); M. H. Ross and L. J. Romrell, *Histology: A Text and Atlas*, 2d ed. (Baltimore: Williams and Wilkins, 1989).
37. A. N. Orekhov, V. V. Tertov, and S. A. Kudryashov, "Trigger-Like Stimulation of Cholesterol Accumulation and DNA and Extracellular Matrix Synthesis Induced by Atherogenic Serum or Low Density Lipoprotein in Cultured Cells," *Circulation Research* 66 (1990): 311; R. H. Davis, G. J. Stewart, and P. J. Bregman, "Aloe Vera and the Inflamed Synovial Pouch Model," *Journal of the American Podiatric Medical Association* 82 (1992): 140.

8

Does Aloe Vera Have a Place in AIDS Therapy?

Background of AIDS

Acquired Immune Deficiency Syndrome (AIDS) is a medical condition characterized by a severe breakdown in the body's immune system. A transmittable virus induces a poorly functioning immune system, which results in life-threatening infections and cancers. The first case of AIDS was reported in 1981. During 1983 Robert Gallo of the National Cancer Institute and Luc Montagnier of the Pasteur Institute in France co-discovered the AIDS virus. Gallo called the virus human T-cell lymphotropic virus type III. The number of HIV-infected individuals in 1986 in the United States was estimated at 1.5 million.[1] The amount of money spent on AIDS research is ten times that spent on diabetes, heart disease, and cancer. Most HIV-infected individuals develop AIDS, with a virtual 100 percent mortality. Many people harbor misconceptions about AIDS, so media coverage generates considerable anxiety. Pneumocystis carinii pneumonia, a parasitic lung infection, and an unusual skin cancer called Kaposi's sarcoma were first documented in the early cases. In 1981–83 patients treated for AIDS were otherwise-healthy homosexual men who had immune deficiencies. Early reports of AIDS among intravenous drug users led scientists to believe that AIDS was caused by an infectious agent transmitted by blood and semen.[2]

How the Virus Functions

Viruses are minute infectious agents that can only be seen under the electron microscope. HIV infects cells of the immune system called helper T-cells, which have a receptor on their cell surface called CD_4. Helper T-cells direct the immune system's response against a foreign AIDS virus. The HIV enters the blood and attacks the helper T-cell using a glycoprotein on the viruses' surface called gp 120, which attaches to the CD_4 receptor on the lymphocyte. After the gp 120 protein hooks onto CD_4, it exposes one of its sections (a string of amino acids called the V-3 loop) to another enzyme receptor on the lymphocyte—the newly isolated CD_{26}. The V-3 loop acts as a biological key unlocking the CD_{26} doorway. HIV then fuses with the lymphocyte membrane and penetrates the lymphocyte, the cytoplasm, and the nucleus. The virus integrates the lymphocyte chromosome and begins to reproduce, severely compromising the body's immune system. Finding a way to inhibit the enzyme called CD_{26} could provide a possible weapon against AIDS.[3]

The retroviruses contain RNA and the enzyme reverse transcriptase, which changes the RNA to produce a DNA strand and then a double DNA strand. The RNA and transcriptase enter the cell, leaving its envelope at the plasma membrane. The viral RNA is copied into DNA by reverse transcriptase. The DNA is then replicated and integrated into the genome of the host cell, causing genetic change in the host. The DNA can remain dormant in the host cell for years without causing disease in monocytes and macrophages. It may alter the normal function of the cell or even cause cell death. After using the cell components to reproduce, the virus moves to the cell membrane and leaves the cell by budding, causing cell death. These retroviruses were isolated and found to kill T-cells as well as cause cancer. The cell death enables the virus to infect other cells. As the virus spreads throughout the body, more T_4 (CD_4) cells are infected and destroyed. Usually lymphocytes (T-cells) are permissive cells and virtually allow the virus to kill the lymphocyte. Macrophages and monocytes are CD_4 cells but have a repressor that results in suppression of the expressor and replication of the integrated HIV viral DNA. This is called a nonpermissive CD_4 cell. Activation can occur by another viral infection, such as herpes. This is why HIV infection is characterized by a decline of CD_4 cells (helper cells) over time and the weakening of cellular immunity. This, in turn, makes the patient susceptible to a variety of opportunistic infections. The immune system breaks down with a loss of CD_4 cells and a rise of viruses in the body. This is the picture of HIV infection that results in the fatal condition called AIDS.[4]

Modes of Transmission

Intercourse appears to be the primary means of HIV transmission. The HIV virus in infected semen can enter the bloodstream through lacerations in the lining of the vagina, rectum, and anus and small cuts in the mouth. The spread of AIDS is by homosexual and/or heterosexual transmission. Wives of hemophiliacs as well as female prostitutes have been found to have antibodies to the virus and can transmit the disease. Thus either sex can pass the HIV by sexual intercourse. Contaminated blood can transmit the HIV virus to persons undergoing transfusion of blood or health care workers coming in contact with blood. However, screening tests have virtually eliminated the transmission of AIDS by transfusion of blood. Infected mothers can pass the virus to infants during or before parturition. The virus quickly attacks the immune system, which is undeveloped in the baby. HIV has been isolated from most fluids of the body, and any body fluid can transmit the disease.[5]

The AIDS Infection

The HIV virus attacks the helper T-cells and severely decreases the lymphocytes. T-cells are a main line of defense against viral, bacterial, fungal, or parasitic infection and make up the cellular immunity. However, the helper T-cells help the B-cells produce antibodies, which is known as humoral immunity. When antigens such as microbes invade the body, they are ingested by macrophages, which fragment the antigens into peptides. These peptides are then displayed on the surface of the macrophage. T-lymphocytes have receptors that recognize and combine with the peptide. The T-cells divide and release lymphokines, which stimulate the B-lymphocyte that secretes antibody proteins. These antibodies are soluble forms of their receptors.[6] By binding to the antigen, the antibodies can neutralize the destructive influence of the antigen. The T- and B-cells can become memory cells that increase the immune system's readiness to eliminate the antigen if it presents itself in the future.[7] There are two kinds of T-cells: the T_4 cells that aid B-cells in antibody production and T_8 cells or "killer" T-cells, whose function is to directly eliminate the infection by killing the virus-infected cell that is displaying the foreign protein.

When the immune system is stimulated by the virus, the lymph nodes enlarge and the person experiences fatigue. These symptoms disappear in a few days, and the person feels fine for years.[8] Other infections, nutritional status, and immune function will determine the progress of disease as well as the susceptibility to the disease. Serious opportunistic infections help to define the AIDS condition.[9] Pneumocystis carinii is a lung parasitic protozoa infection that produces coughing, fever, and shortness of breath. This condition causes death in AIDS patients. Kaposi's sarcoma is a malignant tumor that travels to lymph tissue and appears as purple lesions on the skin. Lymphomas are also seen in AIDS patients. Common symptoms of AIDS include fever, weight loss, weakness, and anemia.[10]

Tests for the Presence of the AIDS Virus

The ELISA (enzyme-linked immunosorbent assay) is a simple blood test to detect for serum antibodies to the AIDS virus (seropositive). A positive ELISA means that the person has been exposed to the virus, as evidenced by the presence of antibodies. A positive result usually requires confirmation testing with the Western blot assay, which is more specific for the antibodies to the virus than the ELISA assay. The ELISA assay is used to screen blood, but a positive result is usually followed by the Western blot because of the possibility of a false positive. These assays help to detect people exposed to AIDS and go far to keep blood transfusions safe.[11]

The Immune System Combats against the AIDS Virus

Cell-mediated immunity involves the T-lymphocyte that originates in the thymus. Humoral immunity involves the B-cells that come from the bone marrow and form antibodies. The T- and B-cell differ in their function but also in the way they locate foreign invaders. The B-cells can recognize antigens because they carry specialized receptors or antibodies on their surface. The T-cell also carries a unique receptor, but unlike the B-cells, the receptor on the T-cell cannot see the entire antigen. Instead the T-cell receptor only recognizes protein fragments of the antigen or peptide chains of amino acids. They form a complex between the peptide and the cell surface. The T- and B-cells are good partners in finding viruses that hide in cells.[12] Antibodies from the B-cells respond to toxins and outer surface antigens, whereas the T-cells discover hidden antigens inside pathogens and those presented to it from macrophages. The viral protein breaks down inside a cell, and peptide chains go to the cell surface. The T-cell receptor forms a complex with the antigen that activates the T-cell to release interleukins that cause the B-cell to form antibodies. Both cells work together in fighting off the virus. The B-cells help process the antigen so that the T-cells can complex the antigen on the cell surface. Thus the B-cells stimulate the T-cells into action. This is a positive and negative feedback system.

The CD_4 (helper) cells recognize the peptide from protein taken up by the macrophage. The CD_8 or "killer" T-cell functions to eliminate the infection, usually by killing the virus-infected cell. These latter cells are called cytotoxic T-cells. When the B-cell is stimulated into action, it can make millions of antibodies in a short period of time. It is essential that the immune system recognize self from nonself. This function is learned early in the organism's development. An autoimmune disease is when the cells can't tell the difference between self and foreign cells.[13]

Observations That Do Not Fit the Current Theory about AIDS

Scientists are afraid to reveal their ignorance and confusion about AIDS. Recorded observations warn us that our understanding about AIDS falls short of the mark. However, this failure does nothing to stop the death toll of AIDS.[14]

1. *HIV AND AIDS GO BACK TO 1872.* Hundreds of AIDS-like cases were described in medical journals prior to the early 1980s. Cases were recorded in the 1930s and 1940s with all the characteristics of AIDS.[15] Kaposi's sarcoma and *Pneumocystis carinii* were observed in the early 1900s. It may be that AIDS itself can be distinct from HIV if this data is correct. Moritz Kaposi first identified the disease in 1872.[16]

2. *IS HIV NECESSARY TO CAUSE AIDS?* The current theory tells us that HIV is necessary and sufficient to cause AIDS. The WHO (World Health Organization) tells us that AIDS does not occur in the absence of HIV. Is there AIDS without HIV? Luc Montagnier found three AIDS patients without HIV. Is this new or have other cases been ignored?[17] Paul Ewald, an evolutionary biologist at Amherst College, suggests that HIV may not be a new and deadly virus, but an old one that has taken on acquired deadly tendencies. He argues that HIV may have been infecting people benignly for centuries before it started causing AIDS.[18]
3. *FOR HIV TO BE TRANSMITTED SEXUALLY IT MUST BE PRESENT IN REPRODUCTIVE FLUIDS.* There are many puzzling observations in this area. Examination of reproductive fluid (semen) does not always reveal HIV virus. The wife of the tennis star Arthur Ashe, who had AIDS as a result of transfusion, was HIV-free.[19]
4. *ONE CAN HAVE HIV EXPOSURE WITHOUT AIDS.* For example, prostitutes can be exposed to HIV sero-positive men and not get AIDS.[20] Drug abuse presents a greater risk of contracting HIV than promiscuity does. A depression of normal T-cells predisposes and is predictive of HIV infections. People with normal immune function are resistant to HIV infections. In fact, HIV infections may not lead to AIDS if other co-factors are lacking such as other infections and immunosuppressant conditions. Consideration must be given to defective HIV viruses.

The current theory states that all or nearly all people infected with HIV will develop AIDS. If you have the antibodies to HIV you will die of the disease. However, the record shows people can lose the HIV positivity accompanied by a normal T-cell count. It appears that those people whose immune systems are impaired will develop the HIV infection. Thus the status of the immune system before, during, and after the HIV exposure is very important. People who have healthy lifestyles after the HIV infection may overcome HIV.[21] In other words, there may be a successful immune response to HIV. People can fight off the infection and remain healthy. Co-factors alongside

HIV aid in the AIDS tragedy. AIDS requires the input of other infections and immune suppression to work with the HIV virus in producing the disease. Immune suppression predisposes people to AIDS, as it predisposes them to other opportunistic diseases. All AIDS patients have multiple causes of immune suppression.[22]

The failure of HIV researchers to explain the basic facts of AIDS is one of the reasons why a treatment has not been forthcoming. In fact, it is not clear how HIV causes AIDS. The "HIV equals AIDS" concept does not explain the facts. It's too easy. It may be that the current concept about AIDS is based upon false assumptions. AIDS researchers may have ignored the accepted criteria for establishing disease. However, concepts that apply to pneumonia, diphtheria, and cholera may not apply to HIV infection. Immune suppression by other infections along with the HIV virus can explain the AIDS disease.

An Alternative for Explaining AIDS

The question whether or not HIV virus is sufficient by itself to cause AIDS requires much consideration. Yes, HIV is highly correlated with AIDS, but is it cause-and-effect? Therefore, HIV is needed for AIDS but requires other conditions be present. Immunosuppression, destruction of T_4 cells, and macrophages as well as multiple infections go hand in hand to produce AIDS.

Co-Factors Associated with AIDS May Provide a Target for Therapeutic Measures

How could so many great scientists be wrong for so long a time? What can be done for people with AIDS that has not been tried? Has the problem of AIDS been oversimplified? Every medical student believes if you are exposed to the HIV virus you get AIDS. We all believe this, do we not? However, our ignorance about AIDS is greater than what we know about the disease. In order to stop AIDS, one must find all the co-factors associated with the disease and stop them. All the infections act synergistically with HIV, which has broad implications. Thus preventing a co-factor infection would decrease the risk of AIDS. Special nutrition, proper hygiene, behavior modification, and other improvements in lifestyle should reduce the risk of AIDS and prevent the development of overt disease.[23] Exposure to drugs and infection must be prevented so that people can have healthy lives. The AIDS risk for blacks and Hispanics is much higher than that for whites. This is directly related to their poor social economic status. Vaccines and medicines may help us in this fight against AIDS, and improved nutrition and lifestyle may reduce the transmission but not eliminate the HIV virus.

Nutritional Influence on AIDS

Undernourished individuals have impaired immune responses.[24] Nutrition deficiencies can act as a major co-factor in the immunodeficient virus infection. The restoration of the immune system by proper nutrient intake must be an important guideline in treating AIDS patients.[25] Since deficiencies of pyridoxine, folic acid, vitamin A, vitamin C, and vitamin E impair cellular and antibody immunity, these nutrients should be monitored in AIDS patients. However, most AIDS treatment centers in the United States do not have a standard nutrition program for AIDS patients.[26] Poor mental image, loneliness, and depression have been shown to contribute to immunosuppression. Some 80 percent of all HIV-infected people worldwide are found in sub-Saharan Africa.[27] If in this area of the world, malnutrition is the most widespread immunosuppressant in the human, it might help explain the high incidence of AIDS in sub-Saharan Africa. This region has economic poverty, malnutrition, and an inadequate safe water supply. Malnutrition (poor diet) causes impaired host resistance, with a greater susceptibility to the HIV infection as well as opportunistic infections. The reduced immune function (reduced T-cell function) coupled with heightened opportunistic infections is the result of AIDS, leading to death. Since normal immune function depends on good nutrition, can malnutrition be a contributor to AIDS in people who have the HIV virus? I am sure some would say, "No." Drug abuse enhances the malnutrition-immunosuppression relationship in HIV-positive people.[28] Health care professionals must establish an adequate nutritional and drug abuse education for HIV-positive individuals to improve the quality of their lives.

Weight loss is very dramatic in AIDS patients. Anti-viral therapy causes some weight gain, but other considerations are needed in this regard. Hyperalimentation leads to some increases in body fat, but there is little or no repletion of protein stores. Anabolic hormone treatment needs to be considered in AIDS patients. Malnutrition in AIDS may be due to malabsorption, diarrhea, and intestinal infection. B_{12} deficiency is a result of malabsorption, and the intrinsic factor is reduced in patients with AIDS. This deficiency may be due to macrophages carrying viruses in the brain.[29] Vitamin C has anti-viral and antioxidant influences that could help control the progress of HIV infection and cellular damage. It also plays an important role in regulating the function of the immune system (cell-mediated immunity). Vitamin C is necessary for the phagocytic function of neutrophils and macrophages.[30] When AIDS patients are malnourished they become protein-depleted. Most of the functions in our bodies are protein-dependent, particularly our defense mechanisms. The major protein content is found in muscle. If muscle protein declines, the muscles become weak, as seen in AIDS patients. Body protein loss may be due to malabsorption, anorexia, muscle atrophy, and hypermetabolism. Malabsorption and diarrhea are frequent in AIDS patients, which can account for the weight loss. Pathologies in the gastrointestinal tract range from infections to neoplasms causing the diarrhea/malabsorption seen in AIDS. Disuse of muscle causes atrophy and is a factor in this wasting disease.[31]

Synthetic Drugs Have Not Solved the Problem

In the early 1980s, when the HIV virus was shown to be the cause of AIDS, it did not take long for pharmaceutical companies to find drugs to destroy the virus, at least in the laboratory. AZT was tried in infected people in 1985, and the results were so promising that the drug was hurried to market for patients to use. A few years later, AZT's therapeutic value began to fade because the virus mutated into new forms that were resistant to AZT's therapeutic action. In fact, HIV has mutated into forms that have evaded every other new drug tested so far. No single drug can do the job. It was then decided to use combined drugs, but deciding exactly what and how these combinations are to be made is difficult. Combinations of drugs were used to attack different steps in the life cycle.[32] For example, AZT was combined with a second drug to attack the reverse transcriptase enzyme that copies viral RNA into DNA that is inserted among the cell's genes. The presence of the second drug makes the virus more susceptible to the action of AZT.

The detection of the transmission of an AZT-resistant strain of HIV was alarming when it was discovered in 1993, because it altered the consequences of treatment strategies. These findings seem to cast doubt on the usefulness of AZT and other drugs in treating HIV. Also, AZT did not delay the onset of AIDS in patients carrying the HIV virus.[33] The results so far seem to indicate that AZT is effective but only for a short period. However, CD_4 lymphocytes of patients receiving AZT rose significantly even though there was no clinical benefit. The CD4 cell count has been considered to be a valuable measure of the AIDS symptoms. However, some feel that it is not a reliable indicator of the effectiveness of drug treatment in HIV infection. The disappointment of believing that infectious diseases are past, the despair of people who have HIV, and the anger of people who represent HIV-infected people may force the direction of AIDS research to go to a place where benefits are not forthcoming. The sense of crisis about AIDS may force investigators to make bad judgments regarding effective treatment.

Therapeutic Uses of the Immune System

Efforts are being made to make vaccines more specific. When it comes to making an AIDS vaccine, almost all researchers ruled out the classical approaches for safety reasons. The live, attenuated approach was dismissed because the vital genetic material in the vaccine could integrate into the host's genes, which might cause cancer. The whole killed strategy was rejected because if some HIV were not killed, the vaccine could cause AIDS. However, instead of using the entire virus, vaccine makers synthesize or cloned certain pieces of the virus, omitting the disease-causing genetic material. These viral pieces or antigens can be presented to the immune system with novel adjuvants, making, in effect, a killed specific vaccine. Components of the immune system as biological mimics may help in the treatment of disease.[34]

Two approaches have been used to employ the immune system to fight disease. Selected T-cells or antibodies respond to a precise target. The T-cell is called cell-mediated, whereas the antibody response is called humoral (antigen-specific reactions). Non-antigen-specific reactions involve the actions of cytokines or anti-bacterial peptides. Vaccines make use of the immune system's memory. They can recognize and destroy nearly all intruders and can remember the intruder over many years. Using molecular methods, scientists can locate the genetic components of a microorganism that causes the disease. They can isolate a specific protein and vaccinate people with this specific compound rather than the whole organism. Also, monoclonal antibodies can be used to discover and neutralize the weakness in viral defenses. The "killer" T-cells cannot destroy an antigen unless it is processed by the macrophage and presented to the T-cell on the surface by means of the major histocompatibility complex. Substances called adjuvants can be used to make sure the T-cell sees the antigen.[35]

Sophisticated methods have been used to manipulate antibodies. Interleukin-4 and interleukin-5 produced by T-cells augment the production of antibodies by B-lymphocytes. Monoclonal antibodies can be directed against a specific cell-mediated part of the immune system. They can be directed against CD_4 or CD_8 molecules of T-cells that bind antigens. Vaccines thus have the potential for protecting "self" from attack. The target therapy for autoimmune diseases is the T-cells that attack tissue. If one can block the activity of the T-cell having a particular antigen-binding receptor, one can have a strategy to eliminate the autoimmune condition.[36]

The desperate and tragic situation of AIDS has led investigators to try to develop therapeutic vaccines. So far, the vaccines have not succeeded clinically but many approaches for research have been found. One approach entails isolating a protein from the virus envelope called gp 160 (composed of gp 120 and gp 41). The gp 160 is injected into HIV-infected patients, causing the person to make antibodies that become available to attack the whole HIV virus. The second approach involves taking CD_4 molecules from T-cells and forming antibodies to the CD_4 molecules that can be used to bind the CD_4 receptor and prevent the virus from entering and destroying the T-cells. The drop in the CD_4 T-cell count has been inhibited by these approaches.[37] Monoclonal antibodies against the amino acid sequence found in the V-3 loop of the gp 120 of the HIV coat protein as well as the CD_{26} have received much consideration in this regard. The CD_{26} is a cell surface protein that helps HIV to enter cells. Other peptides such as 637-666 have been obtained and synthesized that inhibit infection by other HIV-1 strains. This peptide has no detectable toxicity. One wonders if this peptide should be called a drug.[38] It is possible that the Kaposi's sarcoma in AIDS patients can be combated by the immune system. The immune system can attack tumor antigens and increase the probability of wiping out the disease. Also, monoclonal antibodies against molecules could also be used. They could be directed toward interleukin receptors found on cancers to inhibit the disease. However, one wonders if neutralizing antibodies or the cell-mediated arm is the best approach to the AIDs problem.[39] While a prophylactic vaccine against AIDS infection represents the best hope for controlling the devastating worldwide AIDS epidemic, most of the really interesting emphasis has been placed on therapeutic vaccines.

Can Aloe Vera Make a Contribution to the Treatment of AIDS?

ACEMANNAN is a biologically active polysaccharide that was successfully isolated from aloe vera in 1984 by Carrington Laboratories under the leadership of Bill H. McAnalley. Acemannan is a complex polysaccharide consisting of long-chain, beta-linked mannan polymers interspersed with acetyl groups.[40] Acemannan is stable, has a long half-life, is non-toxic, and is not metabolized until it reaches the target cell. Macrophages are phagocytic immune cells that ingest and destroy viruses, bacteria, and tumor cells. These cells secrete a number of important chemicals such as growth factors, enzymes, and cytokines. The tumor necrosis factor (TNF) can destroy tumor cells and stimulate fibroblast cells for wound healing. Macrophages can release interleukins that can enhance inflammation against infection.[41]

Acemannan, an immune stimulant, was licensed by the USDA to aid in the treatment of canine and feline fibrosarcoma.[42] As an adjuvant, Acemannan increases the immune response to an antigen. This ability is important to the effectiveness of a vaccine, as antigens alone sometimes fail to produce an immune response. This immunostimulant and vaccine adjuvant ability would be extremely important in the fight against AIDS. Acemannan was shown to have positive in vitro results against HIV.[43] It was also shown to be synergistic with AZT under double-blind conditions.[44] CD_4 cell counts were stabilized in sixteen to forty-eight weeks by Acemannan. The feline leukemia virus is like HIV. It causes death in cats within eight weeks. However, when infected cats were treated with Acemannan, after twelve weeks 71 percent of the animals were alive and in good health. Also, many studies indicate that Acemannan has a therapeutic benefit for cancers. It showed a positive response against fibrosarcoma in dogs and solid tumors in humans. By increasing the lymphocyte activity, Acemannan may increase the protective immunity (killer cell function, antibody production, and anti-tumor immune response).[45]

Acemannan has both anti-viral and immunomodulating properties with a wide range of treatment applications for viruses, cancer, inflammatory diseases, and wound healing. Acemannan can inhibit viral replication and stimulate cellular immunity, which makes it useful for treating AIDS. The isolation of a known structural polysaccharide from aloe vera can be used to treat major problems that affect mankind. This discovery opens up the field of carbohydrate research for investigators all over the world.[46]

ALOE VERA: The power of the immune system was shown to be remarkable when improved by modern vaccine methodology. The body protects itself by a diversity of cells and molecules whose target is the antigen or the HIV virus. The protein coat of the virus (gp 120) is on the outside, and gp 41 is embedded in the virus membrane. Vaccines against the virus protein coat are under consideration. The HIV virus and Acemannan (Carrisyn) are taken up by the macrophage. The macrophage intends destroying the virus. Acemannan alters the outer viral protein coat so as to alter the binding site so that it does not fit into the T_4 receptor to destroy the T_4 cell (figure 8.1). As a result, the T_4 cell count remains elevated.

If Acemannan can prevent the decline of the T_4 cell, we wonder if aloe vera can do the same thing? One wonders if aloe vera has ever been used as a control in the Acemannan studies. One would think that the array of biological agents surrounding the polysaccharide in aloe vera would be more natural and beneficial to altering the virus so that it would not destroy the T_4 cell. If Acemannan can

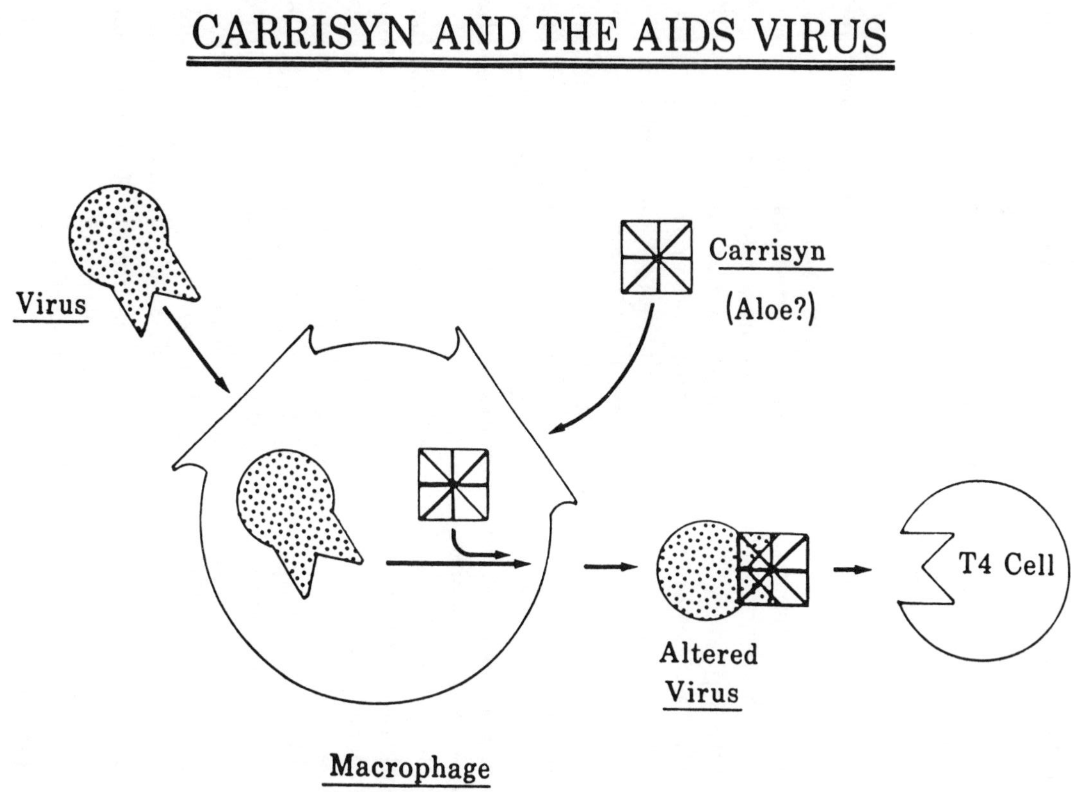
CARRISYN AND THE AIDS VIRUS
Virus
Carrisyn
(Aloe?)
Altered
Virus
T4 Cell
Macrophage

Fig. 8.1.

alter the viral outer protein, possibly so can aloe vera. If the helper T_4 cell is prevented from being destroyed by aloe vera, the bursa cells (B-lymphocytes) can continue to make antibodies (figure 8.2).

We have shown in our laboratory that aloe vera can prevent and regress the development of adjuvant-induced arthritis.[47] Adjuvant arthritis is induced in the laboratory rat by giving *Mycobacterium butyricum.* This is an autoimmune disease that involves both antibody and cellular immunity. The characteristics of this condition in the animal model are virtually identical to those of rheumatoid arthritis. If a therapeutic agent works well in this model, it should work well in the clinical condition. Anecdotally, several people with osteoarthritis and rheumatoid arthritis (six to eight) received great benefit from oral aloe vera gel (4 ounces/day) over several months. As a biological vehicle, Aloe vera has an additive anti-inflammatory influence on hydrocortisone,[48] vitamin C,[49] certain amino acids,[50] aspirin, and other biological activities.[51] The possibility that aloe vera can act as an adjuvant to enhance the immune response to an antigen comes out of the work of R. P. LaBadie. He found that there are two functionally and chemically distinct immunomodulatory compounds in the gel of Aloe vera. One fraction could enhance antibody formation and another could inhibit antibody formation such that LaBadie called aloe vera an immune modulator. He believes that this modulatory activity is common in other plants. LaBadie also showed that aloe vera can inhibit and stimulate phagocytosis as well as "mop up" oxygen radicals.[52] I believe our laboratory first showed that aloe vera could act as an immune stimulator on wound healing as well as an immune inhibitor on inflammation.[53] Aloe vera can inhibit the migration of polymorphonuclear leukocytes into the site of inflammation as well as block the oxygen radicals that produce inflammation.[54] I believe aloe vera or possibly critical fractions might block the HIV virus and improve the clinical condition as well as possibly prevent the destruction of the T_4 cell. I look to aloe vera as a possible help to control these autoimmune inducers, immunosuppressors, and infections that would go against the human organism.

Jeffrey Bland studied the effect of oral aloe vera juice on colonic bacterial activity, protein digestion/absorption, gastrointestinal motility, and pH as well as stool parameters. He found that protein absorption was improved, with no diarrhea, improved bowel regularity, increased energy and well-being, improved gastrointestinal motility,

POSSIBLE EFFECT OF ALOE VERA ON ANTIBODY PRODUCTION IN THE PRESENCE OF THE AIDS VIRUS

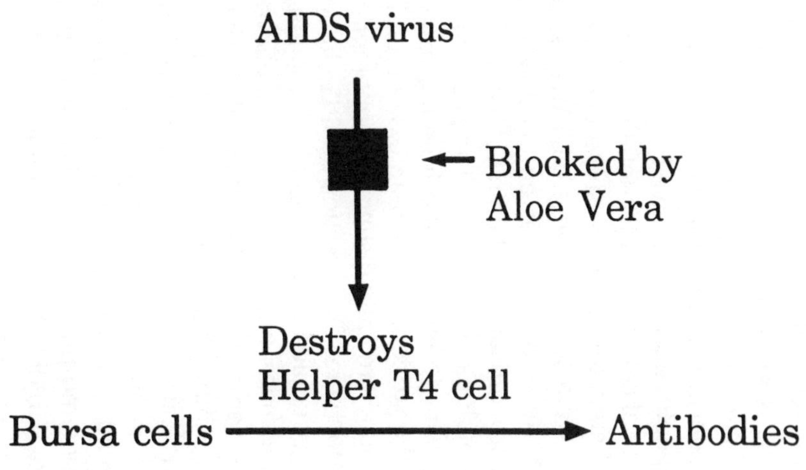

Fig. 8.2.

and a greater water-holding characteristic of the stool. Intestinal yeast and unwanted bacteria were decreased.[55] This suggested that aloe vera contained an agent that was bacteriostatic on improved gastrointestinal function. The bacteriostatic property of aloe vera was also recorded with freeze-dried aloe vera.[56] When AIDS patients are described as malnourished or nutritionally depleted, the inference is that they are protein- and energy-depleted. They lose their energy reserve and total body fat as well as muscle protein. The major site of protein loss is muscle protein.[57] Subcutaneous treatment of mice with 150 mg/kg whole-leaf aloe vera for four days increased the strength of gastrocnemius muscle contraction 38 percent after a 50 mv stimulus. This increased strength of muscle contraction might be transposed to the AIDS patient who suffers from muscle weakness because of the decreased protein-induced muscle mass (figures 8.3 and 8.4). We are aware that the lectins obtained from aloe are anabolic, as revealed by Dr. W. Winters several years ago in a paper presented at the International Aloe Science Council (unpublished).

Deficiencies of pyridoxine, folic acid, vitamin A, and vitamin E result in reduced cell-mediated immunity and reduced antibody responses. Zinc deficiency is associated with lymphoid atrophy and lower thymus activity.[58] These nutritional deficiencies can act as cofactors with the HIV infection. These nutritional deficiencies are found in AIDS patients. The AIDS infection depletes the immune cells and reduces the immune response, but nutritional deficiencies help in the immune depression. Aloe vera possibly may help to improve the immune status because it contains all the needed vitamins and it may correct the energy and protein deficiencies seen in the "HIV Wasting Syndrome." The high nutrient intake of aloe vera may modulate the immune function and enhance resistance to AIDS progression. In the underdeveloped countries such as those of Africa, aloe vera could be distributed from hospitals to combat the WHO-predicted 45 million cases of HIV infections by the year 2000.

Summary

Researchers have seen a disappointing twelve years in their research with AIDS. No curative agent or worthwhile vaccine has been developed, and people continue to die of AIDS. The reason scientists

EFFECT OF ALOE VERA ON THE STRENGTH OF GASTROCNEMIUS MUSCLE CONTRACTION

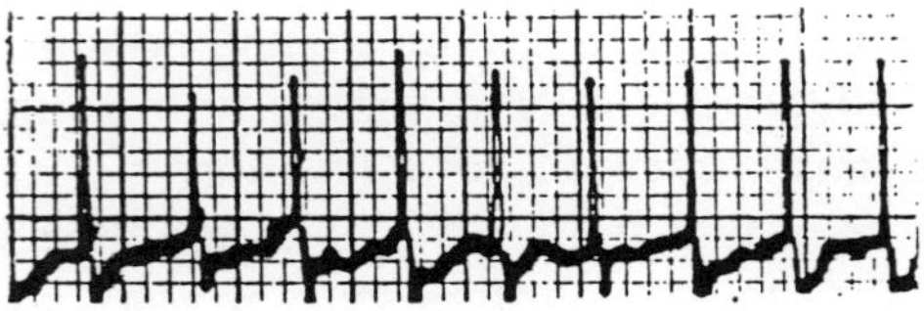

ALOE VERA 150 MG/KG X 4

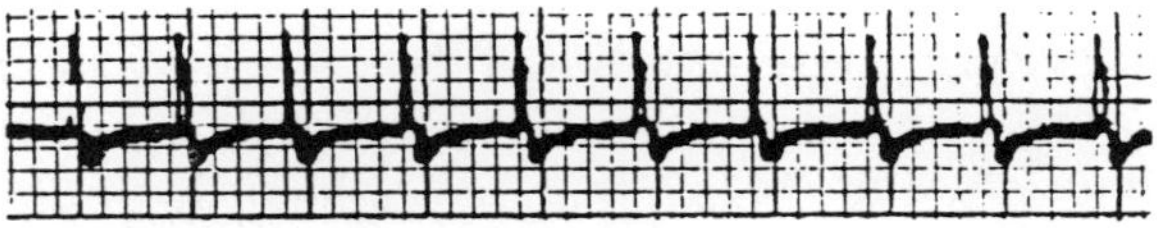

AQ. CONTROL

STIMULUS = 50 mv + 38%

Fig. 8.3.

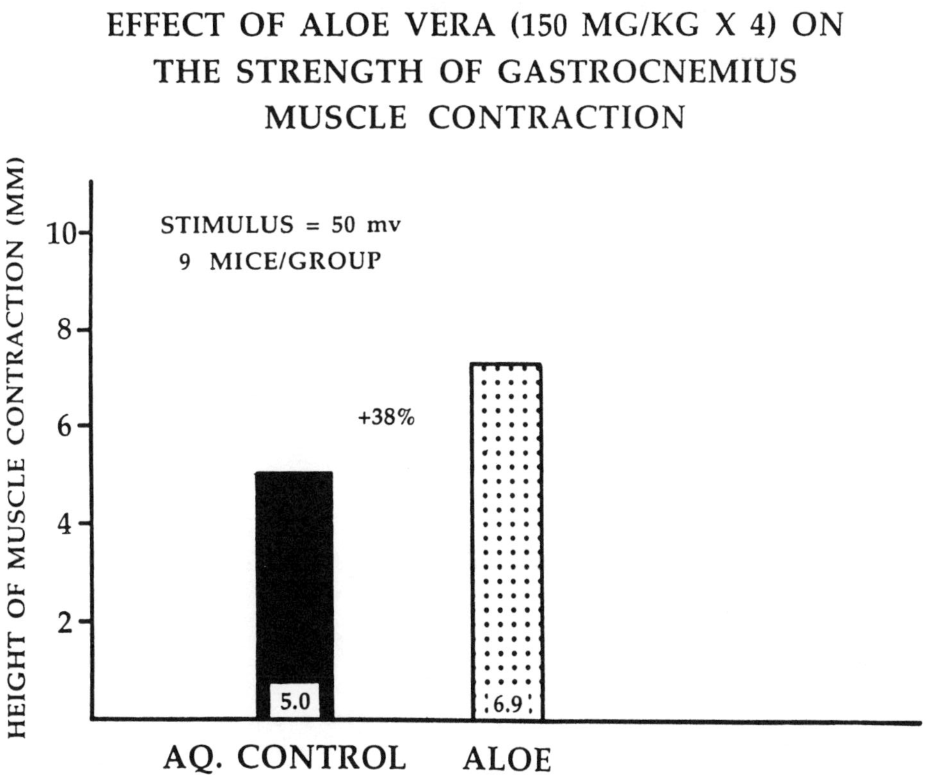
EFFECT OF ALOE VERA (150 MG/KG X 4) ON
THE STRENGTH OF GASTROCNEMIUS
MUSCLE CONTRACTION
HEIGHT OF MUSCLE CONTRACTION (MM)
10
8
6
4
2
STIMULUS = 50 mv
9 MICE/GROUP
+38%
5.0
6.9
AQ. CONTROL
ALOE

Fig. 8.4.

continue to fail in this tragic period of research is that they are holding onto traditional thinking. They continue to look for one compound to knock out the HIV virus. The multitude of factors alongside the HIV virus are not receiving equal attention. Since there are many co-factors, which are immunosuppressant, in the production of the AIDS syndrome, I feel that a treatment of many compounds such as those with aloe vera would be beneficial in the treatment of this multi-factorial syndrome. The worldwide AIDS epidemic is volatile and unstable, and the major impacts are still to come. Global AIDS may be out of control because of poor leadership, lack of coordination, and complacency. A pessimistic picture is painted all around the world, which is not responding to the AIDS crisis. The world is not responding because there is no effective treatment for AIDS. We feel that aloe vera, which is non-toxic, or one of its extracts might be used as an effective treatment for the global AIDS syndrome.

References

1. B. J. Bastian, "AIDS: Education against Fear," *Carolina Tips* 49 (1986): 1.
2. T. J. Coats, "Prevention of HIV-1 Infection: Accomplishments and Priorities," *Journal of the National Institutes of Health* 5 (1993): 73; R. Root-Bernstein,: *Rethinking AIDS* (New York: Free Press, 1993).
3. J. Seligmann and M. Marby, "One More Piece of the Puzzle," *Newsweek,* November 8, 1993, 72.
4. W. E. Paul, "Infectious Diseases and the Immune System," *Scientific American,* September 1993, 91; C. A. Mims, *The Pathogenesis of Infectious Disease* (New York: Academic Press, 1987).
5. Bastian, "AIDS," 1.
6. G. J. Nossal, "Life, Death and the Immune System," *Scientific American,* September 1993, 53.
7. C. A. Janeway, "How the Immune System Recognizes Invaders," *Scientific American,* September 1993, 73.
8. Bastian, "AIDS," 1.
9. Root-Bernstein, *Rethinking AIDS.*
10. P. Furth, "AIDS: The Human Aspects of Care," *Medical Student,* March/April 1987, 17.
11. E. Papadopulos-Eleopulos, V. F. Turner, and J. M. Papadimitriou, "Is a Positive Western Blot Proof of HIV Infection?" *Biotechnology* 11 (1993): 696.
12. Noggal, "Life, Death and the Immune System." 53.
13. Paul, "Infectious Diseases," 91.
14. Root-Bernstein, *Rethinking AIDS.*
15. Ibid.
16. F. A. Ellis, "Multiple Idiopathic Hemorrhagic Sarcoma of Kaposi," *Archives of Dermatological Syphilology* 30 (1934): 706; L. H. Breimer, "Did Moritz Kaposi Describe AIDS in 1872?" *Clinical Medicine* 19 (1984): 156.

17. J. Maddox, "Where the AIDS Virus Hides Away," *Nature* 362 (1993): 287; R. A. Weiss, "How Does HIV Cause AIDS?" *Science* 260 (1993): 1273.
18. G. Cowley, "The Future of AIDS," *Newsweek,* March 1993, 47.
19. Root-Bernstein, *Rethinking AIDS.*
20. Ibid.
21. Ibid.
22. Ibid.; W. Blattner, R. C. Gallo, and H. M. Temin, "HIV Causes AIDS," *Science* 242 (1988): 514; C. Gorman, "Are Some People Immune to AIDS?" *Time,* March 1993, 49.
23. R. R. Watson, *Nutrition and AIDS* (London: CRC Press, 1994).
24. Ibid.
25. V. K. Jain and R. K. Chandra, "Does Nutritional Deficiency Predispose to Acquire Immune Deficiency Syndrome?" *Nutrition Research* 4 (1984): 537.
26. Task Force on Nutritional Support in AIDS, "Guidelines for Nutrition Support in AIDS," *Nutrition Today* 24 (1989): 27.
27. J. C. Caldwell, I. O. Orubuloye, and P. Caldwell, "Underreaction to AIDS in Sub-Saharan Africa," *Society of Scientific Medicine* 34 (1992): 1169.
28. J. P. Van Vugt, *AIDS Prevention and Services Community Based Research.* (Westport, CT: Bergin & Garvey, 1994); M. C. Lopez, D. S. Huang, B. Waltz, G. J. Chen, and R. R. Watson, "Splenocyte Subsets in Normal and Protein Malnourished Mice after Long-Term Exposure to Cocaine or Morphine," *Life Science* 49 (1991): 1253.
29. P. M. Dreyfus, "Diet and Nutrition in Neurologic Disorders," in M. E. Shils and V. R. Yound, eds. *Modern Nutrition in Health and Disease* (Philadelphia: Lea & Febiger, 1988), 1458.
30. W. Prinz, R. Bortz, B. Bregin, and M. Hersch, "The Effect of Ascorbic Acid Supplementation on Some Parameters of the Human Immunological Defense System," *International Journal of Vitamin Nutritional Research* 47 (1977): 248.
31. D. P. Kotler, A. R. Tierney, S. K. Brenner, et al., "Preservation of Short-Term Energy Balance in Clinically Stable Patients with AIDS," *American Journal of Clinical Nutrition* 51 (1990): 7; S. Chandra and R. K. Chandra, "Nutrition, Immune Response and Outcome," *Progress Food Nutritional Science* 10 (1966): 1; R. T. Chlebowski, "Significance of Altered Nutritional Status in Acquired Immune Deficiency Syndrome," *Nutrition and Cancer* 7 (1985): 85.
32. J. Cohen, "Can Combination Therapy Overcome Drug Resistance?" *Science* 260 (1993): 1258.
33. M. Chase, "First Transmission of AZT-Resistant HIV is Reported," *Wall Street Journal* 4 (1993): 22; S. Lehrman, "AIDS Administrators Plan Crisis Meeting over Future of AZT," *Nature* 362 (1993): 483; L. K. Altman, "Drug Resistant Strains of HIV Linked to Tripling of AIDS Deaths," *New York Times,* December 16, 1993.
34. H. Wizzell, "The Immune System as a Therapeutic Agent," *Scientific American,* September 1993, 127.
35. H. S. Ginsberg, *Vaccines 93: Modern Approaches to New Vaccines including Prevention of AIDS* (Cold Spring Harbor Laboratory Press, 1993).
36. J. Klein, *Immunology* (Blackwell Scientific Publications, 1990).
37. Root-Bernstein, *Rethinking AIDS.*
38. S. Jiang, K. Lin, N. Strick, and A. R. Neurath, "HIV-1 Inhibition by a Peptide," *Nature* 365 (1993): 113.
39. Wizzell, "The Immune System." 127.

40. D. Womble and J. H. Helderman, "Enhancement of Allo-Responsiveness of Human Lymphocytes by Acemannan (Carrisyn)," *International Journal of Immunopharmacology* 10 (1988): 967.
41. C. F. Nathan, "Secretory Products of Macrophages," *Journal of Clinical Investigation* 79 (1987): 319.
42. N. C. Pedersen and J. E. Barbough, "Clinical Overview of Feline Immunodeficiency Virus," *Journal of American Veterinarian Medical Association* 199 (1991): 1298.
43. J. B. Kahlon, M. C. Kemp, R. H. Carpenter, Bill H. McAnalley, et al., "Inhibition of AIDS Virus Replication by Acemannan in Vitro," *Molecular Biotherapy* 3 (1991): 127.
44. N. Clumeck, "A Phase II Study of Acemannan Alone and with Zidovudine (AZT) among Symptomatic and Asymptomatic HIV Patients," *Retrospective Analysis,* Carrington Laboratories Rept. 9500.2, June 1992.
45. C. Harris, K. Pierce, G. King, et al., "Efficacy of Acemannan in Treatment of Canine and Feline Spontaneous Neoplasms," *Molecular Biotherapy* 3 (1991): 207.
46. Carrington Laboratories, Inc., *1992 Annual Report: Research and Development* (Dallas, TX: 1992), 6.
47. D.C. Hanley, W. A. Solamon, B. Saffran, and R.H. Davis, "The Evaluation of Natural Substances in the Treatment of Adjuvant Arthritis," *Journal of the American Podiatric Association* 72 (1982): 275.
48. R. H. Davis, W. L. Parker, and D. P. Murdoch, "Aloe Vera as a Biologically Active Vehicle for Hydrocortisone Acetate," *Journal of the American Podiatric Medical Association* 81 (1991): 1.
49. R. H. Davis, "The Anti-Arthritic Activity of Vitamin C," *Pennsylvania Academy of Science* 63 (1989): 42.
50. R. H. Davis, "Topical Influence of Aloe Vera on Adjuvant Arthritis," *Physiologist* 31 (1988): 206.
51. R. H. Davis, M. G. Leitner, J. M. Russo, and M. E. Byrne, "The Biology of Aloe Vera," *Pennsylvania Academy of Science* 62 (1988): 43.
52. L. A. Hart, P. H. Van Enckevort, H. Van Dijk, R. Zaat, K. T. D. De Silva, and R. P. LaBadie, "Two Functionally and Chemically Distinct Immunomodulatory Compounds in the Gel of Aloe Vera," *J. Ethnopharmacology* 23 (1988): 61.
53. R. H. Davis, "Inhibitory and Stimulatory Systems in Aloe Vera," *Aloe Today,* Winter 1992.
54. R. H. Davis, J. M. Kabbani, and N. P. Maro, "Aloe Vera and Inflammation," *Pennsylvania Academy of Science* 60 (1986): 67.
55. Jeffrey Bland, "Effect of Orally Consumed Aloe Vera Juice on Gastrointestinal Function in Normal Humans," *Preventive Medicine*, March/April 1985, 1.
56. J. P. Heggers, G. R. Pineless, and M. C. Robson, "Dermaide Aloe/Aloe Vera Gel: Comparison of the Antimicrobial Effects," *Journal of American Medical Technology* 41 (1979): 293.
57. Watson, *Nutrition and AIDS.*
58. Ibid.

9

Steroids, Sterols, and Aloe Vera

The Nature of Rheumatoid Arthritis

Inflammation means that the body is protecting itself from damage by activating the immune system. This system fights foreign material that the body considers not part of itself. Body cells may be changed by a viral reaction so that they appear foreign to the immune system. This autoimmune response is the developing of an immunity to specific parts of the body such as joints, causing an inflammation called arthritis. Antibodies form in the blood and attack the joint tissue that appears foreign. In the normal joint, cartilage covers the bone ends, which are enclosed by a synovial membrane lubricated with fluid. The synovial lining contains cells that make hyaluronic acid, which it secretes into the synovial fluid. In rheumatoid arthritis, the synovial lining thickens and inflammatory cells as well as protein enter synovial fluid from plasma.[1] This leads to destruction of joint cartilage and bone erosion, which impairs joint function. This is an overgrowing of tissue, which becomes vascularized. The synovial fluid of an inflamed joint swarms with neutrophils and contains products of activated phagocytic cells.[2]

Most of the evidence supports the concept of increased oxygen radicals in synovial fluid of rheumatoid patients.[3] Ascorbic acid levels are below normal, suggesting that oxygen radicals oxidize the ascorbate present. Oxidant damage occurs in inflamed rheumatoid joints. The oxidants are placed in synovial fluid by activated neutrophils.[4] Other agents damage the joint, such as proteolytic enzymes as well as mediators of inflammation released by phagocytes.[5] All these things can cause cartilage destruction. The treatment of arthritis challenges the physician. Some 37 million Americans suffer from some form of inflammatory disease for which no cure exists. An estimated

13 million sufferers take non-steroid anti-inflammatory drugs to relieve the pain and inflammation that accompany arthritis, but many products have harmful side effects.[6] Specific drug levels must be present in the blood to exert a beneficial effect. These drugs only treat the pain and inflammation. No one drug can reverse the progress of arthritis.

The Adjuvant Arthritis Model

Adjuvant arthritis in rats is an animal model that closely resembles human rheumatoid arthritis.[7] Adjuvant arthritis is produced by the injection of heat-killed *Mycobacterium butyricum* in light mineral oil. The mycobacterial antigens are recognized as foreign by the host's immunological system, which starts a stereotyped series of responses.[8] There is a breakdown of connective tissue in the area of the injection. The denatured collagen, then, itself acts as an antigen stimulating the production of autoantibodies. These immunoglobulins then circulate throughout the body, attacking normal collagen.[9] The similarity between human rheumatoid arthritis and adjuvant arthritis makes the latter a valuable research tool. The animal model presents a specific sequence of events. Following injection of the bacteria in mineral oil into the hind paw, an immediate inflammatory response is seen. Within seven to fourteen days, edema develops throughout the body in the other paws, the ears, and the penis, demonstrating the immunological phase.[10] By differentiating between immediate and delayed effects of therapeutic agents tested, anti-inflammatory and immunosuppressive activities can be assigned to them. To be considered anti-inflammatory, the drug must inhibit edema in the injected paw. Agents are considered immunosuppressive if they repress the appearance of the disease in the non-injected paws, with little or no effect on the injected extremity. An agent may possess both anti-inflammatory and immunosuppressive activity.[11]

Effect of Ribonucleic Acid (RNA), Ascorbic Acid, and Aloe Vera on Inhibiting Adjuvant Arthritis

A comparison of ascorbic acid, thymus extract, RNA, and aloe extract administered daily at 150 mg/kg subcutaneously for thirteen days over a twenty-one-day period revealed that aloe (water) extract from a fresh aloe leaf had the best anti-inflammatory (48 percent) and the best anti-arthritic response (72 percent) (table 9.1). This was the first study that was performed in my laboratory with aloe.[12] I was very excited to find that aloe vera had good biological activity. Adjuvant arthritis was inhibited 62 percent by RNA and 29 percent by ascorbic acid. The thymus extract immune inhibition was also good at 67 percent. This response was recorded before the isolation of thymus hormone.

We obtained an RNA salt (type IIS) and an RNA acid (type VI) from Torula Yeast (#6500, Sigma Chemical Corp, St. Louis). Rats were given 150 mg/kg/day × 13 subcutaneously of each RNA, and the hind paw edema of adjuvant arthritic rats was measured on days 7, 14, and 21. On day 21, the anti-arthritic and the anti-inflammatory effects for the RNA salt were both 100 percent. However, both responses obtained with the RNA acid were less than 20 percent (figure 9.1). This represents a clear-cut difference in the effectiveness of the salt and the acid.[13] RNA is used by the cell to send messages from the nucleus to the cytoplasm to control the making of protein antibodies. Possibly the RNA is defective in autoimmune diseases. This is why we focused on RNA against adjuvant arthritis. RNA is known to combine with antigenic fragments invading an animal's immune system. If antigens are complexed with RNA prior to entering the body, there is an enhanced reaction, with a heightened and prolonged response. We feel that the injected RNA may prevent the host's immune system from recognizing the antigen as foreign. Possibly the host may recognize the antigen but is unable to respond to it. The administered RNA may alter the immune cascade after the foreign body identification has occurred. The injected RNA may affect the transfer RNA, the messenger RNA, or the structural ribosomal RNA.

Rheumatoid arthritic patients exhibit a reduced plasma level and a white blood cell concentration of ascorbic acid. Spongy gums and tooth decay are consistent with the vitamin C deficiency of scurvy. Low vitamin C levels may be found in other forms of arthritis.[14] In addition, aspirin, often used as an analgesic and an anti-inflammatory agent, increases the excretion of vitamin C into the urine and inhibits the vitamin C uptake by leukocytes and tissues. In the patient with rheumatoid arthritis, there seems to be an increased demand for vitamin C. This increased demand and a subsequent vitamin C depletion

PREVENTION OF ADJUVANT ARTHRITIS BY ADMINISTERING DAILY 150 MG/KG SUBCUTANEOUSLY FOR 13 DAYS ASCORBIC ACID, THYMIC EXTRACT, ALOE EXTRACT AND DNA OVER A 21 DAY PERIOD.

	EDEMA OF HIND PAWS	
	INFLAMED	IMMUNE
ADJUVANT	23.2	14.7
ASCORBIC ACID	23.0 (0.9)	10.4 (29)
THYMUS EXTRACT	19.4 (16)	4.8 (67)
ALOE EXTRACT	12.1 (48)	4.1 (72)
RNA	15.9 (32)	5.6 (62)

12 RATS/GROUP ± = S.E. ( ) = % INHIBITION

Table 9.1.

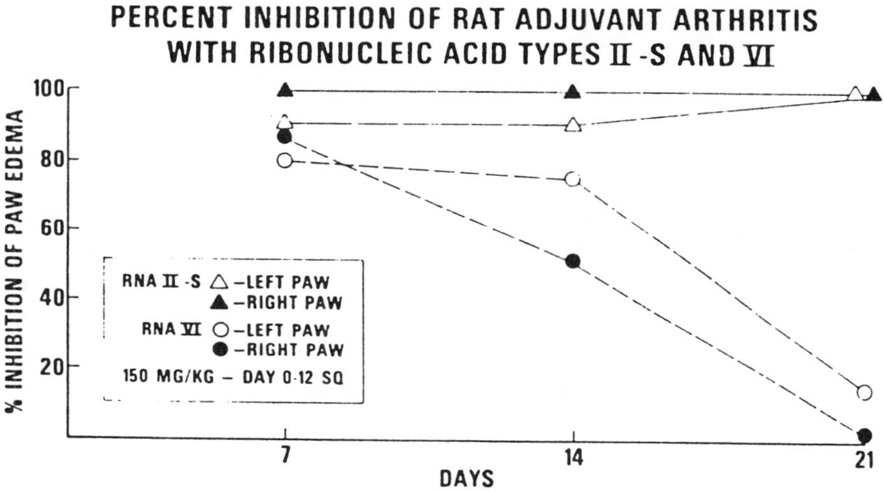
PERCENT INHIBITION OF RAT ADJUVANT ARTHRITIS
WITH RIBONUCLEIC ACID TYPES II -S AND VI
% INHIBITION OF PAW EDEMA
100
80
60
40
20
RNA II -S △ –LEFT PAW
▲ –RIGHT PAW
RNA VI ○ –LEFT PAW
● –RIGHT PAW
150 MG/KG – DAY 0-12 SQ
7
14
21
DAYS

Fig. 9.1.

may be related to the increased number of activated neutrophils producing oxygen radicals at the site of inflammation, which oxidize ascorbate.[15]

Ascorbic acid functions in the conversion of proline to hydroxyproline, a major role in collagen synthesis.[16] Vitamin C also enhances collagen synthesis by promoting the aggregation of ribosomes in the endoplasmic reticulum.[17] This must be related to protein synthesis. The decrease in blood and tissue ascorbic acid would reduce collagen repair and perhaps allow increased collagen destruction. In addition to its role in collagen synthesis, ascorbic acid stimulates the production of corticosteroids. This increased production of glucocorticoids, which are immunosuppressive, could decrease the formation of antigen antibody complexes and the development of autoantibodies. It has been shown that ascorbic acid has mainly an immunosuppressive action, as opposed to an anti-inflammatory activity, in the adjuvant arthritic rat.[18] There is also a decrease of osteogenic changes in the adjuvant arthritic rat following administration of ascorbic acid.[19] As already stated, inflammation is not the only symptom found in the arthritic rat. The adjuvant arthritic rat appears to suffer pain resembling that of humans with rheumatoid arthritis. This was established in part by the observation that in the arthritic rat there is a depression and disruption of normal neural functions. These responses appear to be similar to those found in humans during episodes of chronic pain. The pain seems to be most severe approximately 2 to 3 weeks after the inoculation.[20]

Polymorphonuclear leukocyte infiltration also can be used to help establish the anti-arthritic response of vitamin C. A standard measure for anti-inflammatory agents is the inhibition of polymorphonuclear leukocytes at the site of inflammation.[21] It has been shown that substances such as anthranilic acid, a natural nonsteroidal immunosuppressive agent, decrease the number of lymphocytes and polymorphonulcear leukocytes in the adjuvant arthritic rat.[22]

Administration of *Mycobacterium butyricum* in heavy oil produces a severe localized adjuvant arthritis in which the paw was increased twelvefold over three weeks by autoantibodies. Daily subcutaneous vitamin C at 150 mg/kg/day decreased the edema from 8.1 $\pm$ 2.5 units of edema to 1.6 $\pm$ 1.5 units of edema in arthritic animals. This response represents an 80.3 percent decrease in edema (table 9.2). In rheumatoid arthritis, the synovial lining thickens, permeability of blood vessels increases, and polymorphonuclear leukocytes flood into the inflamed area. Phagocytes in the inflamed joint produce damage to the joint.[23] Ascorbate levels in blood and synovial fluid are below normal in the rheumatoid arthritic patient.[24] Vitamin C may produce beneficial effects, such as the decrease in swelling of the arthritic paw by the antioxidant scavenging, or "mopping up," of reactive oxygen radicals.[25] It is possible that vitamin C works against mediators produced by oxygen radicals, such as prostaglandins, proteolytic enzymes, or leukotrienes.[26] In any event, inhibiting the production of oxygen radicals would be beneficial to the arthritic patient.

The level of analgesia increased from 7.5 $\pm$ 0.7 g to 10.8 $\pm$ 1.5 g in adjuvant arthritic rats ($p = 0.05$) by daily subcutaneous administration of 150 mg/kg of vitamin C (table 9.3). Pain results from the immune reaction that causes tissue damage. Bradykinin and histamine stimulate nerve endings that influence the immune paw. Muscle spasm and the production of lactic acid also may be contributing pain factors. Severe pain was present in adjuvant arthritic rats over the three weeks of the study.[27] Vitamin C produced analgesia in these animals, even in the presence of severe pain.

Since Vitamin C did not reduce the temperature of the paw, it might be assumed that blood flow was not reduced toward normal. Surface skin temperature did not correlate with the beneficial response observed for pain and swelling in the arthritic rat that was given vitamin C.

Infiltration of polymorphonuclear leukocytes into an inflamed area is an important cellular response to injury. Polymorphonuclear leukocytes were significantly reduced in the adjuvant arthritic paw (60 percent) by the administration of vitamin C. The number of polymorphonulcear leukocytes per high power field was reduced from 3.0 $\pm$ 0.4 in arthritic controls to 1.8 $\pm$ 0.2 in vitamin c–treated arthritic rats ($p < 0.02$). These data suggest that vitamin C inhibits the production of oxygen radicals from polymorphonulcear leukocytes. However, future studies must be done to determine if a significant correlation exists between the production of oxygen radicals, polymorphonuclear leukocyte infiltration, and the dose-response relationship with ascorbic acid. The decrease of swelling, pain, and

ANTI-INFLAMMATORY EFFECT OF VITAMIN C ON LOCALIZED ADJUVANT ARTHRITIS

	EDEMA VOLUME (UNITS)
CONTROL	−0.6 ±0.2
ADJUVANT ARTHRITIS	8.1 ±2.5
+VITAMIN C 150MG/KG	1.6 (−80.3%) ±1.5

12 ANIMALS/GROUP. $P<0.05$

Table 9.2.

VITAMIN C INFLUENCE
ON LOCALIZED ADJUVANT ARTHRITIS

	TEMP. (°C)	ANALG. (GM.)	PMN (NO./HPF)
CONTROL	30.0 ± 0.6	11.6 ± 1.1	1.4 ± 0.3
ADJUVANT ARTHRITIS	34.1 ± 0.3	7.5 ± 0.7	3.0 ± 0.4
+ VITAMIN C 150MG/KG	34.7 ± 0.2	10.8* ± 1.5	1.8** ± 0.2
% CHANGE	0.0	+ 44.0	− 60.0

12 ANIMALS/GROUP. *P = 0.05 **P < 0.02

Table 9.3.

inflammation achieved by vitamin C in the adjuvant arthritic rat model could be promising in the treatment of rheumatoid arthritis.

RNA and ascorbic acid are present in aloe vera. We attempted to combine ascorbic acid, RNA salt, and aloe vera at a 5 percent concentration in hydrophilic cream as a topical treatment to regress adjuvant arthritis (table 9.4). Regression of adjuvant arthritis by topically administering daily 5 percent aloe, RNA, and ascorbic acid together in a hydrophilic cream for thirteen days (days 21–33) over a thirty-eight-day period should provide a good topical preparation.[28] This topical treatment to regress adjuvant arthritis came out of the fact that all three preparations had good anti-arthritic activity and that aloe vera was also a good biological vehicle. Aloe has been used to treat skin conditions in many ancient civilizations, and it has anti-inflammatory and anti-arthritic activity. Ribonucleic acid was effective in both prevention and regression of adjuvant arthritis.[29] The immunosuppressive action by RNA was very evident in adjuvant arthritis. Similar observations were demonstrated with ascorbic acid.[30] It seemed reasonable to us to combine all three substances in a cream and apply the preparation topically to regress adjuvant arthritis. The results were as follows: 5 percent aloe + RNA + ascorbic acid regressed adjuvant arthritis 45 percent, and the inflamed paw was inhibited 39 percent. It should be noted that the magnitude of this response is slightly less than the "steroid effect." This type of nonsteroidal topical preparation would be very useful for the physician treating arthritic patients. We feel this entire series of studies represents a major discovery in treating inflammation and arthritis. Our topical treatment should eliminate a great deal of suffering and misery.

Amino Acid and Steroids

All the known amino acids, as well as three sterols and possibly a steroid or so, are present in aloe vera. My laboratory has shown that dietary amino acid supplementation improves survival and liver glycogen deposition in cortisone-treated adrenalectmized rats.[31] The possibility that certain amino acids also exhibit anti-phlogistic effects was suggested. Epsilon-amino caproic acid is a proven anti-inflammatory agent, and the administration of phenylalanine and tryptophane reduces the infiltration of white blood cells and PMNs into an

REGRESSION OF ADJUVANT ARTHRITIS BY ADMINISTERING DAILY 5% ALOE, RNA AND ASCORBIC ACID TOGETHER IN HYDROPHILIC CREAM FOR 13 DAYS TOPICALLY (DAY 21-33) OVER A 38 DAY PERIOD.

	EDEMA OF HIND PAWS	
	INFLAMED	IMMUNE
OIL	4.4	4.9
ADJUVANT	10.2	6.7
CREAM ALONE	3.1	5.6
5% ALOE + RNA + ASCORBIC ACID IN CREAM	6.3 (39)	3.7 (45)

12 RATS/GROUP   ± = S.E.   ( ) = % INHIBITION

Table 9.4.

area of local inflammation. In studies on mustard-induced foot edema in rats, we have detected some anti-inflammatory activity in seven of seventeen amino acids screened.[32]

Since glucocorticoids draw on carcass protein for amino acids and excrete them in a definite pattern in the urine, it is not surprising to find amino acids such as tryptophane, phenylalanine, and isoleucine, which influence the action of cortisone. The combination of lysine, tyrosine, and histidine supplemented into dietary gelatin increase the survival of cortisone-treated rats. Vitamin B_{12} also had a life maintenance value in adrenalectomized animals.[33]

Inflammation can best be described as a necessary series of cellular and immune responses to tissue insult caused by trauma, bacterial invasion, or immune problems. While necessary for wound healing, if uncontrolled, inflammation can lead to serious conditions. Inflammation arising from irritants, surgery, and arthritis can be treated with steroids. Corticosteroids decrease edema by reducing capillary permeability and vasodilation as well as by stabilizing lysosomal membranes. Steroids can increase the spread of infection by inhibiting connective tissue formation. Steroid effectiveness depends on dosage, hormone distribution, absorption rate, and the influence on white blood cells. Glucocorticoids have a poor rate of absorption through the skin. Aloe vera not only aids the absorption of hydrocortisone but also contributes to the biological activity such that we call aloe vera a "biological vehicle." This vehicle effect should enable the physician to lower the steroid dose to reduce the risk of side effects. Possible side effects of glucocorticoids that can possibly be reduced by aloe vera include: adrenal suppression; Cushing's syndrome with localized stria on the abdomen; moon face; dermatitis; acne cysts; and psoriasis. Repeated daily application of steroid does not increase skin absorption but does reduce the clinical effect.

The aloe vera gel consistently inhibits infection and promotes healthy tissue growth.[34] Decolorized aloe vera reduces edema and inflammation in normal rats, and in the diabetic model it was effective in healing wounds, edema, and pain.[35] Our laboratory demonstrated topical and systemic activity of aloe vera in the prevention and inhibition of adjuvant-induced arthritis.[36] Aloe vera blocked irritants such as gelatin, kaolin, carrageenan, mustard, and croton oil.[37] We showed that aloe vera inhibited inflammation but also improved wound healing.[38] Since steroids inhibit wound healing, aloe vera's positive influence on wounds and circulation makes it a natural as a vehicle for corticosteroids.

The quantification of PMN infiltration into a site of tissue damage is a valuable tool for evaluating the acute anti-inflammatory activity of many compounds, including steroids and aloe vera.[39] PMN infiltration is closely linked to the theory of oxygen radical formation in inflammation.[40] The oxygen radical theory provides insight into the mechanisms of inflammation and can be used to understand the activity of aloe vera, which may act as an oxygen radical scavenger. When an injury occurs, vasoactive substances cause an increase in vascular permeability. Edema, pain, and swelling are then observed. PMNs increase their metabolism and cause a production of oxygen radicals.[41] We feel that aloe vera acts as a scavenger and "mops up" the oxygen radicals so that they prevent tissue damage with the production of inflammatory mediators (figure 9.2).[42]

Two weighed cotton pellets were placed under the skin for twelve days (figure 9.3). The granuloma tissue weight was then determined. When 25 mg/kg of L-tryptophane was subcutaneously administered daily for twelve days, the granuloma tissue was inhibited 15.8 percent, as compared to 10.8 percent inhibition for cortisone acetate administered daily for twelve days at 1.0 mg/kg (table 9.5). The combination of each was not additive on granuloma tissue weight. However, the same 25 mg/kg dose of phenylalanine inhibited granuloma tissue weight 29.8 percent (table 9.6). A 1.0 mg/kg dose of cortisone acetate inhibited granuloma tissue 5.9 percent. The combined treatment of 1.0 mg/kg cortisone acetate and 25 mg/kg phenylalanine produced a synergism effect on granuloma tissue (41.7 percent inhibition). A dose-response relationship was recorded with cortisone acetate. Administration of aloe vera subcutaneously up to 400 mg/kg $\times$ 12 had no effect on granuloma weight (table 9.7). In fact, our wound-healing studies indicate that aloe stimulates fibroblasts to produce collagen and proteoglycans. However, there is no evidence that aloe vera produces a chronic inflammatory response. One wonders if aloe vera would help hydrocortisone with its chronic anti-inflammatory activity.

A topical standardization of hydrocortisone acetate was obtained in a mustard-induced paw edema in normal rats (table 9.8). Edema was induced by a 2 percent mustard (Colman's mustard) injection into the plantar surface of the rat's left hind paw. At this time,

OXYGEN RADICALS IN INFLAMMATION

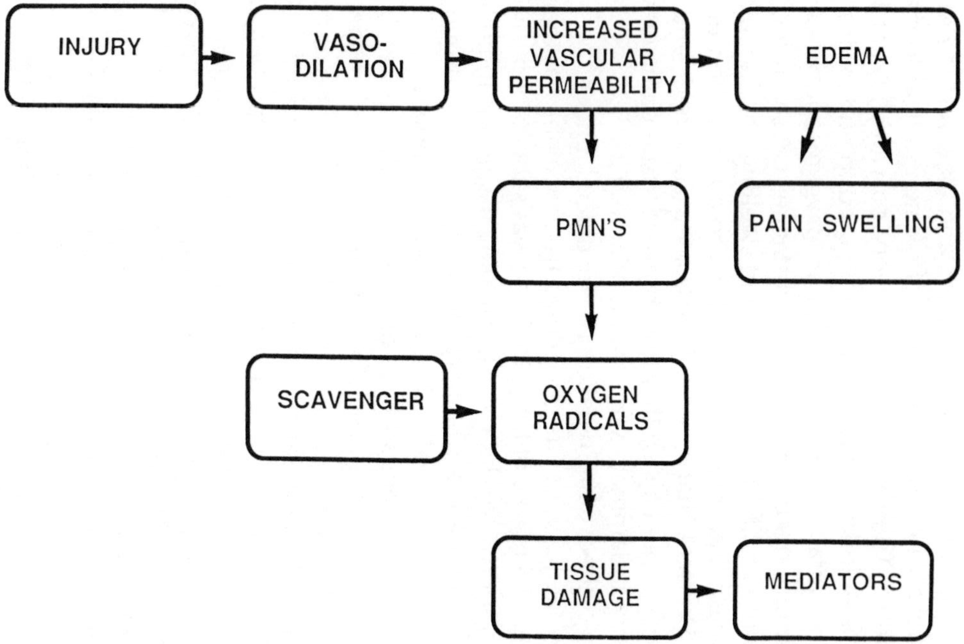

Fig. 9.2.

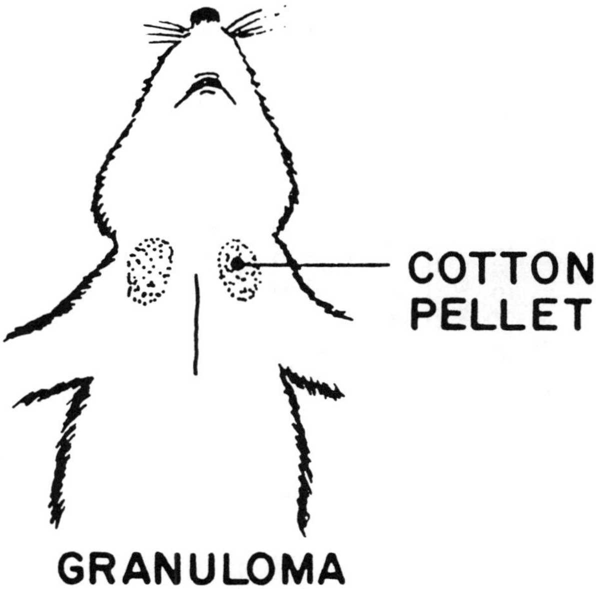

Fig. 9.3.

INFLUENCE OF L–TRYPTOPHANE ON GRANULOMA WEIGHT IN ADRENALECTOMIZED RATS

TREATMENT	DOSE mg/kg	GRANULOMA WEIGHT mg	INHIBITION %
CONTROL	–	66.9 ± 6.0	–
CORTISONE ACETATE	1	59.7 ± 3.5	10.8
L-TRYPTOPHANE	25	56.3 ± 8.7	15.8
COMBINATION	1+25	63.6 ± 5.2	4.9

± STANDARD ERROR 7–9 RATS PER GROUP

Table 9.5.

INFLUENCE OF L-PHENYLALANINE ON GRANULOMA WEIGHT IN ADRENALECTOMIZED RATS

TREATMENT	DOSE mg/kg	GRANULOMA WEIGHT mg	INHIBITION %
CONTROL	—	94.5 ± 12.9	—
CORTISONE ACETATE	1	88.9 ± 13.0	5.9
CORTISONE ACETATE	5	60.4 ± 6.2	36.1
L-PHENYLALANINE	25	66.3 ± 5.1	29.8
COMBINATION	1 + 25	55.1 ± 4.7	41.7

± STANDARD ERROR   7—9 RATS PER GROUP

Table 9.6.

ANTIFIBROSIS EFFECT OF COLORIZED ALOE VERA IN ADULT RATS*

TREATMENT MG/KG X12	NO OF RATS	B.WT. CHANGE ± GM	COTTON PELLET** WT. DIFFERENCE MG
CONTROL	12	±31±2	1413±123
50	12	±12±5	1444±125
200	12	±15±3	1344±55
400	12	±17±5	1499±93

*400 – 500 GMS B.W.T. ; **CONNECTIVE TISSUE WEIGHT

Table 9.7.

LOCAL MUSTARD EDEMA
STANDARDIZATION OF HYDROCORTISONE ACETATE IN PETROLATUM IN NORMAL MALE RATS

HYDROCORTISONE ACETATE mg %	MEAN EDEMA ml.	INHIBITION %
2 % MUSTARD (PETROLATUM)	0.73	—
+1	0.65	11.0
+5	0.58	20.5
+50	0.48	34.2

3 RATS PER GROUP

Table 9.8.

each rat received topical 1, 5, or 50 mg percent hydrocortisone acetate in petrolatum. The paw volumes were recorded using a mercury plethysmograph. Readings were taken immediately after the mustard injection and again six hours later. The difference between the initial measurement and the six-hour measurement was recorded as the induced edema. The percentage of inhibition of 2 percent mustard–induced edema obtained by topical 1, 5, and 50 mg percent hydrocortisone acetate in petrolatum was 11.0, 20.5, and 34.2 percent, respectively. This is a good dose-response curve for hydrocortisone acetate applied topically. The combination of L-phenylalanine (100 mg percent) and hydrocortisone acetate (10 mg percent) topically applied produced a synergistic inhibition against 2 percent mustard–induced edema. The percentage of inhibition recorded for hydrocortisone acetate was 0.5 percent. L-phenylalanine inhibited the 2 percent mustard edema 30.0 percent. The combination of hydrocortisone acetate and L-phenylalanine synergistically inhibited edema 58.2 percent (table 9.9).

Aloe Vera, Hydrocortisone, and Sterol Influence on Wound Tensile Strength and Anti-Inflammation

Aloe vera may be the most powerful, non-toxic, plant-derived treatment of both inflammation and wound healing.[43] Presently, hydrocortisone is a most effective treatment for inflammation.[44] For this reason, physicians often use hydrocortisone clinically. However, while inhibiting inflammation, hydrocortisone blocks wound healing.[45] Therefore, treatments using hydrocortisone to treat inflammation present physicians with a conflicting dilemma. When treating wounds, it becomes necessary to counteract the anti-wound-healing properties of hydrocortisone. What means of treatment are physicians to use when both anti-inflammatory and increased wound-healing effects are desired?

Aloe vera is one of the few substances known to effectively decrease inflammation and promote wound healing.[46] We proved that aloe and hydrocortisone work in an additive and dose-related manner to decrease inflammation. One objective of this work focuses on whether aloe, given with hydrocortisone, would mask or negate hydrocortisone's anti-wound-healing properties. This response would be a major contribution to medical care.

LOCAL ANTI-EDEMA EFFECT OF L-PHENYLALANINE IN PETROLATUM IN NORMAL RATS

TREATMENT	DOSE mg %	MEAN EDEMA ml.	INHIBITION %
2 % MUSTARD CONTROL	–	0.613	–
+ HYDROCORTISONE ACETATE	10	0.610	0.5
+ L-PHENYLALANINE	100	0.430	30.0
+ COMBINATION	10 + 100	0.260	58.2

3 RATS PER GROUP

Table 9.9.

A thorough review of the literature revealed a number of sterol properties. Sterols tend to reduce membrane permeability by increasing membrane viscosity.[47] Y. Shidoji, M. Wantanabae, T. Oku, et al,[48] found that sterols decrease the intestinal absorption of cholesterol. Additionally, certain sterols have been used in the effective treatment of diseases, such as renal osteodystrophy and pathological conditions resulting from calcium malabsorption, such as secondary hyperparathyroidism.[49] Sterols also block cholesterol synthesis within subcutaneous cells by inhibiting HMG-CoA reductase.[50]

Case studies document that whole-plant aloe vera is effective in promoting wound healing. In 1935, C. E. and C. Collins were the first to report that aloe vera had effectively healed a woman's X-ray-induced dermatitis.[51] Aloe also successfully treats burns and irradiation-induced ulcers.[52] Davis et al reported that three aloe containing wound healing promoting agents (growth factors) were evaluated: gibberellin, auxins, and mannose-6-phosphate.[53]

An objective of this study was to determine whether the sterols in aloe contain wound healing properties similar to growth factors. By actively inhibiting cholesterol synthesis, a necessary process required in cell growth and proliferation, sterols may decrease wound healing.[54] Additional literature on sterol wound healing capabilities is lacking. Therefore, sterol activity in aloe as a wound repair promoting agent needs to be evaluated.

As previously mentioned, R. H. Davis, M. G. Leitner, J. Russo, et al., documented that aloe effectively reduces inflammation.[55] The laboratory results have proven that anti-inflammatory activity exists within several individual constituents of aloe vera. It is our goal to determine the specific contributions of aloe's sterols (lupeol, campesterol, and β-sitosterol) on the plant's anti-inflammatory activity as well as to determine their contribution to wound healing.

Pertinent literature reveals that sterols inhibit inflammation. Srivastava, Varma, Tandon, et al., isolated a hexane fraction containing β-sitosterol from the plant *Pluchea lanceolate.* They determined that this fraction was able to reduce edema by as much as 47.9%.[56] From their work, it is clear that sterols are powerful anti-inflammatory agents. Three known sterols present in aloe vera (lupeol, campesterol, and β-sitosterol) were evaluated, and the anti-inflammatory activity of each were measured. Sterol components of aloe are expected to provide anti-inflammatory activity.

The purpose of this study is fourfold. First, the wound-healing effects of hydrocortisone alone were quantitatively determined as compared with hydrocortisone with aloe to determine if aloe vera would block the wound-healing suppression of hydrocortisone. Next, lupeol's effects on wound healing were tested. In the third part of the study, the anti-inflammatory properties of three sterols found in aloe vera (lupeol, campesterol, and β-sitosterol) were quantified. The fourth part revealed whether lupeol inhibited inflammation in a dose-response manner.

Wound-Healing Tensile Strength Assay

Two separate wound tensile strength experiments were performed. Adult HSD-ICR male mice (30 g) were used. On the first day, each mouse was given a one-inch surgical wound on its shaven back. Each wound on the mice was then closed by 9 mm surgical staples placed at half-inch increments, for a total of three staples per wound. In the first experiment, nine groups (seven mice per group) were given subcutaneous injections of hydrocortisone acetate daily over four days at 0.01, 0.1, and 1.0 mg/kg, respectively. Aloe vera was also given with each dose of hydrocortisone acetate at 100 and 300 mg/kg in an attempt to block the steroid's wound-healing inhibition property. Animals receiving only hydrocortisone acetate were steroid controls. One group of seven mice received only water (10 ml/kg basis) and was considered the aqueous control. All combination treatment values were compared with the wound tensile strength values recorded for the corresponding steroid controls.

In the second experiment, four groups (ten mice per group) were used. An aqueous control group was injected on a 10 ml/kg basis. Three treatment groups were injected with different dosages of lupeol: 330 μg/Kg, 100 μg/Kg, and 33 μg/Kg.

All groups were injected daily for a four-day period. On the fourth day, six hours after the final injection of solutions, the wound tensile strength was evaluated by injecting air from a 60 cc syringe into the abdominal cavity until the wounds on the back burst. The syringe was calibrated in millimeters to obtain more precise measurements. The amount of air injected into the abdominal cavity was recorded.

Croton Oil–Induced Ear Swelling Assay

In two experiments, groups (ten mice per group) of adult male HSD-ICR mice were given 10 μl croton oil (2.5 mg/ml) topically to the inner right ear. The left ear was not treated with the croton oil irritant and served as the control.

In the first experiment, three groups were each treated with 10 μl of one of the following sterols: lupeol, β-sitosterol, and campesterol, in 10 μg/μl concentrations. In the second experiment, specific lupeol dosages of 10.0 μg/μl, 3.3 μg/μl, 1.0 μg/μl, and 0.1 μg/μl were applied to four groups of mice and then compared with the croton oil control mice to determine a dose-response curve. For all of the mice, the sterols were applied topically to the croton oil–treated ear half an hour later. In each experiment, one group of animals received only croton oil treatment and, therefore, served as the croton oil control group.

Six hours after treatment, a 6 mm biopsy punch specimen was taken from both the right and left ear of each mouse. These specimens were weighed on the pan balance and the weight difference between the two was compared to determine the amount of inflammation remaining in the right ear. The student's t-test was performed to determine if there was a significant difference between each treated group and the control group.[57]

Results and Discussion

Wound-Healing Activity

Previous experiments by R. H. Davis, W. L. Parker, and D. P. Murdoch proved that aloe vera effectively increases hydrocortisone's anti-inflammatory properties in an additive and dose-response manner.[58] Our present research clearly indicates that aloe also effectively decreases hydrocortisone's anti-wound-healing properties. Researchers strive to determine the compounds within aloe that are the active wound-healing promoters and anti-inflammatory agents and the mechanisms by which these compounds work.

In our first study, aloe vera successfully blocked the inhibitory effects on wound healing of hydrocortisone (figure 9.4; table 9.10).

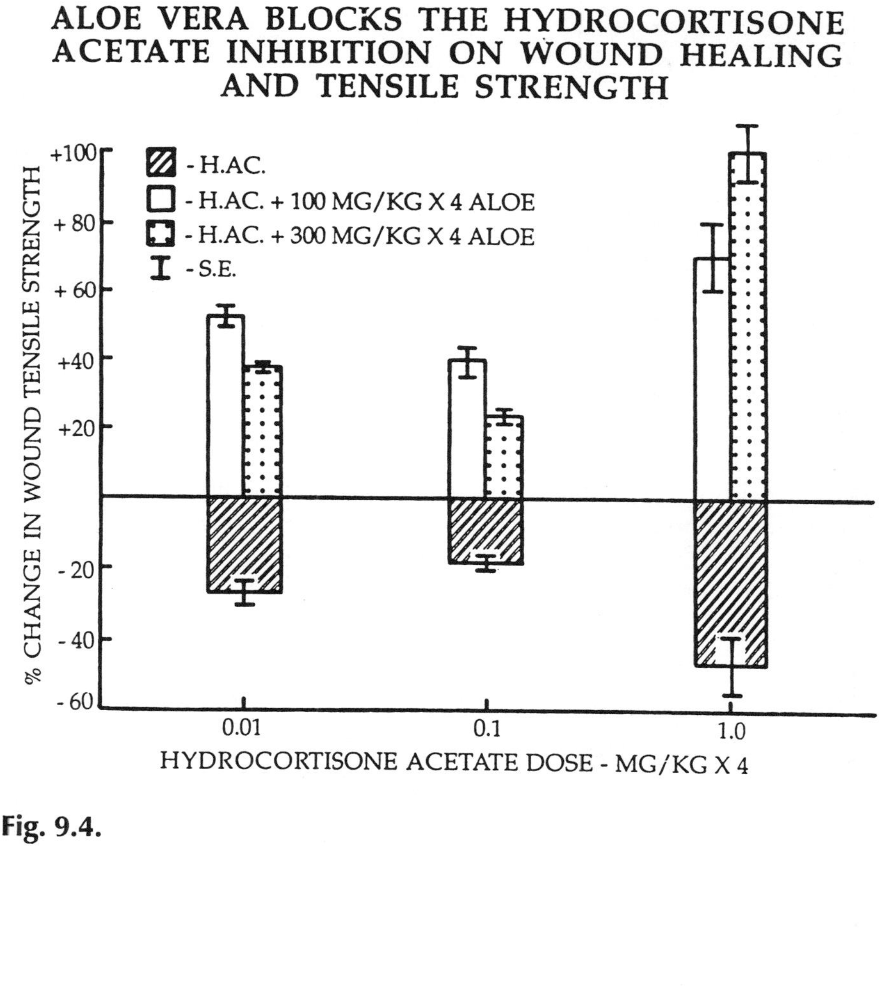
ALOE VERA BLOCKS THE HYDROCORTISONE ACETATE INHIBITION ON WOUND HEALING AND TENSILE STRENGTH
- H.AC.
- H.AC. + 100 MG/KG X 4 ALOE
- H.AC. + 300 MG/KG X 4 ALOE
- S.E.
% CHANGE IN WOUND TENSILE STRENGTH
+100
+ 80
+ 60
+40
+20
- 20
- 40
- 60
0.01
0.1
1.0
HYDROCORTISONE ACETATE DOSE - MG/KG X 4

Fig. 9.4.

ALOE VERA BLOCKS THE HYDROCORTISONE ACETATE INHIBITION ON WOUND HEALING AND TENSILE STRENGTH

TREATMENT MG/KG	% CHANGE IN WOUND TENSILE STRENGTH (- or +)
0.01 H.AC.	- 26.7 ± 2.4
+ 100 ALOE	+ 51.5 ± 3.1
+ 300 ALOE	+ 39.4 ± 1.7
0.1 H.AC.	- 17.8 ± 1.0
+ 100 ALOE	+ 40.5 ± 3.9
+ 300 ALOE	+ 24.3 ± 2.1
1.0 H.AC	- 46.7 ± 6.8
+ 100 ALOE	+ 66.7 ± 6.7
+ 300 ALOE	+ 100.0 ± 7.9

7 MICE/GROUP. ALOE BLOCKS H.AC. AT ALL DOSES - P<0.005

Table 9.10.

As predicted, hydrocortisone acetate caused a significant reduction in wound healing. Mice injected with 0.01 mg/kg hydrocortisone experienced 26.7 percent reduction in wound healing. These animals when also treated with 100 mg/kg and 300 mg/kg aloe showed 51.5 percent and 39.4 percent increase in wound healing, respectively, over the hydrocortisone group alone.

Mice given 1.0 mg/kg hydrocortisone experienced 46.7 percent reduction in wound healing. Aloe-treated mice (100 mg/kg and 300 mg/kg) showed 66.7 percent and 100.0 percent increase in wound healing, respectively, over the hydrocortisone group alone. All groups were significant at $P < 0.005$.

In each of the three hydrocortisone concentrations, aloe vera was highly effective in reversing hydrocortisone's anti-wound-healing properties. Aloe not only inhibited hydrocortisone's anti-wound-healing activity, but also increased wound tensile strength above the aqueous control. Before the mechanism of this response is revealed, the agents participating in this response must be identified.

Steroids are known to reduce wound healing.[59] Macrophages play an important role in decreasing long-term inflammation and stimulating fibroblasts to increase wound healing.[60] Macrophages promote fibroblast activity and wound repair in a number of ways. They undergo phagocytosis-induced secretion of interleukin-1 and tumor necrosis factor–stimulating fibroblast activity.[61] M. H. Ross and L. J. Romrell found that macrophages also release proteases and GAGases, which actively function to increase migration of macrophages through connective tissue to the site of the wound, improving macrophage activity and promoting wound repair.[62] Finally, R. F. Diegelmann, K. I. Cohen, and A. M. Kaplan discussed several other ways macrophages stimulate collagen deposition, fibroblast proliferation, and tissue repair.[63] Therefore, by inhibiting macrophages, hydrocortisone inhibits these processes and wound healing. Research indicates that aloe vera stimulates wound healing even when given concurrently with hydrocortisone. Steroids strongly impair the wound-healing process, and therefore aloe must contain powerful growth-promoting agents to show the effects it did. What then does aloe contain that so effectively stimulates the wound healing while also acting to reduce inflammation? The objective was to determine whether aloe's sterols (specifically lupeol) contribute to the plant's wound-healing capabilities.

In each group, lupeol inhibited the wound-healing process in a dose-response manner compared with the aqueous control group (figure 9.5). The mice injected with 33 μg/kg caused 9.3 percent less wound tensile strength. Animals treated with 100 μg/kg resulted in 17.3 percent decreased wound tensile strength, whereas the 330 μg/kg lupeol dose caused a 21.7 percent decreased wound tensile strength. The results agree with the relevant literature; lupeol does not contribute to aloe vera's cell growth and proliferative property. Lupeol was much milder than hydrocortisone, yet it had a similar response.

Macrophages possess the ability to oxygenate sterols; therefore, the effects of oxygenated sterols can be applied.[64] Oxygenated sterols fit into the anti-estrogen receptor site on non-estrogen target cells such as fibroblasts.[65] Binding of oxysterols at this site causes inhibition at the lanosterol demethylation and HMG-CoA reductase steps of cholesterol synthesis.[66]

Cholesterol is important in DNA synthesis and is a necessary ingredient in cell membranes.[67] Thus cholesterol is required for proper cell growth and proliferation.[68] Fibroblasts require both exogenous and endogenous cholesterol for activity.[69] Sterols, through inhibiting cholesterol synthesis in the fibroblast, reduce fibroblast growth.[70] This consequently results in less cholesterol at the site of the injury and less redistribution of intracellular cholesterol to the plasma membrane. Ultimately, this decreases cell proliferation and growth.[71]

Macrophages also appear to require cholesterol for maximum activity.[72] Since sterols lower the amount of endogenous cholesterol and since fibroblasts require macrophages for activity, this, too, may indirectly participate in decreasing fibroblastic activity and thus diminish wound repair.

Furthermore, while the mechanism of action is not at all understood, mevalanoic acid is required for cell growth and proliferation. Whether mevalanoic acid in itself is active or only serves as a precursor to other growth-promoting compounds in aloe vera remains unknown. Since sterols block HMG-CoA reductase, they inhibit the production of mevalanoic acid, leading to decreased cell growth and proliferation.

The research and past literature refute the idea that the plant sterols of aloe vera promote wound healing and do not, therefore,

INHIBITORY INFLUENCE OF LUPEOL ON WOUND TENSILE STRENGTH

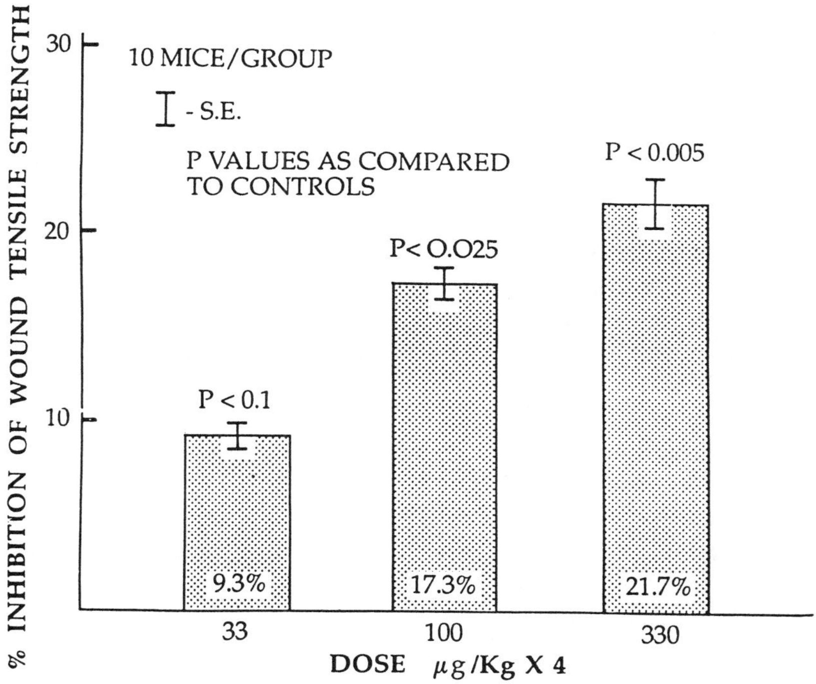

Fig. 9.5.

contribute to aloe in this respect. If aloe vera contains these growth inhibitors, why does the whole plant promote growth so significantly? Is aloe vera a growth modulator? Since sterols make up only a small percentage of the total aloe plant contents, their inhibitory effect must be masked by far more powerful growth promoters.[73] The plant contains numerous strong growth factors, including certain amino acids, gibberellin, and indole-3-acetic acid, which, our work indicates, is most responsible for aloe's wound-healing property.

One theory is that aloe may act to block steroids, thereby stimulating both leukocyte recruitment and macrophage function (figure 9.6). While this possibility is not outlandish, the possibility of aloe inhibiting the steroid would appear to result in decreased anti-inflammatory activity. Research, however, has proven otherwise. R. H. Davis, W. L. Parker, and D. P. Murdoch found that hydrocortisone and aloe together act as a more powerful anti-inflammatory therapy than either hydrocortisone or aloe alone.[74] The most plausible wound-healing explanation is that aloe vera increases wound healing by stimulating macrophages and fibroblasts directly.

I. R. Tizard, R. H. Carpenter, B. H.McAnalley, et al., determined that mannose-containing products increase macrophage activity and promote wound healing.[75] As previously explained, macrophages are essential for proper wound healing to occur. Stimulation of the macrophage will increase cell and tissue growth, fibroblast proliferation, and fibroblast activity.[76] Aloe containing mannose may also promote wound healing in this way.[77]

R. H. Davis, J. J. DiDonato, G.M. Hartman, et al., concluded that fibroblast activation using aloe vera increases collagen and proteoglycan synthesis, thereby promoting tissue repair without a loss of anti-inflammatory activity. They revealed one mechanism to lie in the ability of phosphorylated mannose within aloe (mannose-6-phosphate) to fit into the growth factor receptors on the surface of fibroblasts, initiating or enhancing their activity.[78]

Aloe vera also contains a number of other known growth promoters that probably play an important role in masking hydrocortisone's effects. Experimentally, gibberellin increases wound healing by increasing protein synthesis.[79] It binds to the 5′–dTdA–3′ section of the double-stranded DNA and consequently affects transcription.[80] The exact mechanism of how it effects transcription is unknown. Davis, et al., show that gibberellin significantly improved wound

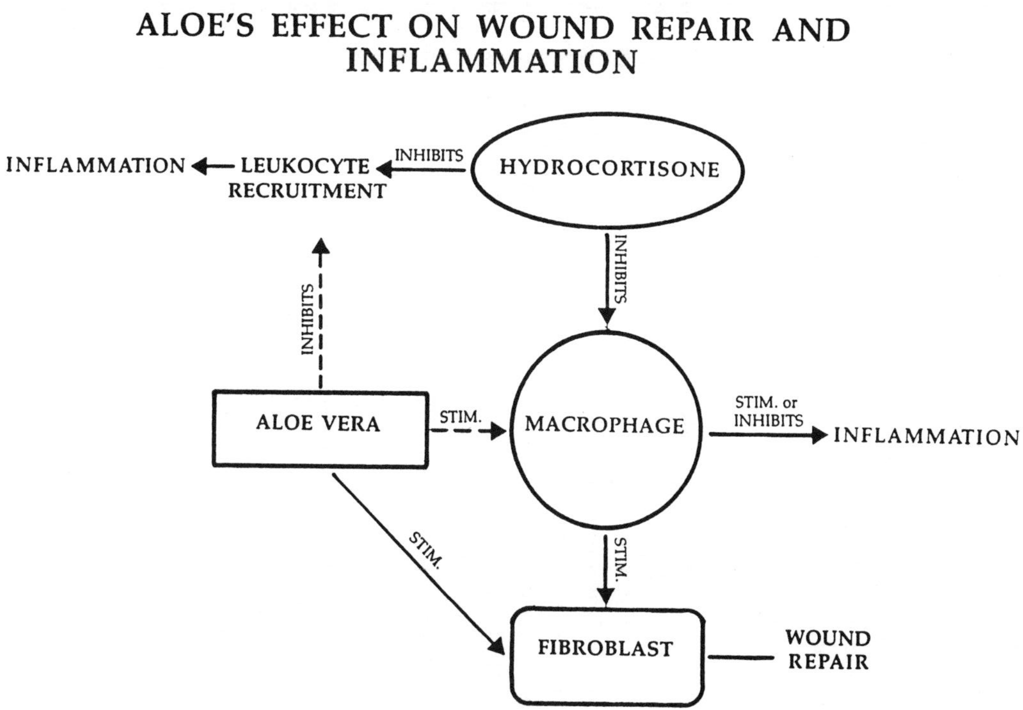
ALOE'S EFFECT ON WOUND REPAIR AND INFLAMMATION
INFLAMMATION
LEUKOCYTE RECRUITMENT
INHIBITS
HYDROCORTISONE
INHIBITS
INHIBITS
ALOE VERA
STIM.
MACROPHAGE
STIM. or INHIBITS
INFLAMMATION
STIM.
STIM.
FIBROBLAST
WOUND REPAIR

Fig. 9.6.

tensile strength more than 100 percent on experimental mice.[81] Indole-3-acetic acid, an auxin, also increases protein synthesis by increasing the uptake of amino acids. These are powerful contributors to aloe's ability to mask hydrocortisone's anti-wound-healing properties. While hydrocortisone reduces fibroblast activity through macrophage inhibition, mannose stimulates the macrophages and fibroblasts, with gibberellin and auxin working diligently to increase protein synthesis. Not barring the possibility that other untested components of aloe also promote wound healing, the overall result of these factors is a powerful increase in wound healing, even in the face of sterols and administered hydrocortisone.

Anti-Inflammatory Activity

Research shows that the sterols in aloe (lupeol, campesterol, and β-sitosterol) are significantly anti-inflammatory (figure 9.7; table 9.11). Of the three sterols, lupeol had the greatest reduction in inflammation at 37.0 percent. β-sitosterol reduced inflammation 31.1 percent, and campesterol reduced inflammation 24.2 percent.

Our final experiment involving lupeol alone revealed dose-dependent anti-inflammatory activity. The mice treated with 0.1 μg/ul lupeol had a 14.8 percent reduction in inflammation. Animals treated with 1.0 μg/ul lupeol showed a 16.9 percent decreased inflammation. Mice treated with 3.3 μg/ul lupeol showed a 28.2 percent reduction in inflammation. The animals treated with 10.0 μg/ul demonstrated 36.2 percent reduced inflammation (figure 9.8). The dose-response curve of lupeol shown in figure 9.8 is similar to the dose-response curve of aloe vera.[82] This implies that the sterols are definitely responsible for a portion of aloe's anti-inflammatory activity.

Hydrocortisone is a well-known anti-inflammatory drug. It acts by suppressing leukocyte recruitment and macrophage activity in the wound area.[83] Leukocytes and macrophages together orchestrate the body's initial inflammatory response.[84] Hydrocortisone thereby inhibits inflammation. These results show that the sterols in aloe also inhibit inflammation.

The structures of the three sterols are shown in addition to the structure of hydrocortisone and cholesterol (figure 9.9). The five compounds are similar in structure. Two functional side groups define

TOPICAL ANTI-INFLAMMATORY ACTIVITY OF THREE STEROLS FOUND IN ALOE VERA APPLIED AT 100 μg DOSES ON CROTON OIL INDUCED EDEMA

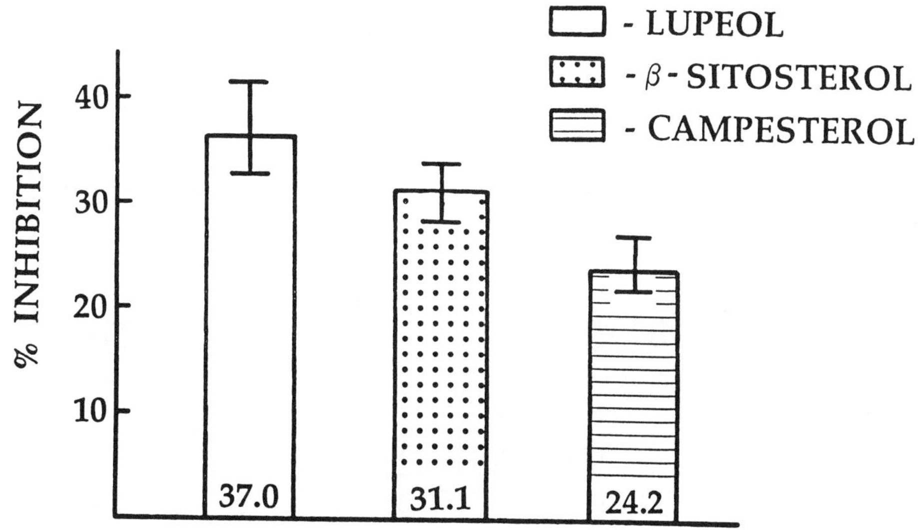

Fig. 9.7.

TOPICAL ANTI-INFLAMMATION ACTIVITY OF THREE STEROLS FOUND IN ALOE VERA APPLIED AT 100 μg DOSES ON CROTON OIL INDUCED EDEMA

STEROLS	INHIBITION
LUPEOL	$37.0 \pm 4.3^{*}$
β - SITOSTEROL	$31.1 \pm 2.9^{+}$
CAMPESTEROL	24.2 ± 1.9

10 MICE/GROUP; 25 μg /10 μl CROTON OIL
$\pm$ = S.E. $^{*}P < 0.02$; $^{+}P = 0.05$.

Table 9.11.

TOPICAL ANTI-INFLAMMATORY ACTIVITY OF LUPEOL

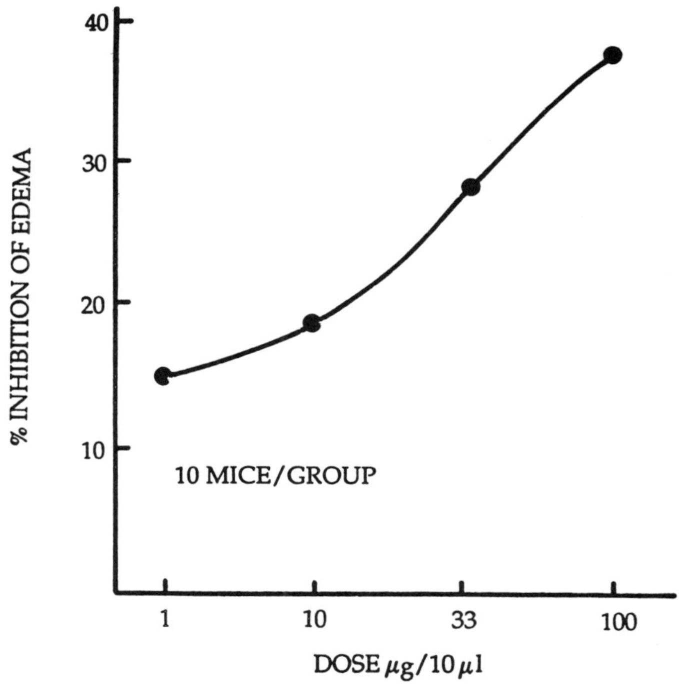

Fig. 9.8.

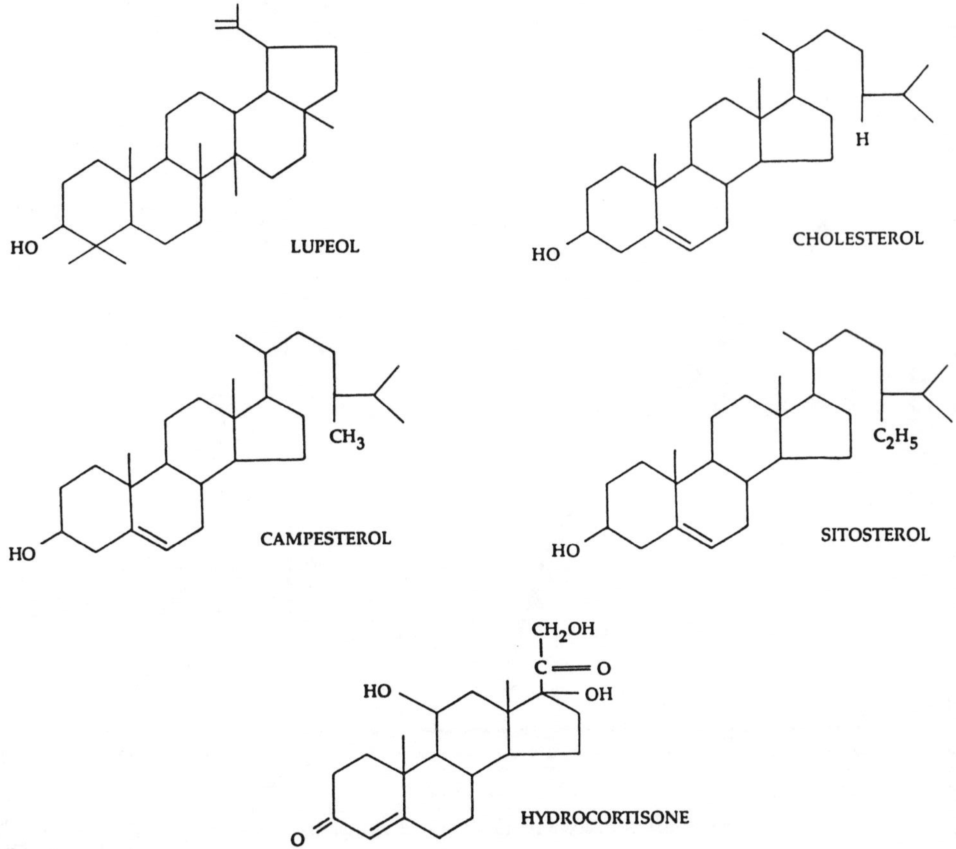
HO
LUPEOL
HO
H
CHOLESTEROL
HO
CH_3
CAMPESTEROL
HO
C_2H_5
SITOSTEROL
CH_2OH
C
O
HO
OH
O
HYDROCORTISONE

Fig. 9.9.

the activity of sterols: the C_4 methyl group and the 3β-OH group. The double bonds within the rings are not necessary for activity. Hydrocortisone and the three sterols all have the C_4 methyl group in common but do not share the 3β-OH group.[85] The sterols' similarity to hydrocortisone (the C_4 group) might be relevant in explaining their anti-inflammatory activity, while their differences (the 3β-OH group and the double bonds) may be the reason for sterols' weaker anti-inflammatory activity. Perhaps of the three sterols, lupeol is the most effective at reducing inflammation because it differs most from cholesterol and is the most similar in structure to hydrocortisone.

Another reason for this anti-inflammatory activity may also lie in sterols' ability to inhibit the cholesterol biosynthetic pathway.[86] Cholesterol stimulates lymphocyte proliferation and granulocyte formation, two factors involved in the inflammatory response.[87] Therefore, reduced cholesterol synthesis decreases inflammation by reducing lymphocyte proliferation and granulocyte formation similar to steroids' mechanism of action. Furthermore, cholesterol stimulates macrophages, which are largely responsible for appropriate lymphocyte activity.[88] Consequently, sterols may lower inflammation by reducing cholesterol availability and decreasing lymphocyte activity.

Aside from the sterols and other compounds in aloe acting to decrease inflammation, the whole-plant aloe appears to have bradykininase activity. Bradykinin causes increased vascular permeability to stimulate inflammation.[89] Bradykininase breaks down bradykinin, reducing inflammation.[90] Aloe vera possesses bradykininase activity and also decreases inflammation in this way.[91]

While it is apparent that sterols contribute to aloe vera's anti-inflammatory activity, they are not the sole active agents involved. Numerous components of aloe have been tested and determined to participate in aloe's wound-healing and anti-inflammatory activity. Continued research will prove aloe to be one of the most clinically useful and safe treatments at a physician's disposal.

Summary

The nature of rheumatoid arthritis can be mimicked by the adjuvant arthritis model. Ascorbic acid, RNA, and aloe extract were found to have good anti-inflammatory and anti-arthritic activity. In fact, the combination in cream at 5 percent concentration regressed adjuvant arthritis 45 percent, and the inflammation was inhibited 39 percent.

The combination of L-phenylalanine (100 mg percent) and hydrocortisone acetate (10 mg percent) topically applied produced a synergistic inhibition against 2 percent mustard–induced edema. Aloe-treated mice block the hydrocortisone acetate wound suppression up to 100 percent. A dose response in reducing wound tensile strength was recorded by hydrocortisone acetate over a dose range of 0.01 to 1.0 mg/kg daily over a period of four days. The aloe vera response had significant value for a physician treating inflammation where wounds were present. Sterols had good anti-inflammatory activity in a dose-related fashion. A thorough discussion of the role of sterols in aloe vera was presented.

References

1. B. Halliwell, J. R. Hoult, and D. R. Blake, "Oxidants, Inflammation and Anti-Inflammatory Drugs," *Federation of the American Society of Experimental Biology* 2 (1988): 2867.
2. B. Henderson and J. C. W. Edwards, *The Synovial Lining in Health and Disease* (London: Chapman and Hall, 1987).
3. J. T. Curnutte and B. M. Babior, "Chronic Granulomatous Disease," *Adv. Human Genetics* 16 (1987): 229.
4. J. F. Rhinehart, L. D. Greenberg, F. Baker, et al., "Metabolism of Vitamin C in Rheumatoid Arthritis," *Archives of Internal Medicine* 61 (1937): 537; P. Robert, H. Hemila, and M. Wikstrom, "Vitamin C and Inflammation," *Medical Biology* 62 (1984): 88; R. S. Panush, J. C. Delafuenti, P. Katz, et al., "Modulation of Certain Immunological Responses by Vitamin C. III Potentiation of in Vitro and in Vivo Lymphocyte Responses," *International Journal of Vitamin Nutritional Research* 23 (1982): 35.
5. Henderson and Edwards, *The Synovial Lining.*
6. J. D. Williams, D. L. Scott, F. B. DeBrito, D. A. Willoughby, and E.C. Huskisson, "Rheumatoid Inflammation and Joint Destruction: Cause and Effect or Parallel Phenomena?" *Agents and Actions* 18 (1986): 538.
7. S. L. Robbins, *Pathologic Basis of Disease* (Philadelphia: W. B. Saunders, 1974).
8. N. A. Burstein and B. H. Waksman, "The Pathogenesis of Adjuvant Disease in the Rat. I. A Histologic Study of Early Lesions in the Joint and Skin," *Yale Journal of Biology Medicine* 37 (1964): 177; E. M. Glenn, "Adjuvant Induced Arthritis: Effect of Standard Drugs on Incidence, Severity and the Underlying Chemical Alteration," *American Journal of Veterinary Research* 27 (1966): 339.
9. L. Katz and S. J. Piliero, "A Study of Adjuvant-Induced Poly-Arthritis in the Rat with Special Reference to Associated Immunological Phenomena," *Annals of the New York Academy of Science* 147 (1969): 515; G. Weissman, "Lysosomes, Autoimmune Phenomena and Diseases of Connective Tissue," *Lancet* 64 (1964): 1373.

10. C. M. Pearson, "Development of Arthritis, Periarthritis and Periostitis in Rats Given Adjuvant," *Proceedings of the Society of Experimental Biology Medicine* 91 (1956): 95.
11. R. J. Perper, B. Alvarez, C. Colombo, et al., "The Use of a Standardized Adjuvant Arthritis Assay to Differentiate Between Anti-Inflammatory and Immunosuppressive Agents," *Proceedings of the Society of Experimental Biology Medicine* 139 (1971): 506; O. Y. Patterson, "Experimental Allergic Encephalomyelitis and Autoimmune Disease," *Advances in Immunology* 5 (1966): 13.
12. R. H. Davis, E. Shapiro, and P. S. Agnew, "Topical Effect of Aloe with RNA and Vitamin C on Adjuvant Arthritis," *Journal of the American Podiatric Medical Association* 75 (1985): 229.
13. R. H. Davis, M. B. Forst, S. A. Rand, and L. Bernhard, "Prevention of Adjuvant Arthritis with Ribonucleic Acid: The Salt versus the Acid," *Journal of the American Podiatric Association* 71 (1981): 482.
14. Rhinehart, Greenberg, Baker, et al., "Metabolism of Vitamin C," 537; Robert, Hemila, and Wikstrom, "Vitamin C," 88; Panush, Delafuenti, Katz, et al., "Modulation of Certain Immunological Responses," 35.
15. Robert, Hemila, and Wikstrom, "Vitamin C," 88; Panush, Delafuenti, Katz, et al., "Modulation of Certain Immunological Responses," 35; M. Raghoeban, J. A. M. Huisman, W. B. Van Den Berg, et al., "Characteristics of the Transport of Ascorbic Acid into Leukocytes," *Life Science* 40 (1987): 449.
16. Burstern and Waksman, "The Pathogenesis of Adjuvant Disease," 177.
17. D. J. McCarty, *Arthritis and Allied Conditions,* 9th ed. (Philadelphia: Lea and Febiger, 1979); D. C. Hanley, W. A. B. Soloman, B. Saffran, et al., "The Evaluation of Natural Substances in the Treatment of Adjuvant Arthritis," *Journal of the American Podiatric Association* 72 (1982): 275.
18. Hanley, Soloman, Saffran, et al., "Evaluation of Natural Substances," 275.
19. Ibid.
20. F. C. Colpaert, "Evidence That Adjuvant Arthritis in the Rat Is Associated with Chronic Pain," *Pain* 28 (1987): 201; R. H. Adler, "Psychotropic Agents in the Management of Chronic Pain," *Journal of Human Stress* 4 (1978): 13; F. C. Colpaert, T. H. Meert, P. H. DeWitt, et al., "Further Evidence Validating Adjuvant Arthritis as an Experimental Mode of Chronic Pain in the Rat," *Life Science* 31 (1982): 67.
21. R. N. Williams and C. A. Paterson, "A Protective Role for Ascorbic Acid during Inflammatory Episodes in the Eye," *Experimental Eye Research* 42 (1986): 211.
22. J. B. Kessel, M. B. Frost, L. R. Corbin, et al., "Effect of Anthranilic Acid on Peritoneal Fluid Cellular Content of Adjuvant Arthritis," *Medical Science* 6 (1978): 209.
23. Halliwell, Hoult, and Blake, "Oxidants, Inflammation, and Anti-Inflammatory Drugs," 2867.
24. J. Lunec, and D. R. Blake, "The Determination of Dehydroascorbic Acid and Ascorbic Acid in the Serum and Synovial Fluid of Patients with Rheumatoid Arthritis," *Free Radical Research Commun* 1 (1985): 31.
25. H. B. Kaplan, H. S. Edelson, and H. M. Korchak, "Effects of Non-Steroidal Anti-Inflammatory Agents on Human Neutrophil Function in Vitro and in Vivo," *Biochemical Pharmacology* 33 (1984): 371.
26. S. J. Weiss, and J. C. W. Edwards, "Collagenolytic Metalloenzymes of the Human Neutrophil., *Biochemical Pharmacology* 35 (1986): 3189.
27. Colpaert, "Evidence," 201; Adler, "Psychotropic Agents," 13; Colpaert, Meert, DeWitte, et al., "Further Evidence," 67.

28. Davis, Shapiro, and Adnew, "Topical Effect of Aloe," 229.
29. Davis, Forst, Rand, and Bernhard, "Prevention," 482.
30. R. H. Davis, K. Y. Rosenthal, L. R. Cesario, et al., "Vitamin C Influence on Localized Adjuvant Arthritis," *Journal of the American Podiatric Medical Association* 80 (1990): 414.
31. R. H. Davis, "Protein Nutrition and Liver Glycogen in Cortisone Maintained Adrenalectomized Rats," *Federation Proceedings* 17 (1958): 33; R. H. Davis, J. S. Fisher, and L. McGowan, "Local Anti-Phlogistic Activity of L-Phenylalamine and L-Tryptophane," *Journal of Endocrinology* 41 (1968): 555.
32. R. H. Davis, J. M. Kabbani, and N. P. Maro, "Aloe Vera and Inflammation," *Pennsylvania Academy of Science* 60 (1986): 67.
33. Davis, "Protein Nutrition," 33; R.H. Davis, *Influence of Nutrition on the Growth and Survival of Cortisone Maintained Adrenalectomized Rats,* Ph.D. thesis, Rutgers University, 1958.
34. B. C. Coats, *The Silent Healer: A Modern Study of Aloe Vera* (Garland, TX: self-published, 1979).
35. Davis, Kabbani, and Maro, "Aloe Vera and Inflammation," 67; R. H. Davis, M. Leitner, and J. Russo, "Aloe Vera: A Natural Approach for Treating Wounds, Edema and Pain in Diabetes," *Journal of the American Podiatric Medical Association* 78 (1988): 60.
36. Davis, Shapiro, and Agnew, "Topical Effect," 229.
37. R. H. Davis, M. Leitner, J. Russo, et al., "Anti-Inflammatory Activity of Aloe vera Against a Spectrum of Irritants," *Journal of the American Podiatric Medical Association* (79 (1989): 263.
38. R. H. Davis, M. G. Leitner, J. M. Russo, et al., "The Biology of Aloe Vera," *Pennsylvania Academy of Science* 62 (1988): 43.
39. Davis, Kabbani, and Maro, "Aloe Vera and Inflammation," 67.
40. Halliwell, Hoult, and Blake, "Oxidants, Inflammation, and Anti-Inflammatory Drugs," 2867.
41. Ibid.
42. R. H. Davis, W. L. Parker, and D. P. Murdoch, "Aloe Vera as a Biologically Active Vehicle for Hydrocortisone Acetate," *Journal of the American Podiatric Medical Association* 81 (1991): 1.
43. R. H. Davis, W. L. Parker, R. T. Samson, et al., "The Isolation of an Active Inhibitory System from an Extract of Aloe Vera," *Journal of the American Podiatric Medical Association* 81 (1991): 258.
44. P. M. Sutton, R. J. Feldmann, and H. I. Maibach, "Vasoconstrictor Potency of Corticoids: Intradermal Infection," *Journal of Investigative Dermatology* 57 (1971): 371; D. L. Berliner, and A. G. Ruhmann, "Comparison of Growth under the Influence of 11-β-Hydroxy and 11-Keto Corticosteroids," *Endocrinology* 78 (1966): 373; H. I. Maibach and R. B. Stoughton, "Topical Corticosteroids," *Medical Clinic of North American* 57(1973): 1253.
45. Sutton, Feldman, and Maibach, "Vasoconstrictor Potency," 371; Berliner and Ruhman, "Comparison of Growth," 376; Maibach and Stoughton, "Topical Corticosteroids," 1253.
46. Davis, Leitner, Russo, et al., "Anti-Inflammatory Activity," 263; L. C. Parish, J. A. Witkoski, and L. E. Millikan, "Aloe Vera: Its Chemical and Therapeutic Properties," *International Journal of Dermatology.* 30 (1991): 679; R. H. Davis, M. G. Leitner, J. M. Russo, et al., "Wound Healing: Oral and Topical Activity of Aloe Vera," *Journal of American Podiatric Medical Association* 79 (1989): 559.

47. F. M. Michelangeli, J. M. East, and A. G. Lee, "Structural Effects on the Interaction of Sterols with the (Ca^2+ Mg^2+) ATPase," *Biochemical Biophysics Acta.* 1025 (1990): 99.
48. Y. Shidoji, M. Watanabae, T. Oku, et al., "Inhibition of β-sitosterol on Intestinal Cholesterol Absorption in Rat Using in Vivo Dual Isotope Ratio Method," *Journal of Nutritional Science Vitaminology* 26 (1980): 183.
49. Parish, Witkoski, and Millikan, "Aloe Vera," 679.
50. B. Cypriani, C. Tabacik, and B. Descomps, "Effect of Estradiol and Antiestrogens on Cholesterol Biosynthesis in Hormone Dependent and Independent Breast Cancer Cell Lines," *Biochemical Biophysics Acta.* 972 (1988): 167; A. K. Gupta, R.C. Sexton, and H. Rudney, "Effect of Vitamin D3 Derivatives in Cholesterol Synthesis and HMG-CoA Reductase Activity in Cultured Cells," *Journal of Lipid Research* 30 (1989): 379; P. A. Dawson, J. E. Metherall, N. D. Ridgway, et al., "Genetic Distinction between Sterol Mediated Transcriptional and Posttranscriptional Control of 3-Hydroxy-3-Methylglutaryl Coenzyme A Reductase," *Journal of Biological Chemistry* 266 (1991): 9128.
51. C. E. Collins and C. Collins, "Roentgen Dermatitis Treated with Fresh Whole Leaf of Aloe Vera," *American Journal of Roentgenology* 33 (1935): 396.
52. T. C. Barnes, "The Healing Action of Extracts of Aloe Vera Leaf on Abrasions of Human Skin," *American Journal of Botany* 34 (1947): 597; C. C. Lushbaugh and D. B. Hale, "Experimental Acute Radiodermatitis Following Beta Irradiation: V.Histopathological Study of the Mode of Action of Therapy with Aloe Vera," *Cancer* 6 (1953): 690.
53. R. H. Davis, J. J. DiDonato, G. M. Hartman, et al., "Anti-Inflammatory and Wound Healing Activity of a Growth Substance in Aloe vera," *Journal of the American Podiatric Medical Association* 84 (1994): 77.
54. M. E. Kazanecki, M. F. Melhem, K. J. Spichty, et al., "Diet Induced Reduction in Serum Lipoproteins Stimulates Cell Proliferation in Weaning Rats," *Pharmacological Research* 21 (1989): 533; A. N. Orekhov, V. V. Tertov, and S. A. Kudryashov, "Triggerlike Stimulation of Cholesterol Accumulation and DNA and Extra-Cellular Matrix Synthesis Induced by Atherogenic Serum or Low Density Lipoprotein in Cultured Cells," *Circulation Research* 66 (1990): 311; M. R. Soma, A. Corsini, and R. Paoletti, "Cholesterol and Mevalonic Acid Modulation in Cell Metabolism and Multiplication," *Toxicology Letter* 1 (1992): 64; B. L. Tang, C. C. Teo, K. Y. Sim, et al., "Cytostatic Effect of Antiestrogens in Lymphoid Cells: Relationship to High Affinity Antiestrogen Binding Sites and Cholesterol," *Biochimical Biophysics Acta* 1014 (1989): 162.
55. Davis, Leitner, Russo, et al., "Anti-Inflammatory Activity," 263.
56. V. Srivastava, N. Varma, J. S. Tandon, et al., "Anti-Inflammatory Activity of Pluchea Lanceolate: Isolation of an Active Principle," *International Journal of Crude Drug Research* 28)1990): 135.
57. G. W. Snedecor, and W. G. Cochran, *Statistical Methods,* 6th ed. (Ames: The Iowa State University Press, 1967).
58. Davis, Parker, "Aloe Vera as a Biologically Active Vehicle," 1.
59. A. G. Gilman, T. W. Rall, A. S. Niew, et al., *Goodman and Gilman's The Pharmacological Basis of Therapeutics,* 8th ed. (New York: Pergamon Press, 1990); J. E. Balow and A. S. Rosenthal, "Glucocorticoid Suppression of Macrophage Migration Inhibitory Factor," *Journal of Experimental Medicine* 137 (1973): 1031.
60. Gilman, Rall, Niew, et al., *The Pharmacological Basis;* Balow and Rosenthal, "Glucocorticoid Suppression," 1031; R. F. Diegelmann, K. I. Cohen, and A.

M. Kaplan, "The Role of Macrophages in Wound Repair: A Review," *Plastic Reconstructive Surgery* 68 (1981): 107; A. C. Guyton, *Textbook of Medical Physiology,* 8th ed. (Philadelphia: W. B. Saunders, 1991); M. H. Ross and L. J. Romrell, *Histology: A Text and Atlas,* 2d ed. (Baltimore: William and Wilkins, 1989).

61. Guyton, *Textbook*, and Ross and Romrell, *Histology*.
62. Ross and Romrell, *Histology*.
63. Diegelmann, Cohen, and Kaplan, "The Role of Macrophages", 107.
64. K. L. Carpenter, C. E. Brabbs, and M. J. Mitchinson, "Oxygen Radicals and Atherosclerosis," *Klin. Wochenschr.* 69 (1991): 1039.
65. Cypriani, Tabacik, and Desomps, "Effect of Estradiol and Antiestrogens," 197.
66. Ibid.; Dawson, Metherall, Ridgway, et al., "Benetic Distinction," 9128; Tang, Tea, Sim, et al., "Cytostatic Effect," 162.
67. Oreknov, Tertov, and Kuydryashov, "Triggerlike Stimulation," 311; Soma, Corsini, and Paoletti, "Cholesterol," 64.
68. Kazanecki, Melhem, Spichty, et al., "Diet Induced Reduction," 533; Orekhov, Tertor, and Kuydryashov, "Triggerlike Stimulation," 311; Soma, Corsini, and Paoletti, "Cholesterol," 64; Tang, Teo, Sim, et al., "Cytostatic Effect," 162.
69. Soma, Corsini, and Paoletti, "Cholesterol," 64.
70. Ibid.; N. Gerst, A. Duriatti, F. Schuber, et al., "Potent Inhibition of Cholesterol Biosynthesis in 3T3 Fibroblasts by N: [(1, 5, 9)- Trimethyldecyl]-4 Alpha, 10-Dimethyl-8-Aza-Trans-Decal-3 Betaol, a New 2, 3-Oxidosqualene Cyclase Inhibitor," *Biochemical Pharmacology* 37 (1988): 1955.
71. T. Mazzone, and L. Pustelnikas, "Growth Related Modulation of Human Skin Fibroblast Cholesterol Distribution and Metabolism," *Biochimical Biophysics Acta.* 1047 (1990): 180.
72. D. A. Hughes and P. L. Haslam, "Effect of Smoking on the Lipid Composition of Lung Lining Fluid and Relationship between Immunostimulatory Lipids, Inflammatory Cells and Foamy Macrophages in Extrinsic Allergic Alveolitis," *European Respiratory J* 3 (1990): 1128; J. Oiknine and M. Aviram, "Increased Susceptibility to Activation and Increased Uptake of Low Density Lipoprotein by Cholesterol-Loaded Macrophages," *Arteriosclerosis Thrombosis* 12 (992): 745.
73. Parish, Witkowski, and Millikan, "Aloe Vera," 679.
74. Davis, Parker, and Murdoch, "Aloe Vera," 1.
75. I. R. Tizard, R.H. Carpenter, B. H. McAnalley, et al., "The Biological Activities of Mannans and Related Complex Carbohydrates," *Molecular Biotherapy* 1 (1989): 290.
76. Diegelmann, Cohen, and Kaplan, "The Role of Macrophages," 107; Guyton, *Textbook;* Ross and Romrell, *Histology*.
77. Davis, DiDonato, Hartman, et al., "Anti-Inflammatory and Wound Healing Activity," 77; A. D. Klein, and N. S. Penneys, "Aloe Vera," *Journal of the American Academy of Dermatology* 18 (1988): 714.
78. Davis, DiDonato, Hartman, et al., "Anti-Inflammatory and Wound Healing Activity," 77.
79. E. Davis and A. MacLachlan, "Effect of Indole-acetic Acid on Intracellular Distribution of β-Glucanase Activities in Pea Epicotyl," *Archives of Biochemical Biophysics* 128 (1968): 595.
80. F. H. Witham and L. B. Hendry, "Computer Modeling of Gibberellin-DNA Binding," *J. Theropeutic Biology* 155 (1992): 55.
81. Davis, DiDonato, Hartman, et al., "Anti-Inflammatory and Wound-Healing Activity," 77.

82. R. H. Davis, "The Biological Standardization of Aloe Vera," *Aloe Today*, Fall/Winter 1993, 12.
83. Gilman, Rall, Niew, et al., *The Pharmacological Basis.*
84. Guyton, *Textbook;* Ross and Romrell, *Histology.*
85. W. D. Nes, G. G. Janssen, F.G. Crumley, et al., "The Structural Requirements of Sterols for Membrane Function in Saccharomyces Cerevisiae," *Archives of Biochemical Biophysics* 300 (1993): 724.
86. Cypriani, Tabacik, and Descomps, "Effect of Estradrol and Estrogens," 167; Gupta, Sexton, and Rudney, "Effect of Vitamin B3," 379; Dawson, Metherall, Ridgway, et al., "Genetic Distinction," 9128.
87. D. Owens, P. Collins, A. Johnson, et al., "Cellular Cholesterol Metabolism in Mitogen-Stimulated Lymphocytes: Requirement for De Novo Synthesis," *Biochemical Biophysics Acta.* 1051 (1990): 138; Q. Xu, E. Buhler, A. Steinmetz, et al., "A High Density Lipoprotein Receptor Appears to Mediate the Transfer of Essential Fatty Acids from High-Density Lipoprotein to Lymphocytes," *Biochemistry Journal* 287 (1992): 395; D. A. Hughes, P. J. Townsend, and P. L. Haslam, "Enhancement of the Antigen-Presenting Function of Monocytes by Cholesterol: Possible Relevance to Inflammatory Mechanisms in Extrinsic Allergic Alveolitis and Atherosclerosis," *Clinical Experimental Immunology* 87 (1982): 279; R. Ieki, S. Kudoh, H. Kimura, et al., "Human Granulocyte Colony Formation in Serum Free Cultures Stimulated with Purified Recumbinant Granulocyte Colony-Stimulating Factor," *Experimental Hematology* 18 (1990): 883.
88. Hughes and Haslam, "Effect of Smoking," 1128.
89. X. F. Qu, M. Hayashi, K. Yamaki, et al., "Assessment of Vascular Permeability Increase in the Mouse by Dye Leakage during Paw Edema," *Japanese Journal of Pharmacology* 52 (1990): 500.
90. G. R. Waller, S. Mangiafico, and C. R. Ritchey, "A Chemical Investigation of Aloe Barbadensis Miller," *Proceedings of the Oklahoma Academy of Science* 58 (1978): 69.
91. Robert, Hemila, and Wikstrom, "Vitamin C," 88.

10
Aspirin and Aloe

Aspirin prevents heart attacks and stroke as well as clumping of blood in arteries.[1] The role of aspirin in preventing heart attacks is probably its strongest credential as a biological therapeutic. People who take aspirin have fewer heart attacks than those who seldom take aspirin.[2] How does aspirin work? It prevents prostaglandin synthesis throughout the body. Platelets exposed to aspirin can never make prostaglandin again until they are replaced, in about five days or so. Clotting and hardening of the arteries, or atherosclerosis, is caused by prostaglandin release from platelets that contribute to heart attacks and strokes. In the United States all acetylsalicylic acid is called aspirin, which has been in use for more than eighty years. Aspirin (325 mg per tablet) taken every other day caused 44 percent fewer heart attacks than occurred in people who were fed sugar pills (placebos). Pain, fever, and inflammation are symptoms that aspirin best relieves. It relieves the red, swollen joints of arthritis and restores mobility while reducing pain. Many mothers use aspirin to lower high fevers in their children. Those who take aspirin over a long period of time should be wary of irritation and stomach bleeding. Two tablets every four hours give maximum benefit while decreasing the risk.[3] One should not normally take more than twelve aspirins a day and not without water. One should not take aspirin when not needed. Stomach ulcers, bleeding, irritation, allergy, and drug interactions are definite side effects of aspirin. The faster the aspirin disintegrates, the more soluble the aspirin, the less the stomach irritation. Intestinal bleeding, hearing problems, and liver damage have been reported due to long-term use of aspirin at recommended doses. These effects are reversed a few weeks after discontinued use of aspirin.

Prostaglandins are released at the site of pain or inflammation. It is at this site that aspirin blocks the production of prostaglandin to inhibit pain and inflammation.[4] Prostaglandin causes platelets to become sticky to form clots that stop blood flow in the heart and brain. Some prostaglandins constrict blood vessels to further dampen blood flow. Aspirin reduces the stickiness of platelets and causes blood thinning. It blocks a constricting prostaglandin called thromboxane, and at small doses aspirin has no impeding effect on prostacyclin—a prostaglandin that dilates blood vessels and inhibits platelet stickiness. Obviously, aspirin at high doses could upset the yin-yang balance and produce side effects. In fact, small aspirin doses produce greater heart benefits. Some evidence suggests that aspirin by its prostaglandin-blocking action protects or reduces colon and rectal cancer. Some salicylates block prostaglandin in the brain and not at the site of pain as aspirin does. This is why some salicylates relieve pain and fever but have no anti-inflammatory effect. Some drugs are sold without anyone knowing how the drug works. The more beneficial a drug is, the more side effects it has. It is not true that continuing doses of aspirin results in tolerance to aspirin or that aspirin causes drug addiction.

The discovery of aspirin was the result of efforts to isolate a painkiller from willow bark.[5] Today aspirin is synthesized in a pure, inexpensive form. Salicylic acid is the substance from which aspirin is made. Bayer A.G. learned to make aspirin in tablet form. One wonders if aspirin were discovered today, would it be approved for use by the FDA? It probably would wind up as a prescription drug. Aspirin is the most widely used, safest, and cheapest drug ever made. Most drugs, which have specific biological effects, have more side effects. While aspirin is an exception to this rule, it does have significant side effects.

Aspirin is widely used as an analgesic and an anti-inflammatory agent. However, since the absorption of salicylates by tissue is low, the effective dose required to produce a therapeutic response is relatively high. Also, the half-life of aspirin is very short. Aspirin inhibits prostaglandin synthesis in response to pain by blocking the enzyme cyclo-oxygenase, which converts the arachadonic acid into prostaglandin.[6] Pain-inducing stimuli, trauma, immunoglobulins, and oxygen radicals convert membrane phospholipid into arachidonic acid in the presence of phospholipase (figure 10.1). Our previous work suggests that aloe vera may block the formation of arachidonic acid as well as the synthesis or action of prostaglandin.[7] Bradykinin and

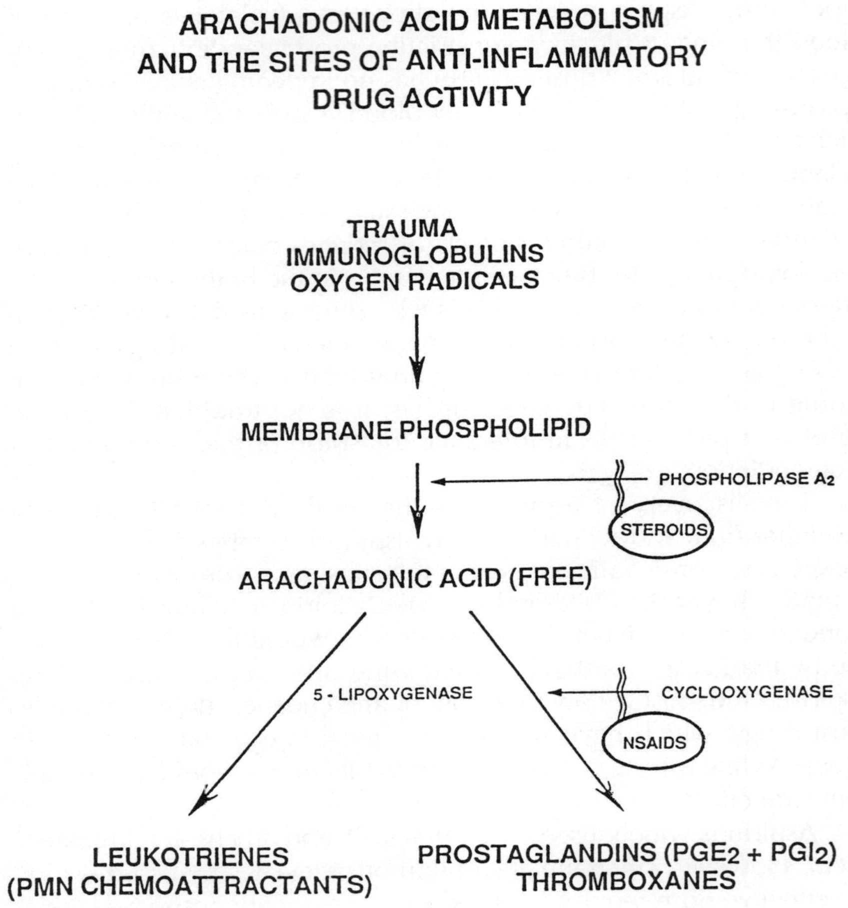
ARACHADONIC ACID METABOLISM
AND THE SITES OF ANTI-INFLAMMATORY
DRUG ACTIVITY
TRAUMA
IMMUNOGLOBULINS
OXYGEN RADICALS
MEMBRANE PHOSPHOLIPID
PHOSPHOLIPASE A2
STEROIDS
ARACHADONIC ACID (FREE)
5 - LIPOXYGENASE
CYCLOOXYGENASE
NSAIDS
LEUKOTRIENES
(PMN CHEMOATTRACTANTS)
PROSTAGLANDINS (PGE2 + PGI2)
THROMBOXANES

Fig. 10.1.

histamine, which are found in inflammation sites, serve to initiate pain. These stimuli of inflammation and pain are inhibited by aspirin and aloe vera. Aspirin's acetyl group destroys the cyclo-oxygenase rather than inhibiting the enzyme so that the cyclo-oxygenase cannot make prostaglandin. Aspirin is best absorbed when administered in solution. Small increases in urinary pH increase the renal clearance of salicylates and thus decrease the plasma levels of the drug. The dissociation of aspirin plays an important role in renal clearance.[8]

Salicylates have been used in the treatment of rheumatoid arthritis to reduce pain and inflammation for almost one hundred years. Oral doses of 4gm/day of aspirin are needed to attain blood levels necessary for an anti-inflammatory response.[9] However, side effects are recorded at this dose level. Ultraviolet light–induced erythema was inhibited by topically applied 5 percent aspirin in cream.[10] Since aloe vera alone has been shown to inhibit the ultraviolet light inflammation, one wonders if aloe vera would improve this response. Aspirin and aloe vera inhibit oxygen radicals and the infiltration of PMNs into an inflammation site. Salicylic acid, the hydrolysis product of aspirin, may be responsible for the anti-inflammatory activity, but also the toxic effects. Aloe vera contains aspirin-like compounds. The mechanism of aspirin's action may be related to: interference with oxidative phosphorylation; endogenous anti-inflammatory peptides from plasma protein; inhibition of leukocyte migration; stabilization of lysosomal membranes; hyperpolarization of neuronal membranes; and the inhibition of the synthesis of prostaglandins. Three grams of aspirin daily reduced by 98 percent the urinary output of prostaglandin metabolite.[11]

The purpose of this study was to determine if aloe vera would improve the efficacy of aspirin. If aloe vera was additive or synergistic with aspirin on inflammation or analgesia, we could use aloe as a "biological vehicle" for aspirin. The dosage of aspirin could be reduced to eliminate the side effects as well as increase the absorption of aspirin. We evaluated the therapeutic background of aspirin relative to the cardiovascular influence, inflammation, analgesia, fever, and arthritis. The topical and systemic anti-inflammatory influence of aspirin in aloe vera will be presented, as well as aspirin's analgestic effect in aloe. The latter analgesic data will be compared with a normal analgesic dose-response curve for aspirin alone. The prospects of using aloe with aspirin on arthritis will be presented. We will discuss the topical influence of aloe vera on foot blood flow and its relation to the entire cardiovascular system. Every effort will be made to discuss the mechanism of action of aloe vera and aspirin as related to inflammation, analgesia, arthritis, and blood flow.

Cardiovascular Disease and Aspirin

Aspirin works by preventing the body's production of prostaglandin. Trauma, immunoglobulins, and oxygen radicals in the presence of phospholipase convert membrane phospholipid into arachidonic acid (free). Hydrocortisone blocks the action of phospholipase and prevents the formation of arachidonic acid and prostaglandin. Aspirin blocks the cyclo-oxygenase enzyme and prevents the formation of prostaglandin. Aloe vera inhibits the infiltration of PMNs into an inflamed area by blocking the leukotrienes, and our work suggests that it blocks the other pathway into the formation of prostaglandins.[12] Possibly aloe vera blocks the formation of arachidonic acid. Aspirin increases the amount of time blood takes to clot by decreasing the rate at which prostaglandins are produced. Prostaglandins contribute to the clotting process by allowing platelets in the blood to stick more easily to each other and to the blood vessel walls. Platelets form the basis of clots in blood vessels. It only takes a small stimulus to form a platelet plug, such as a small irritation of the vascular wall. Aspirins block prostaglandin formation and inhibit clot formation.[13] Clots play a major role in heart attacks and strokes. Aspirin can reduce clot formation and prevent heart attacks and strokes.

Half of all deaths after fifty years of age are due to cardiovascular disease. Therefore, the pharmaceutical industry continues to look for a drug that can eliminate heart attacks and strokes with little or no side effects. The control of CV disease takes years of treatment, so it is difficult to imagine a drug or combination of drugs that can reduce the death toll in this area. When a small cut occurs in a blood vessel, a platelet plug forms to plug the hole and aids the growth of a new vessel wall at the injury site. When the clotting process is not functioning properly, it forms unneeded and dangerous clots, which can block a healthy blood vessel. When a vessel is injured, clotting begins immediately. The vessel wall contracts, and the platelets form a plug. A permanent blood clot forms on top of the platelet clot. These fibrin clots dissolve and are replaced by new vessel wall tissue. Platelet plugs are seen more often in high-pressure arteries, because fibrin clots are usually washed away. However, in veins where blood pressure is low and blood is slow-moving, fibrin clots are formed and are not washed away. Clots are not the cause of CV disease but are a major contributing factor. The formation of clots in healthy vessels may be due to excess body weight, smoking, or a lack of exercise. CV disease causes half the natural deaths in the United States each year.

Heart attacks and strokes primarily involve disturbances of the arterial blood vessels. Full strokes involve death of brain tissue caused by decreased blood supply. Death to heart tissue produces scar tissue called myocardial infarctions. Atherosclerosis (hardening of the arteries) is clot-related and narrows veins and arteries to reduce blood flow, which kills brain and heart tissue. Atherosclerosis plays a role in all heart attacks and strokes. Platelets gather in blood vessels with fat deposits and trigger strokes. Aspirin prevents platelets from sticking together by blocking prostaglandin production. Prostaglandins are key in platelet plug formation. Aspirin stops the platelets from making prostaglandin and thus prevents plug formation. It therefore reduces the risk of heart attack.

Foot Blood Flow (Plantar Surface)

Blood flow leaves the heart at a high velocity of flow and under high blood pressure. As the blood vessels divide in the small arteries and arterioles, the cross-sectional area of the combined vessels increases, causing a decrease in the velocity of flow and decrease in blood pressure. These decreases in flow and pressure occur in the arterioles due to a reduction in total peripheral resistance. The arterioles protect the capillaries, which have little flow, pressure, and small numbers of red blood cells not arranged in layers. The feet have high blood pressure (+90 mm Hg) primarily due to the gravity weight of the column of blood on the venous side.

The arteriole pulse pressure represents the difference between systole and diastolic pressures. As the pulse pressure moves ahead of the flow, it is dampened by the resistance of the arterioles. Pulse pressure increases with age because of the hardening of the vessels that cause a decrease in vessel compliance. In the capillaries, blood flow is reduced so nutrient, gas, and hormone exchange can occur with cells. The velocity of flow in peripheral circulation is slow and is controlled by hormones, the sympathetic nervous system, and metabolic factors. The tightness of blood in peripheral circulation is called central filling pressure (7 mm Hg). It determines and controls venous return, heart contraction, and cardiac output. In older people, the hardening of vessels in peripheral circulation reduces blood flow, as evidenced by cold feet. Cold constricts and heat dilates small vessels. The lack of exercise by older people reduces metabolic metabolites so that vessels do not dilate but remain constricted. Standing severely activates the sympathetic nervous system to cause vasoconstriction. As a result, the temperature and blood flow to the foot tissue are decreased and the tissue becomes hard.

Jess F. Clarke, Jr., president of Miracle of Aloe of Westport, Connecticut, made a 60 percent aloe foot preparation called Miracle Foot Repair. This cream preparation when applied to the plantar surface of the foot is quickly absorbed while it lubricates and softens the skin. The purpose of this study was to determine if "Miracle Foot Repair," or 60 percent aloe vera, applied to the plantar surface would increase peripheral blood flow (vasodilation) so as to increase the nutrient supply to tissue and make tissue soft and healthy. This effect would go far to increase venous return and cardiac output in older people. A future study will focus on the combination of aspirin and aloe vera to determine foot plantar surface perfusion and blood flow.

Measurement of Foot Blood Flow

Five subjects were selected from a white suburban middle-income population who were in good health and free of vascular disease or related medical conditions, i.e., hypertension, diabetes, etc. The subjects ranged in age from twenty-eight to fifty-seven years, with an age mean of forty-one. Three males and two females participated in the study. The MD-35 Procord Vascular Recorder (D. E. Hokanson, Inc.) measured and recorded peripheral vascular circulation. The photoplethysmograph was used to directly measure small vessel/capillary circulation and patency. It is a good indicator of skin profusion. The photoplethysmograph uses infrared sensors to detect skin color changes that occur with each heartbeat. The small and sensitive transducer is strapped to a digit. The output of the photoplethysmograph is a wave form showing volume changes in the measurement area.

The subjects were instructed to apply one tablespoon of 60 percent aloe cream (Miracle Foot Repair) to the bottom of both feet and gently rub it into the skin. They did this every day from December 11 to December 31, 1993. Two baseline studies were conducted on December 3 and December 10 in which no treatment was applied during this baseline period. These two reading periods served as baseline controls (Theory of Internal Control). The subjects were not informed of the purpose of the study and were directed to maintain consistency in application. Waveforms were recorded using the photoplethysmograph on the MD-35 Procord on December 3, 10, 17, 24 and 31. The chart recorder was set at 24 mm/sec, with the range at 0.05. All waveforms were recorded on the subject's right foot, large toe. During the waveform recording, the subjects sat in a chair in a well-heated room.

Three continuous chart recordings for each day were measured for height. Three heights were measured in mm and averaged. The procedure was done for the five testing sessions. Two baseline measurements were obtained to establish a before-treatment baseline level. The three measurements recorded during treatment were compared with the baseline measurements (controls) to obtain the percentage of increase in foot plantar surface blood flow over pretreatment controls.

The Aloe Vera Preparation Increases Foot Blood Flow

Four out of five subjects (80 percent) showed an increase in foot skin profusion. The mean wave length heights (mm) for the two pretreatment baseline measurements were 7.3 ± 1.1 and 6.1 ± 3.9, respectively (table 10.1 and figure 10.2). Applying the 60 percent aloe cream preparation increased the mean wave length heights (mm) to 8.1 ± 3.5, 9.7 ± 0.5 and 12.4 ± 2.3 for weeks 3, 4, and 5. These treatment values represent a 20.5 ± 8.9, 45.2 ± 2.3, and 85.1 ± 15.8 respective percent increases in foot blood flow over pretreatment controls. Possible extraneous factors include room temperature variation, fluctuations in metabolic rate, and ingestion of stimulants

EFFECT OF TOPICAL APPLICATION OF "MIRACLE FOOT REPAIR" ON THE FOOT PLANTAR SURFACE BLOOD FLOW

Pre - Treatment (Weeks)	Peripheral Blood Flow of Foot Skin Wave Height (MM)	%
1	7.3 ± 1.1	-
2	6.1 ± 3.9	-
Treatment * (Weeks)		
3	8.1 ± 3.5	+ 20.5 ± 8.9
4	9.7 ± 0.5	+ 45.2 ± 2.3
5	12.4 ± 2.3	+ 85.1 ± 15.8

5 Healthy volunteers per group. * 1 Tablespoon of miracle foot repair was gently rubbed on the plantar surface of both feet each day.

Tablel 10.1.

TOPICAL ANTI-INFLAMMATORY ACTIVITY OF WHOLE LEAF ALOE AS A VEHICLE (ADDITIVE EFFECT) FOR ASPIRIN.

TREATMENT μg	INHIBITION %
Aloe - 200	18.7 ± 1.6^{A}
Aspirin - 100	23.7 ± 3.1^{B}
Combination - 200 + 100	42.4 ± 3.0^{C}

9 Mice/Group; *Micronized Aspirin; A + B = C ($P > 0.5$)

Fig. 10.2.

(coffee), which are present in the control measurements. However, we feel that this preliminary study suggests that the 60 percent aloe cream preparation increases peripheral blood flow. The 60 percent aloe cream preparation (Miracle Foot Repair) increased foot blood flow 85.1 percent possibly by increasing the local metabolic substances or by directly causing the vasodilation of the small blood vessels to increase foot blood flow. These preliminary results are optimistic for an increase in peripheral vascular circulation by the 60 percent aloe cream preparation. Peripheral foot blood flow may be reduced in older people by a hardening of vessels or a lack in the production of metabolites, which causes vasoconstriction. This vasoconstriction may be overcome by the 60 percent aloe cream preparation, producing healthier feet and a better venous return. An increased venous return increases heart contraction and improves cardiac output. Our thesis is that increased peripheral circulation caused by Miracle Foot Repair would improve heart function and cardiac output in elderly people.

Inflammation

Inflammation has been described as being caused by the release of chemicals from tissues and migrating cells. For example, prostaglandin, histamine, bradykinin, and interleukins play a part in the inflammation process.[14] Also, phagocytic cells can release oxygen radicals and proteolytic enzymes that can produce inflammation. Inflammation is a response of living tissue to injury or injurious agents. There is a train of events in the tissue leading to a homeostatic normal situation. The tissues tend to balance tissue and fluids within a short period of time.[15] A short-term inflammation is characterized by edema, swelling, vasodilation, presence of plasma cells, and the infiltration of PMNs: chronic inflammation is seen when the body cannot get rid of the irritant, so it forms granuloma tissue around the irritant. If one places a cotton pellet under the skin, granuloma tissue forms around the pellet. Hydrocortisone inhibits the granuloma tissue and is, therefore, active against chronic inflammation. Aloe vera has no effect on chronic inflammation in that it does not reduce granuloma tissue around the cotton pellet. However, since aloe vera is a good "biological vehicle" for hydrocortisone against acute inflammation, one wonders if aloe would aid the steroid in blocking chronic inflammation.[16] Steroids inhibit inflammation, but because they decrease connective tissue, they also prevent wound healing. Aloe vera is unique in that it inhibits inflammation and improves wound healing. Aspirin inhibits inflammation, but at high doses that produce side effects. We attempt to determine in this study if aloe vera can act as a "biological vehicle" for aspirin when given topically or systemically. Does aloe vera act in an additive or synergistic fashion with aspirin on topical and systemic inflammation?

Topical Anti-Inflammatory Activity of Whole-Leaf Aloe as a Vehicle (Additive Effect) for Aspirin

Topical Anti-Inflammatory Assay

Adult male ICR-HSD mice (Sprague Dawley Colony, Frederick, Maryland; ten mice/group) were given topically 10 μl of 25 μg/10 μl croton oil solutions. The irritant was applied to the inner surface of the animal's right ear. The left ear was not treated and used as a control. One half hour after the application of the irritant, treatment solutions were added topically to reduce inflammation. One hundred μg of aspirin, 200 μg aloe vera, and a combination of aspirin plus aloe were applied to the same ear. Each solution was given to a different group of animals.[17]

The Results and Discussion

This study proves that aloe and aspirin given topically had an additive (vehicle effect) on inhibiting the croton oil–induced ear swelling. Aloe and aspirin given separately produced a response that was equal to the combination response of aloe plus aspirin: $A+B=C$ ($P>0.5$). The values were identical. These results confirm our previous topical anti-inflammatory data using aloe as a vehicle for aspirin. The use of micronized aspirin helped us to mix the aspirin into the aloe vera (table 10.2 and figure 10.3).

We believe that aloe vera solubilizes the micronized aspirin as well as hydrates and softens the skin so that one can observe the

EFFECT OF TOPICAL APPLICATION OF "MIRACLE FOOT REPAIR" ON THE FOOT PLANTAR SURFACE BLOOD FLOW

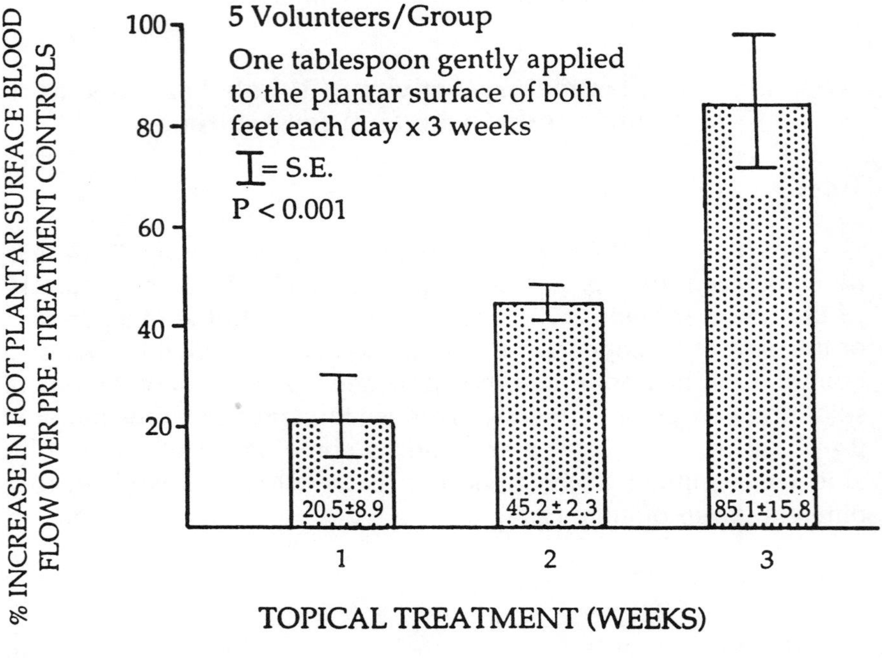

Table 10.2.

TOPICAL ANTI-INFLAMMATORY ACTIVITY OF WHOLE LEAF ALOE AS A VEHICLE (ADDITIVE EFFECT) FOR ASPIRIN.

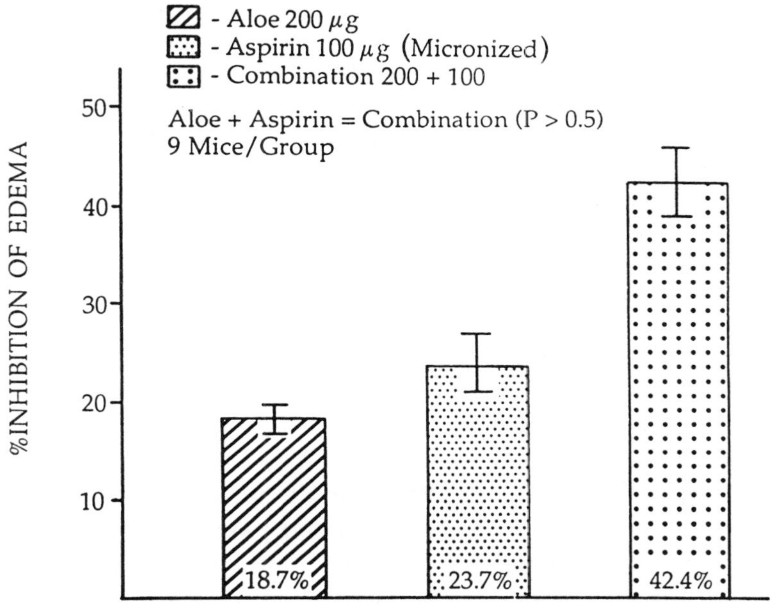

Fig. 10.3.

additive topical anti-inflammatory response. Both aloe vera and aspirin block inflammatory mediators as well as pain. However, aspirin needs aloe as a vehicle to produce the topical anti-inflammatory response.

Anti-Inflammatory Activity of Subcutaneous Aloe Vera and Aspirin on Two Percent Carrageenan–Induced Paw Edema

The Paw Edema Assay

Sprague Dawley male rats (175–200 g; 10 rats/group) were given subcutaneous 250 mg/kg whole-plant aloe, 100 mg/kg aspirin, or the combination on day 1. On day 2 at zero time, rats received 0.1 ml 2 percent carrageenan into the plantar surface of the paw with a 27-gauge needle as well as subcutaneous saline (on basis of 10 ml/kg) with a 22-gauge needle. Control rats received 0.1 ml saline into the paw plantar surface and a subcutaneous injection of saline (10 ml/kg). Volumetric paw readings were obtained by the water plethysmograph at time zero and six hours later.

The Results and Discussion

Administration of 250 mg/kg of whole-plant (leaf) aloe vera reduced the 2 percent carrageenan–induced paw edema 14 percent (figure 10.4). The 2 percent carrageenan–induced paw edema is a maximum inflammatory response designed to prevent the biological activity of both aloe and aspirin. Aspirin at 100 mg/kg inhibited the paw edema 21 percent. Both these anti-inflammatory responses are positive responses. Combining the aspirin and aloe vera produced a 31 percent anti-inflammatory effect. This response would be at least doubled or even tripled in magnitude if the 1 percent carrageenan was used. Nevertheless, the combination exhibited an additive effect, proving that aloe vera is a good vehicle for aspirin, as was recorded for hydrocortisone and ascorbic acid (vitamin C). We feel that aloe vera would protect the aspirin from causing stomach ulcers as well as enhancing its biological activity and tissue absorption. Aloe vera gave us an excellent dose-response curve on analgesia over the dose

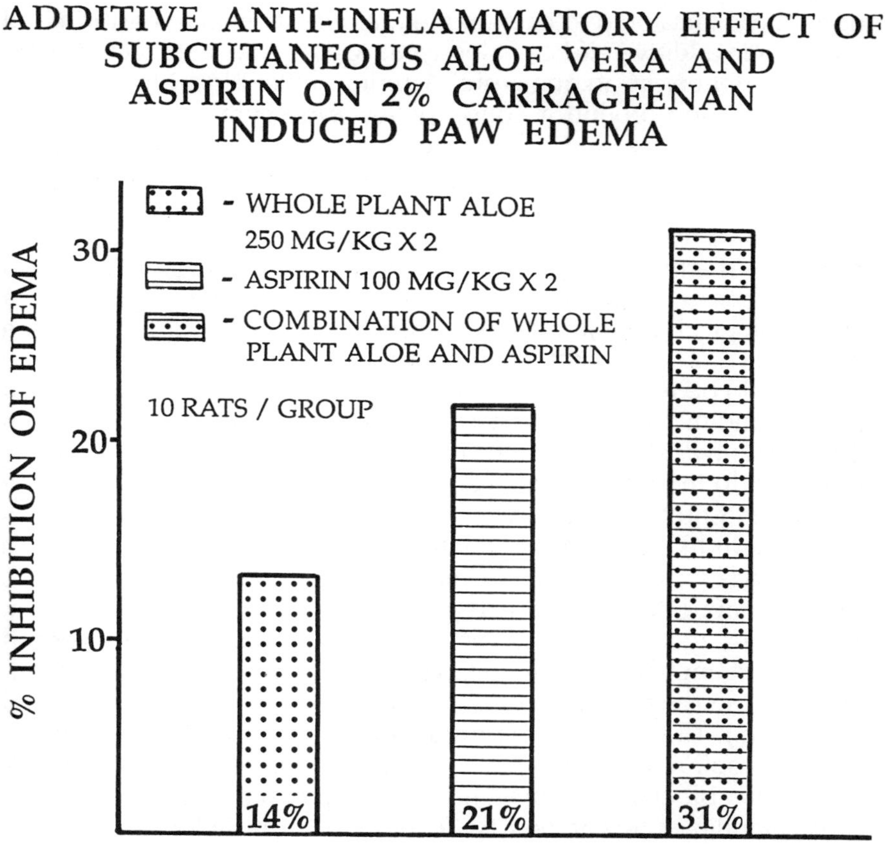
ADDITIVE ANTI-INFLAMMATORY EFFECT OF SUBCUTANEOUS ALOE VERA AND ASPIRIN ON 2% CARRAGEENAN INDUCED PAW EDEMA
- WHOLE PLANT ALOE 250 MG/KG X 2
- ASPIRIN 100 MG/KG X 2
- COMBINATION OF WHOLE PLANT ALOE AND ASPIRIN
10 RATS / GROUP
% INHIBITION OF EDEMA
30
20
10
14%
21%
31%

Fig. 10.4.

range of 5 to 50 mg/kg. Further increases in dosage up to 300 mg/kg produced no further increase in analgesic response.

Prostaglandin, bradykinin, histamine, and 5-hydroxy-tryptamine increase vascular permeability by inducing vascular leakage.[18] They cause edema when injected into the hind paws of rats. Prostaglandin added to the carrageenan injection can enhance the edema formation. These facts help to explain the anti-edema effect of aspirin and the vehicle additive effect of aloe vera. Aspirin, like aloe, acts mainly at the periphery as an analgesic. Aspirin, unlike aloe, blocks granuloma formation around a cotton pellet. Aloe vera stimulates fibroblasts but is not toxic or inflammatory even at massive doses. Aspirin prevents heart attacks and strokes as well as clumping of blood in vessels. For example, one aspirin a day can reduce heart attacks 44 percent and two to six aspirins a day can reduce joint swelling in rheumatoid arthritis. However, the blockage of prostaglandin at high aspirin doses and the irritation cause stomach problems. Aloe vera as a biological vehicle acts as a carrier, which would increase the availability of salicylates by increasing the absorption so that the dose could be reduced. Bioavailability of aspirin is needed to inhibit prostaglandin. Its distribution can be altered by enzymes, albumin binding, and acetylation. Aloe vera would increase the bioavailability of aspirin to increase aspirin's effectiveness. The antioxidants in aloe vera offer a protective effect.

Aspirin-like drugs act as analgesics peripherally by blocking the generation of impulses at the receptors for pain.[19] Narcotic analgesics block synaptic transmission of pain in the central nervous system. Aloe vera's action, at the present time, is considered to be a peripheral one. It appears to have no CNS effect even at high doses. Prostaglandins sensitize pain receptors to mechanical and chemical stimulation. The synthesis of prostaglandin is inhibited by therapeutic doses of aspirin. (Aloe may help here.) The pain response of bradykinin is also blocked. In some models of inflammation, a release of prostaglandin occurs at the CNS level so that aspirin has a CNS component. An ideal analgesic such as aspirin with aloe vera should have a high peripheral activity with little central effect.

Fever and Inflammation

Inflammation tells us that our body's defense mechanisms are functioning to maintain homeostasis in the presence of a damaging irritant or invader. One of the symptoms of chronic inflammation is fever. White blood cells are destroyed by an invading organism releasing pyrogens that elevate body temperature. The pyrogens go to the hypothalamus (controls temperature) to increase body temperature, which helps the white blood cells fight off infection. Aspirin resets the hypothalamus and blocks the incoming pyrogens to reduce the body temperature to normal.[20] Possibly aloe vera could help aspirin control body temperature because of its beneficial preventive influence on systemic and topical inflammation. Aloe vera also does a good job fighting off infection. The combined influence of aspirin and aloe on migraine, tension, and sinus headaches needs to be evaluated.

Side Effects and Treatment with Aspirin

When aspirin is taken for one biological effect and produces an undesired effect, this is called a side effect. All therapeutic drugs have side effects, which depend on the doses administered. The most common side effect for aspirin is stomach upset and bleeding.[21] Most people who need to take aspirin over a prolonged period experience stomach bleeding. A daily dose of twelve aspirins is fifty times as likely to cause side effects as a daily dose of four tablets. Since aspirin is a weak acid, it is likely to upset the gastrointestinal system, which always tries to maintain a balance between acids and bases. Aspirin adheres to the stomach wall and causes patches of the stomach lining to come off. The loss of stomach lining is called an ulcer, which causes bleeding and pain. Since aspirin inhibits prostaglandin synthesis, it breaks down the stomach barrier. Prostaglandin protects the mucosa from its own acid.[22] Aspirin can cause allergic attacks—hives, swollen face, and asthmatic breathing. Overdoses of aspirin (salicylism) can disrupt the central nervous system, causing ringing ears. Other symptoms include vomiting, headaches, confusion, and depression. Our feeling is that aloe vera taken with aspirin would buffer some of the aspirin side effects. Certainly aloe vera would counteract the stomach irritation and bleeding. It would also modulate some of the overdose symptoms.

Aspirin inhibits the synthesis of prostaglandin by inhibiting the prostaglandin synthetase. The relative potency against the sheep seminal vesicle synthetase is as follows: aspirin = 1; phenylbutazone =

7; indomethacin = 185 (table 10.3). The anti-inflammatory dose of indomethacin based on this data would be far less than aspirin.[23] Stomach irritation and bleeding are almost always seen when the high 3200 mg aspirin dose is given to people with rheumatoid arthritis over a long period of time. The drug dose is reduced to 200 mg/day for indomethacin and 600 mg/day for phenylbutazone. For gold and steroid treatment the dose is reduced to 50 mg/week and 5 mg/day, respectively. Of all the non-steroidal anti-inflammatory drugs, aspirin has the shortest half-life, 0.25, as compared to 68 for phenylbutazone (tables 10.4 and 10.5).[24] This data shows us why a relatively large dose of aspirin is required to treat inflammation and arthritis. Our data show that putting aspirin in aloe vera would not only buffer the toxicity and improve penetration, but also could reduce the dosage of aspirin. As a biological vehicle for aspirin, aloe vera would improve absorption of aspirin as well as contribute to its biological effectiveness. In the treatment of rheumatoid arthritis, one starts out by using high doses of aspirin along with physical therapy and education. The aspirin dose could be reduced if given with aloe vera. One goes up the treatment ladder as follows: low-dose steroids; gold salts; methotrexate; high-dose steroids; and experimental therapy (table 10.6). All these harsh treatments could be benefited by using aloe vera as a biological vehicle. We have shown that aloe vera alone can prevent and regress adjuvant arthritis—an experimental model of rheumatoid arthritis.

Mechanism of Action of Aspirin

The inhibition of prostaglandin biosynthesis is clearly achieved by therapeutic doses of aspirin-like drugs. High concentration of salicylates is needed to uncouple oxidative phosphorylation, but this event does not appear to be related to anti-inflammatory activity. Aspirin stabilizes lysosomal membranes, which is inversely correlated with anti-inflammatory activity. L-tryptophan is displaced from serum protein binding sites by anti-inflammatory drugs. These drugs act by displacing peptides from their binding sites on serum protein, and the free form of the peptide protects connective tissues from the effects of inflammatory insults (table 10.7). Inhibition of PMNs is used as an assay for anti-inflammation. Possibly the inhibition is related

RELATIVE POTENCY AGAINST PROSTAGLANDIN SYNTHETASE *

Aspirin	1
Phenylbutazone	7
Indomethacin	185

* Sheep seminal vesicles - Vane, 1974

Table 10.3.

DRUG DOSAGE FOR RHEUMATOID ARTHRITIS

SALICYLATES	3200MG/DAY
INDOMETHACIN	200MG/DAY
PHENYLBUTAZONE	600MG/DAY
GOLD	50MG/WK
STEROID	5MG/DAY

Table 10.4.

NON-STEROIDAL ANTI-INFLAMMATORY DRUGS

	HALF LIFE
PHENYLBUTAZONE	68
SALICYLATE	15
INDOMETHACIN	5
IBUPROFEN	2
ASPIRIN	0.25

Table 10.5.

TREATMENT FOR RHEUMATOID ARTHRITIS

EXPERIMENT TREATMENTS

↑

HIGH DOSE STEROIDS

↑

METHOTREXATE

↑

GOLD SALTS

↑

NSAIDS AND LOW DOSE STEROID

↑

EDUCATION, PHYSICAL THERAPY
AND HIGH DOSE ASPIRIN

Table 10.6.

MECHANISM OF ACTION OF ASPIRIN

1. Inhibits prostaglandin synthesis
2. Displaces anti-inflammatory peptides from plasma protein
3. Blocks migration of leukocytes (?)
4. Stabilizes lysosome membranes
5. Inhibits membrane lipoperoxidation

Table 10.7.

to the blockage of leukotrienes. This entire area has questions that need answers. Drugs that inhibit membrane peroxidation prevent the arachidonic acid cascade from occurring and thus prevent or inhibit inflammation. The prostaglandin phase of inflammation edema coincides with the infiltration of PMNs. Both aspects are inhibited by aspirin. Aspirin has a peripheral effect: By preventing prostaglandin release in inflammation, aspirin prevents the sensitization of pain receptors to mechanical or chemical stimulation. Aspirin may be ineffective as an analgesic in non-inflamed tissue where prostaglandin formation is not occurring. The "biological vehicle" action of aloe vera would influence every aspect on how aspirin works to reduce inflammation and pain.[25]

A two-compartment system for aspirin[26] following an intravenous administration shows that the central compartment distribution is in equilibrium with the peripheral compartment. The rate of elimination of aspirin by the kidney depends upon the pH and dissociation within the tubules and the dose administered, as well as the equilibrium distribution between the central and peripheral compartments (figure 10.5). Systemic bioavailability ranges from 46 to 51 percent of an oral dose of aspirin. Aspirin is hydrolyzed to salicylic acid, a weak inhibitor of the cyclo-oxygenase enzyme, by intestinal, hepatic, and plasma esterases. This suggests the possibility of a dose-dependent absorption kinetics. All kinetics of aspirin appear to be dose-dependent. This could be modified by aloe vera. The distribution of aspirin could be altered by cumulative acetylation that occurs with repeated doses. The bioavailability of aspirin is constant over a wide dose range and appears to be unaltered by long-term administration.

Analgesia

Pain can be pricking and aching pain. Pricking pain is a sharp pain felt in the muscle, skin, and bones. It throbs like a toothache or a headache. Aching pain is not throbbing and is sensed in the internal organs but is not limited to the specific area of its origin. Pain is perceived physically at nerve endings and is interpreted in the brain. When cells are stimulated by a chemical, they release bradykinin to stimulate a nerve ending. An impulse (messae) goes through the nerve to the spinal cord. The pain impulse goes up the spinal cord to a

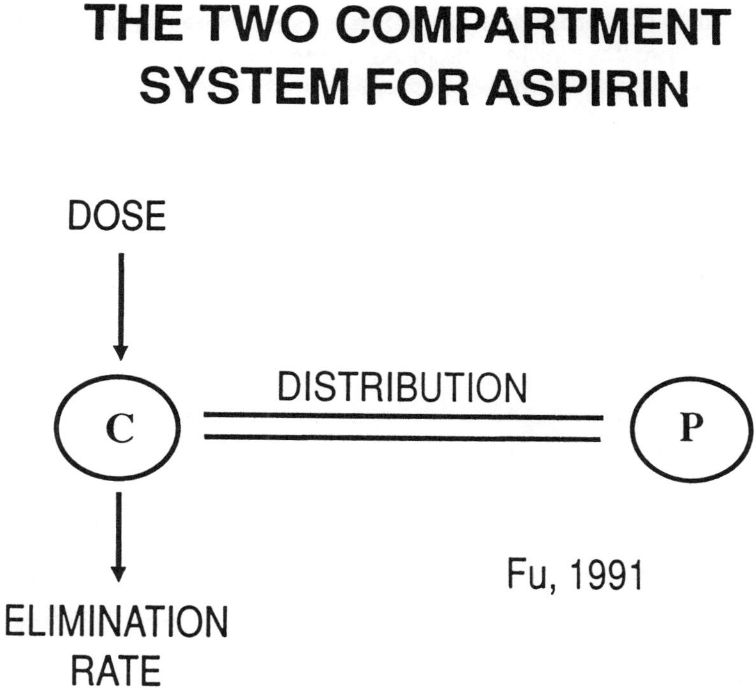
THE TWO COMPARTMENT
SYSTEM FOR ASPIRIN
DOSE
DISTRIBUTION
C
P
ELIMINATION
RATE
Fu, 1991

Fig. 10.5.

"pain gate" mechanism, which can cut off the pain impulse or let it go through to the thalamus. The thalamus determines the origin and severity of pain and then sends the information to the cortex. The cortex will choose a variety of reactions to the pain. Pain is caused by bradykinin and prostaglandin as a result of an injury stimulus. Aspirin can block prostaglandin at the nerve ending and at the thalamus, where prostaglandin aids in pain interpretation. Prostaglandins are present in the hypothalamus, where they play a regulatory function on pain and fever. Aspirin can halt prostaglandin production and can control the sensation of pain. The relationship between prostaglandin and aspirin is a most promising area of research concerning inflammation and pain.[27]

By preventing prostaglandin release in inflammation, aspirin prevents the sensitization of the pain receptors to chemical stimulation. Fatty acid hydroperoxides cause pain whose intensity appears to be greater than that caused by bradykinin, histamine, or prostaglandin E_1. These peroxides may be important precursors of prostaglandins. All pain-inducing substances produce some degree of inflammatory response. Some pain inducers produce vascular changes leading to edema, but others produce inflammation by stimulation of sensory nerves. This type of response is called "neurogenic." Agents that induce pain release substances that enhance the edema response. Sensory nerve terminals may prove to be an important link between pain induced by mediators and the magnitude of the inflammatory response.

The effect of aspirin on pain was considered to be a peripheral action, whereas morphine's analgesic action was thought to be a central nervous system effect.[28] Prostaglandins are released at inflammatory sites that cause pain. Aspirin blocks prostaglandin at the peripheral site and the central site.[29] The relationship between prostaglandin and aspirin helps us to interpret the mechanism of action of various painkillers (figures 10.6 and 10.7).

Salicylates have been used in the treatment of rheumatoid arthritis to reduce pain for many years. High oral doses of aspirin (4gm/day) are needed to attain therapeutic blood levels for the anti-inflammatory and analgesic responses. However, at this dosage, the gastrointestinal symptoms were observed. Ultraviolet light–induced erythema was inhibited by topically applied 5 percent aspirin in cream.[30] Since aloe vera inhibits the ultraviolet light inflammation,

ANALGESIC ACTION OF ASPIRIN

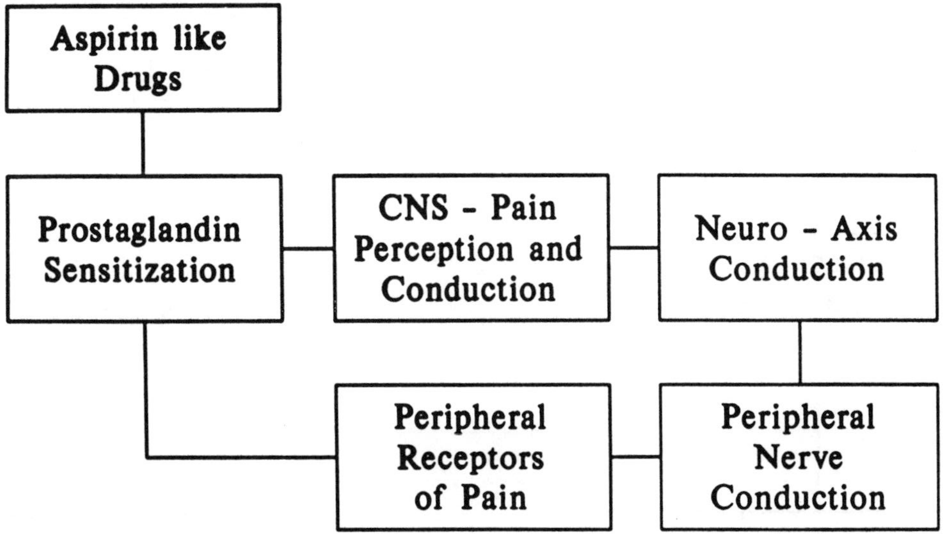

Ferreira, 1979

Fig. 10.6.

EFFECT OF ASPIRIN ON PAIN

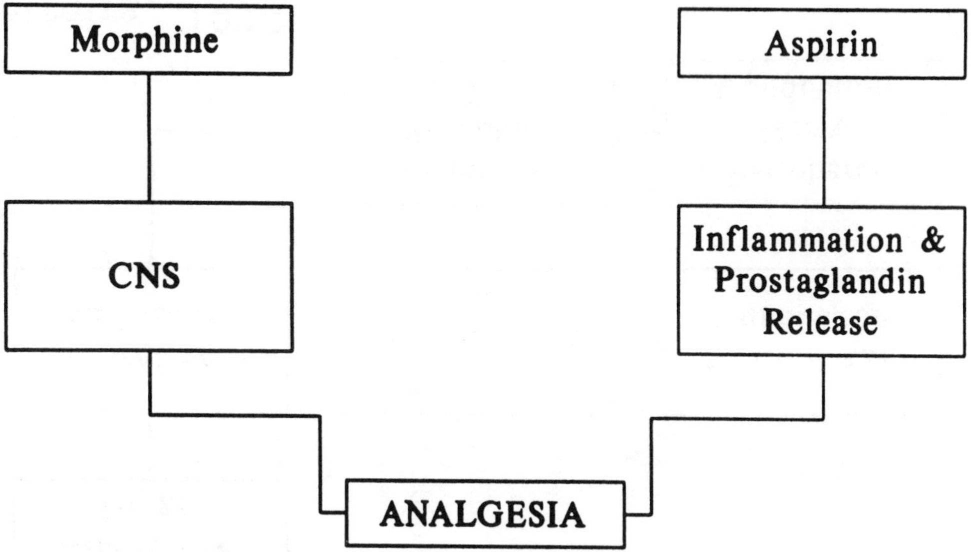

Ferreira, 1974

Fig. 10.7.

would aloe improve the aspirin response? The purpose of this study was to determine if aloe vera has an analgesic response and, also, to determine if this response was additive or synergistic, with the analgesic response seen with aspirin using the hot plate method. An analgesic dose-response curve with aspirin as a test agent standard will also be presented.

The Analgesic Assay

Adult male Sprague Dawley mice (HSD-ICR; 30 gm; 12 animals/group) were given 250 mg/kg aloe vera subcutaneously each day for two days. Another group of mice were treated with 100 mg/kg of aspirin subcutaneously for two days. A third group of mice received the combination of 250 mg/kg aloe and 100 mg/kg aspirin in a similar manner. Control animals received saline alone, 10 ml/kg. Two hours after the last injection, each mouse was tested for the pain response. Using a hot plate set at 48°C, the pain response was characterized by the animal licking its front paws (praying hands response) or lifting its back feet. The time required for the pain response was recorded in seconds. The mean and standard error were calculated as well as the student's "t" test.[31]

The Results and Discussion

Saline-treated mice (controls) exhibited a pain response in 7.9 ± 0.9 seconds (table 10.8, figure 10.8). Subcutaneous administration of 250 mg/kg × 2 of whole-plant aloe vera increased the analgesia time to 9.1 ± 0.9 seconds. As a result of the aloe vera, the mice were able to experience the hot plate–induced pain 15.2 ± 1.4 percent greater than controls. Aspirin-treated mice (100 mg/kg × 2) showed a 10.8 ± 1.3 seconds analgesia time, which was 36.7 ± 4.4 percent greater than that of the controls. However, when the aloe vera and aspirin were combined, the analgesia response (seconds) was increased to 16.1 ± 0.8 ($P<0.001$). This response represented a 102.5 ± 5.2 percent increase over saline controls in analgesia time. Furthermore, the combined response of aloe and aspirin was synergistic, meaning the combined response was greater than the

ALOE VERA INFLUENCE ON THE ANALGESIA RESPONSE OF ASPIRIN

	DOSE	ANALGESIA	
	(MG/KGx2)	TIME (SEC.)	%INC.
SALINE	-	7.9 ± 0.9	-
ALOE VERA	250	9.1 ± 0.9	15.2 ± 1.4
ASPIRIN	100	10.8 ± 1.3	36.7 ± 4.4
COMBINATION	250+100	16.1 ± 0.8	$102.5 \pm 5.2^{*}$

12 MICE/GROUP $\pm$ = S.E. $^{*}P < 0.001$

Table 10.8.

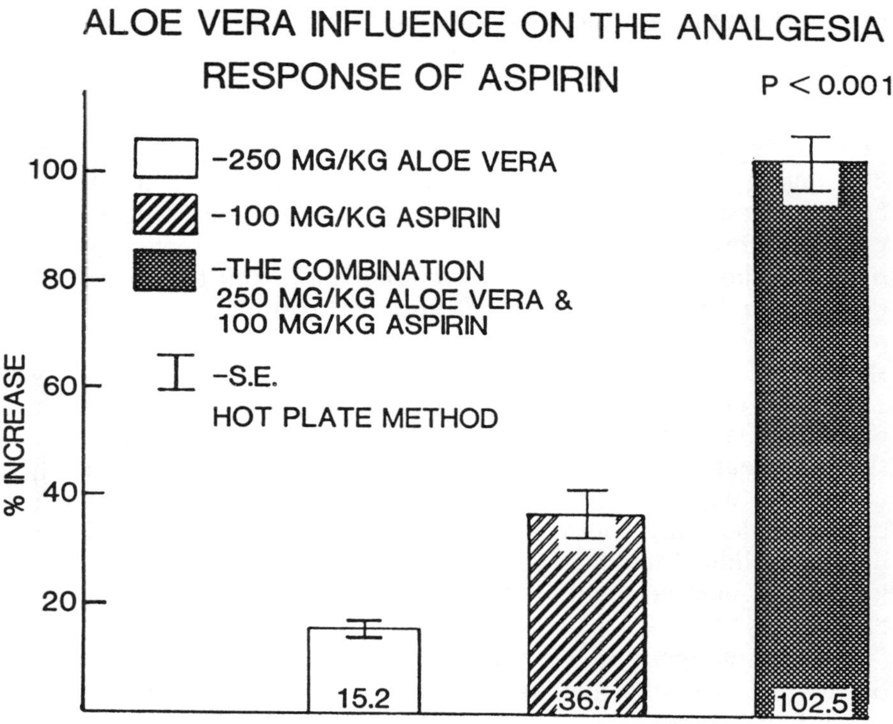

ALOE VERA INFLUENCE ON THE ANALGESIA
RESPONSE OF ASPIRIN
P < 0.001
% INCREASE
100
80
60
40
20
-250 MG/KG ALOE VERA
-100 MG/KG ASPIRIN
-THE COMBINATION
250 MG/KG ALOE VERA &
100 MG/KG ASPIRIN
-S.E.
HOT PLATE METHOD
15.2
36.7
102.5

Fig. 10.8.

sum of both the aspirin and aloe. This synergistic response on analgesia proves that aloe vera is a good vehicle for aspirin. Either aloe vera increased the availability of aspirin to the tissues or the combined analgesic activity united to produce a greater response than the sum of each. Possibly both factors are involved in the synergistic response. An analgesic dose-response curve for aspirin shows that aspirin given without aloe vera produced only a 35.4 percent increase in analgesia over saline controls and the 300 mg/kg dose yielded a 59.5 percent increase (figure 10.9). In fact, we estimate that a dose greater than 450 mg/kg of aspirin would be required to produce a maximum analgesia response. This dosage relationship shows how much aloe vera can reduce the amount of aspirin administered. An attempt was made to alter the dosages of the combination, but to do this the design would have to be changed. Also, in this study an attempt was made to increase the time factor, but here again, the design of the study would have to be altered.

Aloe vera can increase the analgesic activity of aspirin by: protecting its half-life in the blood; increasing its availability to the tissues; increasing its mechanism of action; and synergistically combining with the analgesic activity of aspirin. This achievement can alleviate a large number of side effects of aspirin and have tremendous clinical significance. The amount of aspirin needed to eliminate pain must be multiplied many times to ensure its delivery to the tissues.

S. Grisola reported that salicylate is rapidly distributed throughout the extra-cellular matrixes of the body, but its concentration is *cut* in half in most tissues of the body.[32] This reduction in salicylate concentration makes it necessary to increase the aspirin dosage, which produces side effects. The synergistic effect we observed with Aloe vera would maintain tissue concentration, increase the analgesic response of aspirin, and thus provide a major vehicle tool for medicine in dealing with pain and inflammation. The work of Pedersen shows that orally administered aspirin gave systemic bioavailability at a range of 46 to 51 percent of single oral doses up to 1,300 mg.[33] Somewhere above 450 mg/kg an analgesic plateau is reached where further increases in dosages produce no further increase in response. A possible cause for this finding is that leukotriene B_4, in conjunction with a substance released by polymorphonuclear leukocytes, sensitizes the pain receptors. Leukotrienes play a role in the attracting of polymorphonuclear leukocytes to an injury site.

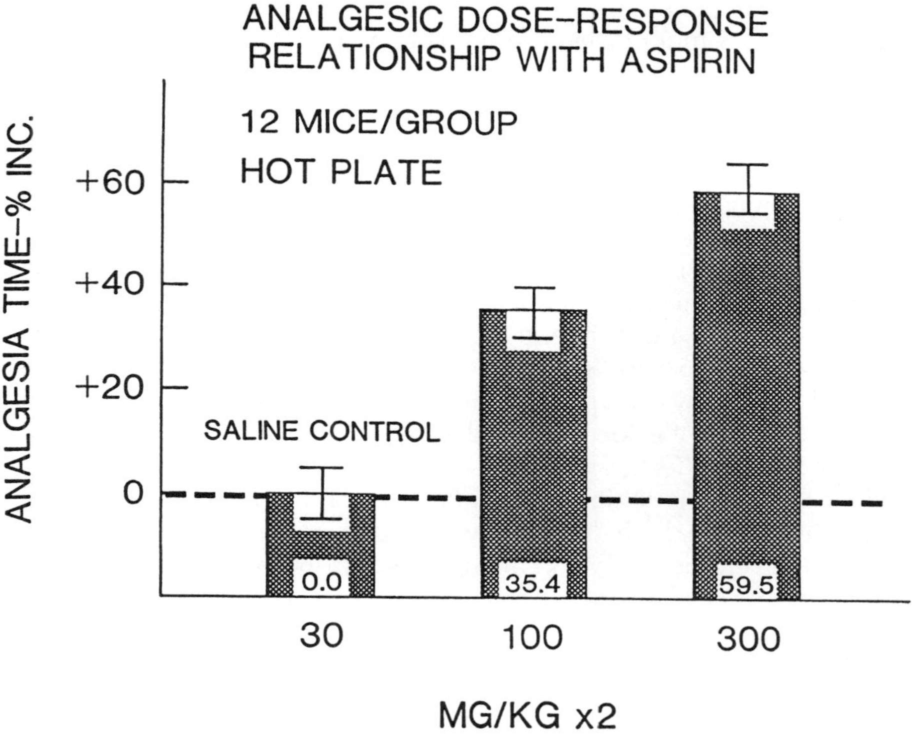
ANALGESIC DOSE–RESPONSE
RELATIONSHIP WITH ASPIRIN
12 MICE/GROUP
HOT PLATE
ANALGESIA TIME–% INC.
+60
+40
+20
0
SALINE CONTROL
0.0
35.4
59.5
30
100
300
MG/KG x2

Fig. 10.9.

The reduction in analgesic activity of aspirin with time is proportional to increased temperature. Thus, in fever, this effect must receive consideration. However, we have shown that aloe vera reduces temperature and improves aspirin's pharmacological effect in lowering body temperature. We feel that the vehicle effect of aloe vera with aspirin is multi-faceted in influencing pain, inflammation, and toxicity.

Aspirin-like drugs act as analgesics peripherally by blocking the generation of impulses at the receptors for pain.[34] Prostaglandins and other products of cyclo-oxygenation of arachidonic acid mediate inflammation, vasodilation, and pain. Aspirin inhibits cyclo-oxygenase activity and thereby decreases prostaglandin synthesis and free radical generation. Prostaglandins sensitize pain receptors to mechanical and chemical stimulation, and its synthesis is inhibited by aspirin. Aspirin also has a central anti-algesic action as well as a peripheral one (figures 10.6 and 10.7). If prostaglandin is released within the central nervous system, parallel to its release at the inflammatory site, it will enhance the local hyperalgesia. In this case, aspirin would have a central effect as well as a local one.[35] In fact, aspirin can act within the brain to inhibit acute inflammation in the periphery. Aloe vera given at very high doses showed no central nervous effect. However, aloe vera does have an analgesic effect in normal and diabetic animals.[36] Since aloe blocks irritant induced edema, one could speculate that its analgesic effect is by way of inhibiting prostaglandin. However, this mechanism of action of aloe vera needs to be worked out. In any event, aloe vera synergistically enhances the analgesic response of aspirin. Aspirin with aloe vera may be a fundamental way to prevent problems before they occur.

Summary

Aspirin prevents heart attacks, stroke, blockage of blood vessels, and inflammation seen in rheumatic fever and rheumatoid arthritis. Mediators released from tissue such as prostaglandin, histamine, and bradykinin produce inflammation and pain. Aspirin blocks these compounds to block inflammation and pain. It blocks prostaglandin synthesis as a mechanism of action. The large dose of aspirin needed to produce a biological response produces stomach irritation. Aloe vera given with aspirin increases the biological activity and absorption of aspirin such that the aspirin dose can be reduced. This decreases aspirin toxicity. The topical biological activity of aloe vera was additive with aspirin on reducing topical croton oil edema. A value of 69.2 percent was recorded, which is a maximum value for the assay. Also, aloe vera given with aspirin subcutaneously was additive on inhibiting carrageenan-induced paw edema. The 2 percent carrageenan was designed to inhibit biological anti-inflammatory activity. An analgesic dose-response curve was presented for aloe vera between 5 and 50 mg/kg. The reduction of pain was achieved by blocking bradykinin and prostaglandin. When aspirin was given with aloe vera to inhibit pain, a synergistic analgesic response between the two was recorded. These data prove that aloe vera enhances the analgesic and anti-inflammatory activity of aspirin and is a good vehicle for salicylates. The dose of aspirin can be reduced to get the therapeutic effect with reduced toxicity.

References

1. G. Weissmann, "Aspirin," *Scientific American,* January 1991, 84.
2. D. Schoonmaker, "The Amazing Power of Aspirin," *Men's Health* 7 (1991): 1.
3. P. E. Schindler, *Aspirin Therapy* (New York: Waller, 1978).
4. T. Thompson, "Taking Aspirin Seriously," *The Remedy Report,* Sept. 1992, 25.
5. H. Dreser, "The Pharmacology of Aspirin," *Pflugers Archives of Gestalt Physiology,* 1899.
6. J. R. Vane, "Inhibition of Prostaglandin Synthesis as a Mechanism of Action for Aspirin-like Drugs," *Nature* 231 (1971): 232.
7. R. H. Davis, J. M. Kabbani, and N. P. Maro, "Aloe Vera and Inflammation," *Proceedings of the Pennsylvania Academy Science* 60 (1990): 67.
8. J. B. West, *Best and Taylor's Physiological Basis of Medical Practice,* 12th ed. (Baltimore: Williams and Wilkins, 1990).
9. S. B. Abramson and G. Weissmann, "The Mechanisms of Action of Non-Steroidal Anti-Inflammatory Drugs," *Arthritis and Rheumatism* 32 (1989): 1.
10. A. Vaananen and M. Hannuksela, "UVB Erythema Inhibited by Topically Applied Substances," *Acta. Dermatological Venereology (Stockh.)* 69 (1989): 12.
11. S. H. Ferreira and J. R. Vane, "New Aspects of the Mode of Action of Nonsteroid Anti-Inflammatory Drugs," *Annual Reviews of Pharmacology* 14 (1974): 57; B. Halliwell, J. R. Hoult, and D. R. Blake, "Oxidant, Inflammation and Anti-Inflammation Drugs," *Federation of the American Society Experimental Biology* 2 (1988): 2874.
12. Davis, Kabbani, and Maro, "Aloe Vera," 667.
13. Schindler, *Aspirin Therapy.*
14. H. Z. Movat, *Inflammation, Immunity and Hypersensitivity,* 2d ed. (New York: Harper and Row, 1979).

15. Helliwell, Hoult, and Blake, "Oxidant, Inflammation and Anti-Inflammation Drugs," 2874.
16. R. H. Davis, W. L. Parker, and D. P. Murdoch, "Aloe Vera as a Biologically Active Vehicle for Hydrocortisone Acetate," *Journal of the American Podiatric Medical Association* 81 (1991): 1.
17. K. Swingle, M. Reitner, and D. Schwartzmiller, "Comparison of Croton Oil and Cantharidin-Induced Inflammation of the Mouse Ear and Their Modification by Topically Applied Drugs," *Archives of International Pharmacodynamic Therapy* 254 (1981): 168.
18. Abramson and Weissman, "The Mechanisms of Action," 1.
19. A Catina, A. Macaluso, A. Hietz, and J. M. Lipton, "Inhibition of Acute Inflammation in the Periphery by Central Action of Salicylates," *Proceedings of the Society of the Natural Academy* 88 (1991): 8544.
20. Schndler, *Aspirin Therapy.*
21. Thompson, "Taking Aspirin Seriously," 25.
22. A. C. Guyton, *Textbook of Medical Physiology,* 8th ed., (Philadelphia: W. B. Saunders, 1991).
23. Ferreira and Vane, "New Aspects," 57.
24. G. G. Graham, "Pharmacokinetics and Metabolism of Non-Steroidal Anti-Inflammatory Drugs," *Medical Journal of Australia* 147 (1987): 597.
25. Catina, Macaluso, Hietz, and Lipton, "Inhibition of Acute Inflammation," 8544; S. Abramson, H. Korchak, and R. Ludewig, "Modes of Action of Aspirin-like Drugs," *Proceedings of the National Academy of Science* 82 (1985): 7227.
26. C. J. Fu, S.Melethil, and W. D. Mason, "The Pharmacokinetics of Aspirin in Rats and the Effect of Buffer," *Journal of Pharmacokinetics and Biopharmaceutics* 19 (1991): 157.
27. Schindler, *Aspirin Therapy;* Guyton, *Textbook.*
28. S. H. Ferreira, "The Site of Analgesic Action of Aspirin-like Drugs and Opioids," in R. F. Beers and E. G. Bassett, *Mechanism of Pain and Analgesic Compounds* (New York: Raven Press, 1979).
29. Ferreira and Vane, "New Aspects," 57.
30. Ibid.
31. Vaananen and Hannuksela, "UVB Erythema," 12.
32. S. Grisola, "Inactivation of Enzymes by Therapeutic Concentration of Aspirin and Salicylates," *Nature* 223 (1969): 80.
33. A. K. Pedersen and G. A. Fitzgerald, "Dose-Related Kinetics of Aspirin," *New Jersey Medical Association* 311 (1984): 1206.
34. Catina, Macaluso, Heitz, and Lipton, "Inhibition of Acute Inflammation," 8544.
35. Ferreira and Vane, "New Aspects," 57.
36. R. H. Davis, J. M. Russo, and M. G. Leitner, "Aloe Vera: A Natural Approach for Treating Wounds, Edema and Pain in Diabetes," *Journal of the American Podiatric Medical Association* 78 (1988): 60.

11

Biological Standardization of Aloe Vera

Our efforts to establish a reliable unit for aloe vera standardization have centered on the results of biological assay. The biological assay results demonstrate the therapeutic possibilities of aloe vera as a whole as well as the effectiveness of substances in aloe on living animals or tissues. When one fractionates active components in aloe vera, the biological assay can be used to help characterize over two hundred biologically active agents in the plant. These components do not act in a random fashion, but they unite and synergize in a specific beneficial way. Adulteration of aloe products is a major concern for the aloe industry. Adulteration occurs by adding maltodextrin or simply diluting aloe with water. In fact, some have just added preservatives to water and call it aloe vera. These practices mislead the consumer and cost the industry a great deal of money each year due to a lack of confidence in aloe vera. Leaders in the aloe industry have a responsibility to encourage purity of aloe vera, which will project a great credibility to the industry. When aloe vera is pure, the consumer will know it and have confidence in aloe. The biological assay can evaluate how genuine (standardization) the aloe vera really is.

Purpose of This Work

1. To describe various biological assays that can be used by the industry to standardize aloe vera and its fractions. Every effort must be employed to obtain a biological reference standard to define an aloe unit so as to evaluate the activity of aloe vera obtained from different sources and manufacturing processes. The reference standard can be made available

to the IASC and the major companies involved in the research and development of aloe vera. The biological assays will be presented with some specific detail so that they can be used by the industry to evaluate the aloe vera. These results can be correlated with chemical evaluations. Some consideration will be given to chemical standardization, but the main consideration will be given to the biological assay.

2. To discuss the "aloe vera molecule" (the polysaccharide) as it relates to the standardization of aloe and its relationship to the many active agents functioning around the polysaccharide. The "conductor-orchestra" concept plays a major role in the biological activity of aloe vera. How the various orchestra players synergize around the conductor will contribute to the potency of the reference standard and the definition of the aloe unit.
3. To present aloe vera's most up-to-date mechanism of action as it relates to such things as wound healing, inflammation, analgesia, etc. Concepts about growth factors, mediators, oxygen radicals, modulation, tissue repair, and inflammation will receive some attention, because aloe vera involves these mechanisms in its therapeutic influence.

Biological Assay for Aloe Vera

In the in vivo assay, aloe vera is tested in the living organism and its biological activity (effectiveness) is assessed among a variety of tissues and cells. In other words, the assay is made at the multicellular level in an attempt to model or mimic the human situation. This method of assay is demanded by regulatory agencies for any evaluation of toxicity and efficacy. When aloe is tested outside the organism, its effectiveness is assessed by a limited number of cells and tissues, which is called an in vitro assay. The in vitro assay is less expensive, faster, and more accurate, but the results may be more apparent than real. However, human tissue models have been designed in a number of areas of biological research that have proven to be very valuable. For example, human tissue models have been successfully used to evaluate the absorption of therapeutic agents through the skin.

When biological and chemical assays on aloe vera agree, this is strong evidence for specific aloe vera activity. If the biological assay differs from the chemical method, the difference is not due to error, as the biological method is usually right. This may occur in fractionation work. However, chemical methods may be preferred when available. The best biological, active preparation for anti-inflammation, analgesia, wound healing, immunity, and so on, must be individually obtained for biological standardization. We then can obtain a unit for each activity such that each standard preparation can be called a reference standard. In the process of fractionating aloe vera, unknown fractions can then be compared to the appropriate reference standard. If the unknown becomes more active than the reference standard, it becomes the new reference standard. Accurate biological assays are possible only when the active principle is identical with the active principle of the unknown preparation compared with it. The slopes of each dose-response curve must be parallel in order to make a comparison of biological activity.

The sensitivity of a biological assay is defined as the smallest amount of aloe vera that produces a specific biological response. The accuracy of an assay refers to the variation in the response to aloe vera with each increasing dose of aloe. At some dose, the response reaches a plateau in which increasing the aloe dose does not produce a further increase in response. The length and slope of the dose-response curve will be specific for each biological activity in aloe vera and will determine how well one can assay each biological activity in aloe vera. Our experience with most of the dose-response curves for the different therapeutic activities in aloe vera suggests that each curve can be used to explore the depths of aloe vera.

Biological Error of an Assay

The best way to estimate biological error is to repeat a measurement several times to see if the results agree with each other. Whenever a measurement is repeated many times, an amount of variation will occur that is characteristic for that certain biological activity. The larger the number of measurements, the smaller the variation responsible for most of the error. A mean value is recorded by making a number of measurements in an assay and obtaining an added total of the measurements that can be divided by the number of observations. How the individual values disperse around the mean value is called the standard deviation. If the variance of a large number of samples in aloe vera is obtained, one can record the standard error. However, the estimated standard error can be obtained from a random sample, so that we can compare population values instead of sample values. We can obtain for aloe vera's biological activity a 95 percent or 99 percent confidence limit. That is, if we did 100 experiments with aloe vera, we could expect the true result to occur, within a certain limit, 95 or 99 times out of the 100 experiments. If the biologist determines the biological response of an aloe vera sample for anti-inflammation, wound healing, analgesia, or immunity, it is impossible to "fool" a certification agency as to whether or not the preparation is aloe or a fraudulent substance that looks like aloe vera. One cannot "mimic" the sensitivity, slope, and plateau of a dose-response curve for a specific activity of aloe vera. Thus a well-defined unit of specific aloe vera activity provides a good standardization for aloe vera.

Monitoring of Aloe Vera for Fraudulent Products

The IASC has been given the job of making sure that what is sold in the marketplace is really the true aloe that the producer says it is. They provide valuable information and advice on how to process aloe. The IASC encourages developing methods of standardization and identification as well as exploring aloe vera for its active components. Our laboratory has obtained good dose-response curves on the major end points of aloe's biological activity. These assays can measure (standardize) as well as determine the absence of aloe in a preparation. The slope of the biological dose-response curve is a precise value that can act as a "fingerprint" for aloe vera and its fractions. We therefore feel we can obtain a reference standard with a defined unit for each biological activity. The various companies could process their aloe vera in different ways and compare them with the reference standard to determine the strength or units of aloe vera. The reference aloe standard could also be used to evaluate fractionated samples from aloe vera. This assumes that the slopes of the dose-response curves are similar. The slope of the curve must not be too steep or too flat. The bioassay must be fast, simple, and accurate. Aloe vera can be standardized and used to monitor aloe vera using the bioassay.

A Proposed Chemical-Biological Assessment of Aloe Vera Being Considered by the Science Committee of the IASC

A. Percent Polysaccharide in Aloe Vera—the Alcohol Precipitation of Polysaccharide from Aloe; Phenol Sulfuric Acid Colorimetric Method for Carbohydrate Determination.

The total percent polysaccharide method was conceived by D. C. Gowda of India[1] and modified by R. P. Pelley of the University of Texas Medical Branch, Galveston.[2] The aloe vera gel is composed of polysaccharide, which can be precipitated with ethanol followed by centrifugation to separate alcohol-soluble materials. The phenol-sulfuric acid method for determining carbohydrates is known as the Dubois assay. It accurately determines the amount of polysaccharide hexose present in the precipitate. R. Pelley, Y. T. Wang, and T. A. Waller assayed the polysaccharide content of commercial samples of aloe and found that samples were adulterated with maltodextrin.[3] The chemical characteristics of aloe polysaccharide are different from those of non-aloe polysaccharide. A large number of companies have implemented the Pelley percentage polysaccharide assay in their laboratories. This method provides a standard by which to purify and characterize molecules in aloe vera. At present, some laboratories are using total solids, calcium, magnesium, and the HPLC profile ("E peak"). While these methods are valuable, the percent polysaccharide presents a reliable indicator to detect "fake aloe vera."

B. Micrograms of Glucose per Milligram of Solid

We propose to use μg of glucose/mg solid of aloe vera as an activity criteria assessment for aloe. Also, the ratio of μg glucose/mg solid to the percent polysaccharide presents a ratio that is very difficult to mimic by someone attempting to adulterate aloe. Samples of the aloe leaf were taken at constant intervals from the leaf tip to the base and the amount of aloe vera increased in a straight-line fashion over the entire leaf. The slope, least squares, and "no evidence of plateau" make this aloe leaf assay ideal to evaluate plant production of aloe. We have shown that the wind could increase the production of aloe in the leaf some 2300 percent. The control leaf had a relative glucose of 7.7±0.4 μg/mg of solid.

In our opinion, assaying the amount of glucose (μg) per mg of solid presents a good estimate of the amount of aloe vera in the leaf, and it seems to agree with the biological activity of aloe vera. The relative glucose of a leaf exposed to wind was 10.5±0.7 μg glucose/mg solid. Our results seem to indicate that we can assay the amount of aloe vera by using the specific activity of glucose. The increase in leaf production by 2300 percent of aloe gel by wind corresponds somewhat with the increase in specific activity of glucose. The amount of aloe gel and the amount of glucose seem to increase as one goes from the tip of the leaf to the leaf base. Our studies demonstrated that this nourishment is carried toward the center of the plant by long tubes from vascular bundles to the "pup leaves" in the center of the plant. Wind moves the leaves and causes the gel to move inward. We once thought that mucilage moved aloe from the rind to the other parts of the leaf. Now we know that the wind moves the leaves and provides the momentum to move the gel inward. Increasing the movement appears to increase the production of aloe vera. Mucilage consists of long chain polysaccharides that act as a container for the enclosed gel fillet found in the large parenchyma cells that store water and large amounts of carbohydrate.

C. The Croton Oil–Induced Ear-Swelling Assay

Swingle showed that non-steroidal drugs can block the inflammation induced by croton oil, which is a very strong dermal irritant that produces vasodilation, PMN infiltration, and intercellular edema.[4] Non-steroidal agents block this vascular inflammation.

The assay is accurate, specific, reproducible, rapid, predictable, and easy to operate. We have improved the sensitivity and accuracy of the older croton oil–induced edema assays by using a 6 mm biopsy punch specimen. Adult male mice were given 25 μg/10ul croton oil topically to the outer and inner surface of each animal's right ear, while the left ear was not treated and used as a control. Control mice were given croton oil alone on their right ear. Treated animals had specific whole-leaf aloe applied to the top of the croton oil, in doses ranging from 20 to 1,800 micrograms, thirty minutes after the croton oil application. Six hours later, a 6 mm punch specimen was taken from the right and left ear. The specimens were weighed on a pan balance and the weight differences were compared to determine the amount of inflammation remaining on the right ear. Figure 11.1 shows a dose-response curve with a good slope and a large area on which we can assay small amounts of aloe vera. The coefficient of standard error variation is about 12 percent, which is a rough index of experimental error, and we estimate the plateau of the dose-response curve to be around 80 percent inhibition of edema. At small doses, steroids can push the response to 95 percent inhibition. This assay is one of the most accurate topical anti-inflammatory assays developed and should be ideal for "breaking down" aloe vera (figure 11.1).

The croton oil–induced edema assay revealed that processed aloe inhibited inflammation as well as fresh aloe. When aloe vera was administered orally (100 mg/kg per day), it progressively reduced edema from 25.0 percent on day 7 to 51.9 percent on day 21.[5] Aloe vera has a unique biological property in that it can reduce inflammation and improve wound healing as well. Steroids, on the other hand, inhibit inflammation but also inhibit wound healing. We feel that aloe vera can synergize with hydrocortisone to reduce inflammation and can block hydrocortisone's wound-healing inhibition. Aloe vera reduces acute inflammation but has no effect on chronic inflammation.

When fractions of aloe vera are assayed for topical anti-inflammatory activity, we frequently assay at about 100 μg dosage. However, the small variance characteristic of this assay permits us to go even lower in dosage. Some anti-inflammatory agents (the polysaccharide) reach a maximum response and then take a "nose-dive" on the dose-response curve. This response of polysaccharides is probably due to the release of interleukins that cause inflammation. This kind of response is not recorded by the whole-leaf aloe vera. This "dropoff" at the top of the dose-response curve is characteristic of many fine anti-inflammatory agents. Figure 11.2 shows the topical

ANTI-INFLAMMATORY ACTIVITY OF WHOLE PLANT ALOE IN THE CROTON OIL-INDUCED EAR SWELLING ASSAY

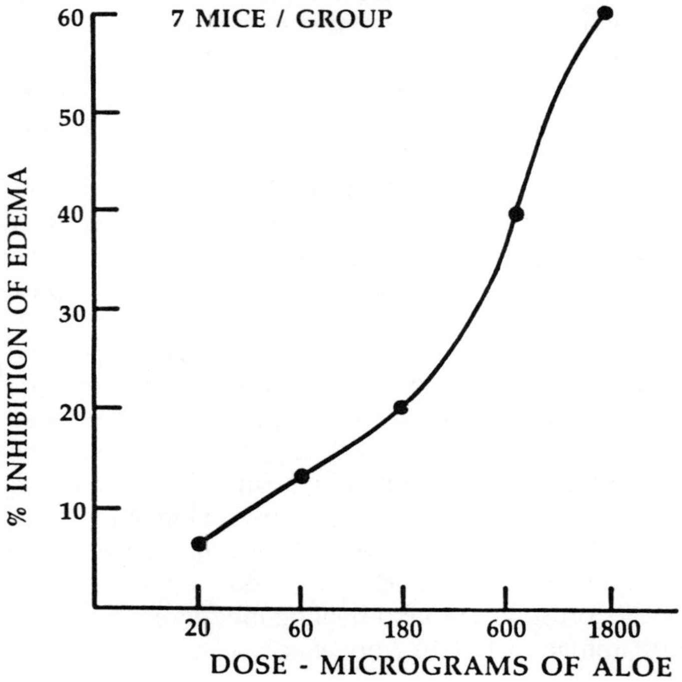

Fig. 11.1.

TOPICAL ANTI-INFLAMMATORY ASSAY OF LIQUID WHOLE LEAF ALOE GEL (LOT 920801) AND BRAND X ALOE VERA JUICE AT 600 MICROGRAMS AGAINST CROTON OIL INDUCED EDEMA.

	LIQUID WHOLE LEAF ALOE GEL (920801)	BRAND X ALOE VERA JUICE
% INHIBITION	46.1 ± 4.9 **	8.4 ± 0.4 *
% SOLID (TOTAL)	1.4	0.3

* Not Significantly Different From Controls (P greater than 0.05).
** Significant Inhibition From Controls (P less than 0.001).

Fig. 11.2.

anti-inflammatory assay of liquid whole-leaf aloe gel and a brand X aloe vera juice assayed at 600μg against croton oil–induced edema. The percent inhibition of liquid whole-leaf aloe gel was 46.1±4.9 which is about right on the dose-response curve where it belongs. However, brand X aloe vera juice was only 8.4±0.4 percent inhibition, which is not significantly different from the control value. Also, the percent total solid for the whole-leaf aloe gel was 1.4, as compared to 0.3 for brand X. The value for brand X represents just preservative and is truly "fake aloe vera." We have assayed a few samples of suspected aloe and have obtained the same results as now reported. We have also assayed aloe of different quality and have been able to make the proper assessment of biological activity. A "unit" of aloe vera using this method has been tentatively defined as that amount of aloe vera that can inhibit croton oil–induced edema 30 percent.

Mechanism of Action of Aloe Vera

Aloe vera contains growth factors that will improve wound healing and repair. It also contains components that will inhibit pain (aspirin-like compounds) and inflammation (amino acids and sterols). Aloe vera by means of components such as growth factors can stimulate fibroblasts to produce collagen and proteoglycans that increase wound tensile strength. The newly formed collagen forms bonds between the margins of wounds to increase the wound tensile strength. If aloe increases tensile strength, it is assumed that the collagen production is also increased. When skin is injured, fibroblasts migrate into the wound to produce collagen and proteoglycans that form the ground substance that holds the collagen fibers together. The collagen acts as steel girders in the proteoglycans' "cement."

The "Danhof response" of aloe vera on the uptake of tritiated thymidine represents an increase in fibroblast numbers but not necessarily a functional increase in collagen or proteoglycans.[6] This response may only be an anatomical but not a functional influence of aloe vera. The measurement of tensile strength is a functional end point. Cells in the wound area communicate with each other by growth factors that stimulate the IGF receptor to produce collagen and proteoglycans to increase tensile strength. Collagen, like aloe, has large complex chains of modified sugars that form the framework for collagen. The proteoglycans form around the collagen and hold water, which gives connective tissue the flexibility and strength necessary for wound healing. Connective tissue can be formed only if the necessary sugars and amino acids are stimulated by the fibroblast to improve wound healing. Aloe vera can stimulate macrophages, which can inhibit inflammation and, at the same time, stimulate fibroblasts to cause wound repair. This is a wonderful effect of aloe vera not seen by any other biological agent that we are aware of.

The many components in aloe vera make it possible to attack a wide variety of irritants, injuries, and insults. We have shown that certain amino acids such as phenylalanine and tryptophan inhibit gelatin-induced inflammation.[7] Aloe vera prevents and regresses adjuvant-induced arthritis with its inflammation.[8] We were able to measure the immune arthritis as well as the inflammation response. Both of these end points were inhibited by aloe vera. Some twenty amino acids are present in aloe vera. Approximately half of the amino acids were shown to have topical and/or systemic anti-inflammatory activity.[9] They include: tryptophan, phenylalanine, alanine, cystine, hydroxyproline, citrulline, and valine, to mention a few. Some amino acids influence survival and liver glycogen deposition of cortisone-maintained adrenalectomized rats.[10] Since both of these biological functions are properties of adrenal steroids, which are known to exhibit anti-inflammatory activity, the possibility exists that amino acids mimic these anti-inflammatory effects. Some of these amino acids were shown to inhibit gelatin-induced abdominal inflammation using peritoneal fluid cytology as the diagnostic tool. Dipeptide of some of these amino acids was also anti-inflammatory.[11] One wonders if aloe vera could inhibit the inflammation within the peritoneal cavity found in women. Inflammation of the abdominal cavity is a major problem in women, especially after menopause.[12]

Aloe vera stimulates fibroblast growth in wound healing but shows no anti-fibrosis activity, suggesting that it does not act like a steroid. The infiltration of PMNs induced by irritants can be blocked by aloe vera, suggesting that it inhibits leukotrienes.[13] Croton oil, a strong irritant, was used to show that aloe vera has oral and topical anti-inflammatory activity. Irritants can release vasoactive substances from mast cells, which cause vasodilation and edema. Prostaglandins and histamine are examples of mediators released by irritants. We used kaolin, carrageenan, albumin, dextran, and mustard to produce acute inflammation.[14] Aloe was especially active against gelatin (76.9 percent inhibition) and kaolin (61.8 percent) but was less active against dextran (22.7 percent). The wide variety of irritants tested helped us to characterize the activity of aloe vera (figure 11.3). Each of the irritants work through a different biochemical pathway to produce inflammation. The fact that aloe vera inhibits inflammation of these different irritants to a different degree says something about "how aloe works." Aloe's many components attack many irritants in various ways.

Oxygen radicals, produced by PMNs, damage tissue and produce inflammation. PMNs also produce mediators that work with oxidants to establish inflammation and encourage the recruitment of inflammatory cells. Aloe vera influences oxygen radical and mediator production. When challenged to phagocytosis, the PMN exhibits a burst of oxygen consumption. They produce several oxygen radicals that have bactericidal activity[15] and are highly reactive. They are generated by PMNs during phagocytic activity at sites of acute inflammation. While free radicals have beneficial anti-bacterial activity, they can further insult vascular endothelium and other tissues. Oxygen radicals have been implicated in phospholipid membrane damage, connective tissue and synovial fluid degradation, increased vascular permeability, and cell death. The influence of aloe vera on inflammation and arthritis can be explained in the light of what we know about oxygen radicals produced by phagocytic cells.

The complexity of aloe vera's components makes the study of its anti-inflammatory activity a difficult task, yet several points can be discussed with regard to mechanisms. Aloe vera does not have a single mechanism of action. Aloe vera contains amino acids that have anti-inflammatory activity,[16] and the salicyclic acid in aloe prevents the biosynthesis of prostaglandins from arachidonic acid. This explains, in part, how aloe reduces vasodilation and decreases the vascular effects of histamine, serotonin, and other mediators of inflammation.

Since prostaglandins play an integral role in regulating both inflammatory and immune reactions, aloe vera can affect both of these systems by blocking prostaglandin synthesis. Aloe also contains bradykinase, which breaks down bradykinin, a vasodilator, and at the same time influences angiotensin, a potent vasoconstrictor.

% INHIBITION OF COLORIZED ALOE VERA (150 mg/kg)
ON 2% IRRITANT-INDUCED EDEMA IN RATS

	% INHIBITION BY ALOE
GELATIN	76.9
KAOLIN	61.8
ALBUMIN	55.9
CARRAGEENAN	55.8
MUSTARD	44.2
DEXTRAN	22.7

10 ANIMALS/GROUP ( ) = % INHIBITION

Fig. 11.3.

Both stimulatory and inhibitory components have been identified in aloe, which means that aloe can act as a modulator of both immune and inflammatory reactions. Aloe vera has been shown to have an immune-suppressive action in adjuvant-induced arthritis.[17] On the other hand, aloe can also act as a stimulator of wound healing and antibody production[18] as well as acting as a prostaglandin blocker. Aloe acts as an immune-modulator by influencing the production of lymphocyte- and macrophage-derived mediators (lymphokinins), including migration inhibitory factor, interleukins, and interferon.[19]

Besides aloe's effects on inflammatory and immune reactions, it is likely that it also acts as a scavenger of free oxygen radicals. Vitamin C in aloe has both a topical and systemic influence against the inflammation seen in adjuvant arthritis.[20] The vitamin C probably "picks up" or scavenges oxygen radicals to reduce inflammation. It has long been recognized that vitamin E, a known anti-oxidant, is a component of aloe vera. Catalase has also been identified in aloe, which, as already described, catalyzes the conversion of H_2O_2 to H_2O and O_2.[21]

The aloe vera molecule is a conductor that leads a symphony of biologically active components. The protein at one end directs the polysaccharide chain into the insulin-like growth factor receptor of the fibroblast. The mannose phosphate at the other end is the effector that fits into the receptor to stimulate the fibroblast to function (make collagen and proteoglycans).

However, in this union with the fibroblast or macrophage the aloe vera molecule leads an orchestra of compounds that synergize with each other to produce a symphony of biological therapeutic effects.

The Analgesic Dose-Response Curve for Aloe Vera

Aloe vera has analgesic as well as wound-healing and anti-inflammatory activity. It reduces pain by blocking the synthesis of bradykinin and prostaglandin. Pain-inducing stimuli such as trauma, immunoglobulins, and oxygen radicals convert membrane phospholipid into arachidonic acid. Our previous work with aloe vera and hydrocortisone suggests that aloe vera blocks the formation of arachidonic acid and prostaglandin.

To demonstrate, mice were given 5, 15, 50, and 300 mg/kg aloe subcutaneously each day for four days, while control mice were injected with distilled water on the basis of 10 ml/kg. Six hours after the injections on day 4, we placed the mice on a hot plate set at 48°C and noted that their pain response was characterized by the animals licking their front paws (praying hands response) or lifting their back feet. The time required for the pain response was recorded in seconds. Aqueous controls exhibited a pain response in 5.3 seconds. Subcutaneous administration of 5 mg/Kg × 4 of aloe increased analgesia to 6.7 seconds—a 26 percent increase. A 15 mg/kg aloe dose increased the time to 8.3 seconds, or a 57 percent increase. A 50 mg/kg and 200 mg/kg aloe dose increased the time on the hot plate to 11.3 seconds, or a 112 percent increase (figure 11.4).

Our results indicate a dose-response relationship of aloe vera on analgesia as the responses climbed with an increase in the aloe concentration. The maximum plateau response of 112 percent occurred at 50 and 200 mg/kg. The curve exhibits a good slope and a dose range from 5 to 50 mg/kg upon which to assay unknown aloe vera samples or fractions. We should note that high doses of aloe vera showed no central nervous effect, so the analgesic response is likely peripheral rather than central involving prostaglandin. Aloe vera provides a major vehicle tool for medicine in dealing with pain and inflammation. Aloe's action mechanism regarding analgesia needs to be worked out through further experiments. However, we do have a method of standardization of aloe vera on analgesia to provide another "fingerprint" of this most complex substance.

Computerized O_2/CO_2 Respirometer (Micro-Oxymax)

Three samples of aloe gel were obtained from a live aloe barbadensis plant, with weights of the samples being one, three, and nine grams, respectively. Each sample was placed in a glass flask, and the temperature of each sample was held constant at 30° C. Oxygen consumption and carbon dioxide production were measured at four-hour intervals. When removed from the plant, the gel was clear. The oxygen rate (μl/min) for one, three, and nine grams of aloe gel was

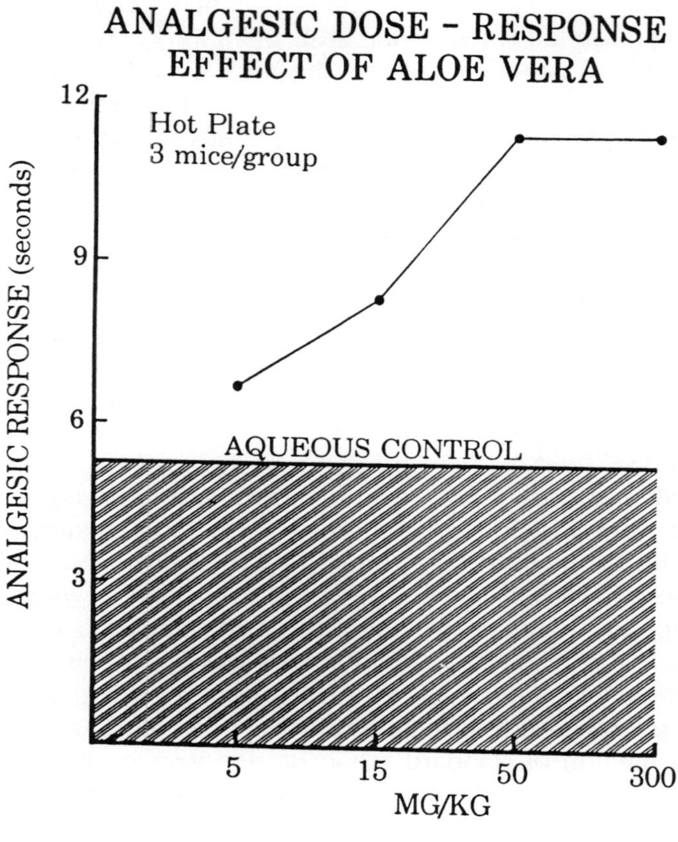
ANALGESIC DOSE - RESPONSE
EFFECT OF ALOE VERA
Hot Plate
3 mice/group
ANALGESIC RESPONSE (seconds)
12
9
6
3
AQUEOUS CONTROL
5
15
50
300
MG/KG

Fig. 11.4.

0.4, 1.1, and 1.8 consumption, while the CO_2 rate (μl/min) production for the same amount of gel was 0.3, 1.1, and 1.8, the oxygen consumption being inverse to the CO_2 production (figure 11.5). The micro-oxymax measures O_2/CO_2 consumption/production in one to eighty measuring chambers using a single set of sensors and has a superior sensitivity over either the old Warburg or the Scholander apparatus. The instrument is fully automated and easy to operate. It is suitable for a wide range of applications for both liquids, solids, and living organisms. The O_2/CO_2 respirometer can be used for bioremediation of oil spills, plants such as aloe, small mammals, fish, insects, bacteria, fungi, and tissue cultures.

The dose-response relationship of aloe gel on oxygen and carbon dioxide rates can be used to measure the microorganism status before, during, and after aloe processing and is much faster than bacteria culturing. The fungus from scalp, feet, and groin that have been treated with aloe vera could utilize the micro-oxymax to see if the aloe treatment was effective. The data thus far seems to suggest that aloe vera modulates phagocytes to control microorganism infections. This procedure is sensitive enough to determine the influence aloe has directly on bacteria and fungus. Possibly the micro-oxymax could give us a tool to deal with the oxidation recorded by the small amounts of aloin present in processed aloe vera. It could help evaluate procedures aimed at removing aloin or assessing the effectiveness of anti-oxidants, such as ascorbic acid, used to "box out" the small amounts of aloin present in aloe vera. The dose-response curves recorded by aloe gel are such that we could easily evaluate the status of aloe quickly after processing.

The Open Wound Assay

We used a 6 mm Baker punch to remove a circular piece of skin from both shaven sides of adult mice. The mice were anesthetized with ether, and a vernier caliper was used to measure diameters as evidence of wound healing. The mice were injected subcutaneously with decolorized aloe at 1.0, 10,and 100 mg/kg for seven days. The controls received aqueous injections on a 10 ml/kg basis. A perfect dose-response curve from 2.36 mm at 1.0 mg/kg was increased to 3.4 mm at 10 mg/kg and 4.33 mm at 100 mg/kg of aloe vera. The

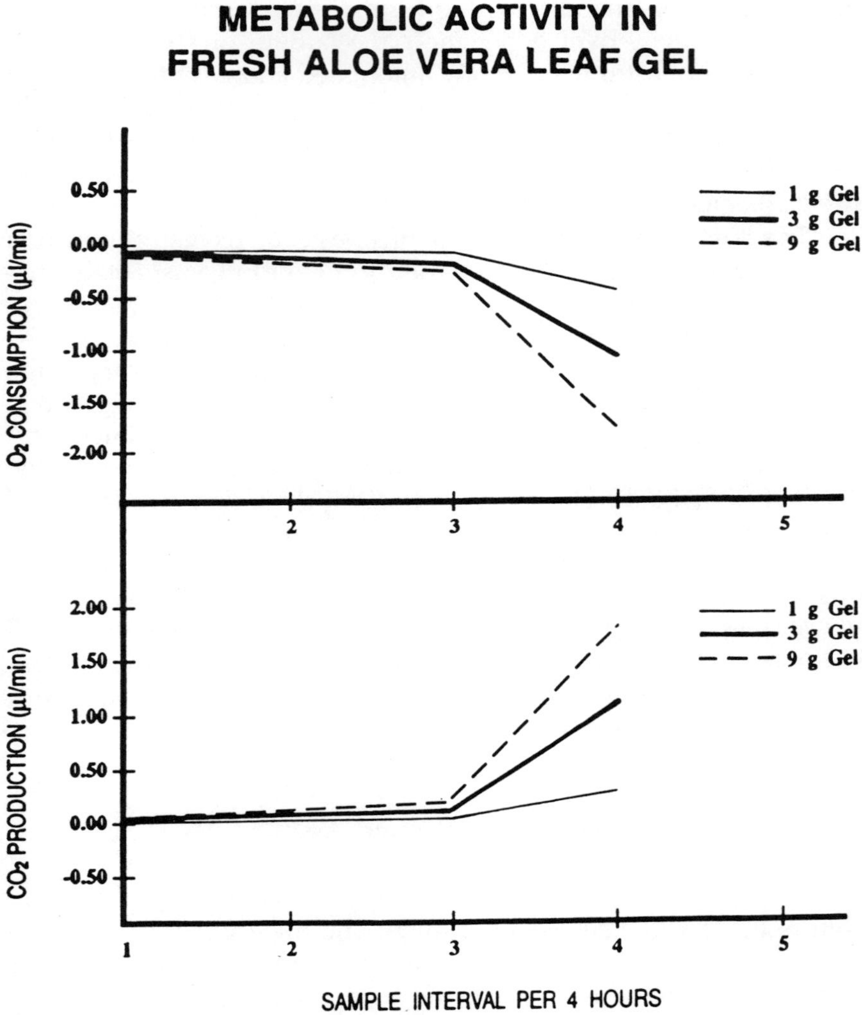
METABOLIC ACTIVITY IN
FRESH ALOE VERA LEAF GEL
0.50
0.00
-0.50
-1.00
-1.50
-2.00
O2 CONSUMPTION (µl/min)
1 g Gel
3 g Gel
9 g Gel
2
3
4
5
2.00
1.50
1.00
0.50
0.00
-0.50
CO2 PRODUCTION (µl/min)
1 g Gel
3 g Gel
9 g Gel
1
2
3
4
5
SAMPLE INTERVAL PER 4 HOURS

Fig. 11.5.

variation in response was almost negligible.[22] We observed that aloe vera, which was colorized, gave no dose-response curve because of the presence of anthraquinones (figure 11.6).

The formula for a straight line may be written as $Y = a + bx$. Y is the response, a is the intercept on Y, x is the dose, and b is the slope of the line. The greater the value of the constant b, the more rapid the increase in the regression line. The slope of the regression line characterizes the aloe or the aloe fraction. The variance of the slope can be calculated and then used to identify aloe. When $Y = X$, the better the slope of the line for biological standardization. Any deviation from this relationship lessens the value of the curve for assaying unknown aloes.

The regression line recorded for the open wound assay is ideal for measuring the wound-healing activity of aloe vera. It has a good slope with a line that best describes the data, and the difference (least squares) between the actual values and the predicted values is very small. The assay is quite sensitive and accurate, and it can be used to assay aloe vera over a wide dose range. This assay agrees well with the wound tensile strength assay. While the open wound assay for wound healing may be a bit more sensitive, the wound tensile strength assay may be more accurate.

We have developed an open wound micro-assay for aloe vera (figure 11.7). Small amounts of aloe vera are administered under the wound cover over four days. The preliminary dose-response curve has a dose range from 30 to about 300 μg. A similar microassay is being developed for the wound tensile strength assay. Microassays are needed when small amounts of aloe fractions are being evaluated.

The Wound Tensile Strength Assay

Adult male Sprague Dawley mice had a one-inch surgical incision placed on their shaven back under ether anesthesia. Each wound was closed with a 9 mm wound clip at quarter-inch spacings, for a total of three fastens per wound. Mice were daily subcutaneously injected for four days starting on the day of surgery at 50 and 200 mg/kg with whole-plant aloe.

Six hours after the four-day injection, the tensile strength of wounds was measured. We injected air into the peritoneal cavity

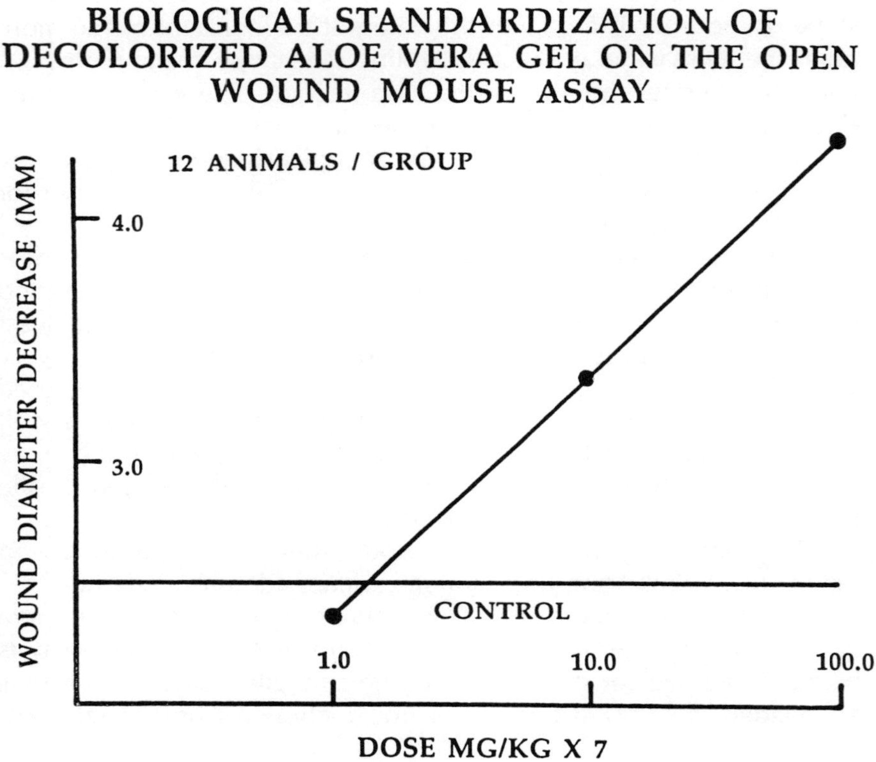
BIOLOGICAL STANDARDIZATION OF DECOLORIZED ALOE VERA GEL ON THE OPEN WOUND MOUSE ASSAY
12 ANIMALS / GROUP
WOUND DIAMETER DECREASE (MM)
4.0
3.0
CONTROL
1.0
10.0
100.0
DOSE MG/KG X 7

Fig. 11.6.

ALOE VERA OPEN WOUND HEALING MICRO - ASSAY

10μl Injections Made Under Scab Daily from Day 1 to 7.
Measure Length on Day 8.

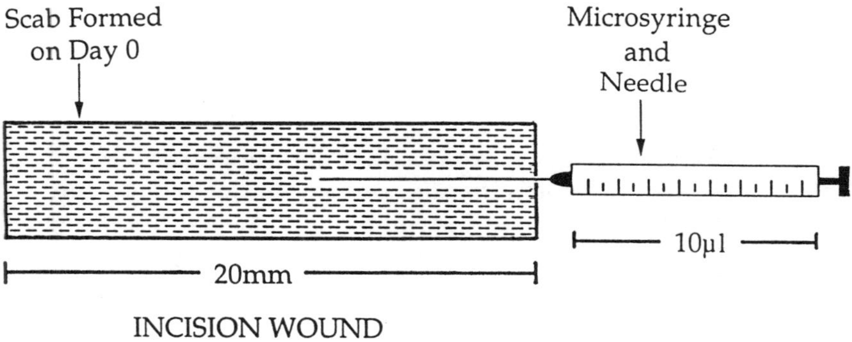

Fig. 11.7.

using a 60 ml syringe with a 22-gauge needle, which was calibrated in millimeters for more precise measurement. The rate of air injection was one mm of air per second until the wound on the animal's back burst or pulled apart.

The air was injected under two conditions:

1. Rubber bands (one-sixteenth inch thick and two-inch diameter) were placed around the neck and anterior to the hind legs to reduce error involving underlying tissue of the peritoneal cavity.
2. When the air was being injected into the abdominal cavity, the animal's skin was pinched closed around the needle to ensure no leakage, and the amount of air injected into the abdominal cavity was recorded. We feel that our newly developed wound tensile strength assay is the most accurate so far developed and can be used to standardize aloe vera regarding wound healing (figure 11.8 and 11.9).

In developing the assay, we obtained the proper time requirements to test for aloe vera tensile strength inducing activity of wounds. We obtained a curve in which aloe vera had room going up the curve to improve tensile strength before reaching the plateau. We considered that the best time to assess the ability of aloe vera to increase wound tensile strength (figures 11.8 and 11.9) was after the surgery on day 4.

We evaluated wound tensile strength over a ten-day period postsurgery and found the tensile strength ranged from 10 mm air on day 3 to a maximum of 35 mm air on day 10 (Figures 11.8 and 11.9). We evaluated the dose-response relationship of aloe vera on wound tensile strength at two days' treatment at 50 and 200 mg/kg and noted that aloe vera increased the wound tensile strength 13.1 and 31.2 percent at 50 and 200 mg/kg over a two-day treatment. The four-day treatment increased the wound tensile strength 6.1 and 61.5 percent, respectively. Based on the postsurgery data, we estimated that aloe vera could possibly increase the wound tensile strength up to 85 percent or more, and we chose the four-day treatment curve as the standardization for aloe vera regarding wound tensile strength (figures 11.8 and 11.9).

Aloe vera heals wounds and reduces inflammation due to the

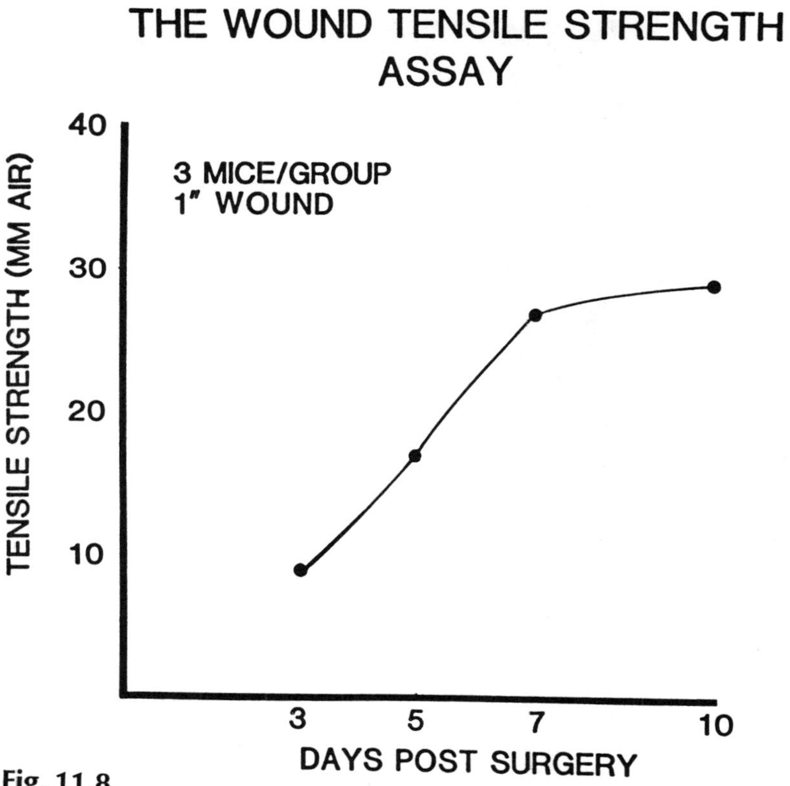
THE WOUND TENSILE STRENGTH
ASSAY
40
30
20
10
TENSILE STRENGTH (MM AIR)
3 MICE/GROUP
1" WOUND
3
5
7
10
DAYS POST SURGERY

Fig. 11.8.

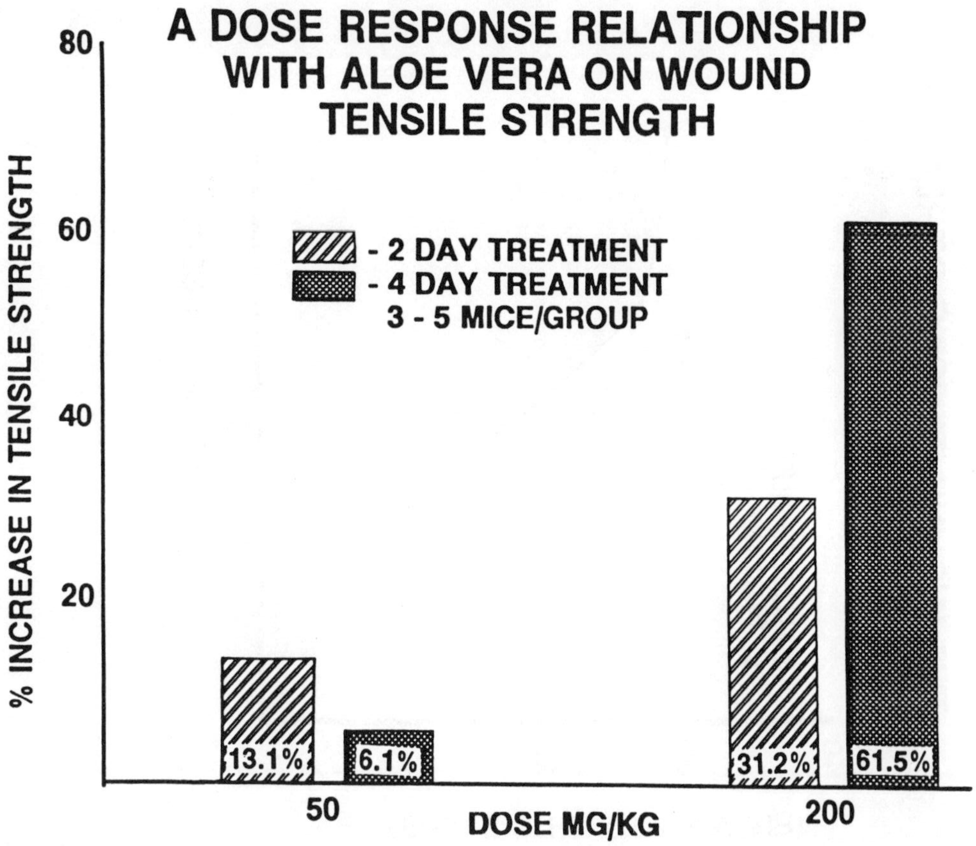
A DOSE RESPONSE RELATIONSHIP
WITH ALOE VERA ON WOUND
TENSILE STRENGTH
- 2 DAY TREATMENT
- 4 DAY TREATMENT
3 - 5 MICE/GROUP
% INCREASE IN TENSILE STRENGTH
80
60
40
20
13.1%
6.1%
31.2%
61.5%
50
200
DOSE MG/KG

Fig. 11.9.

growth factor–like substances in the plant. Gibberellin, auxin, and mannose phosphate are analgesic and can heal wounds and decrease inflammation.[23] In fact these biological actions may be used to characterize growth factors as well as to mark and standardize aloe vera.

An inflammatory process is the first of several stages in wound healing. During this phase, the tissues respond to injury by vasoconstriction and by increasing the vascular permeability. In addition, plasma cells produce specific antibodies to foreign antigens, and PMNs enter the wound to clear away bacteria.

During the proliferative phase, epidermal cells grow under the dry wound surface. Fibroblasts proliferate and synthesize collagen. Poor vascular supply of oxygen slows down collagen synthesis.

In the remodeling phase, collagen fibers undergo extensive reorientation as cross-linking these fibers increases the tensile strength of the wound connective tissue. Mannose-6-phosphate can stimulate the IGF receptor in the fibroblast to improve wound healing and decrease inflammation in a dose-response fashion. This action can activate fibroblasts to synthesize collagen and proteoglycans for tissue repair.

Summary

We have described some of the biological assays that can be used to standardize aloe vera and its fractions. We have also shown how a reference standard and an aloe vera unit can be made. The in vivo and in vitro assay was discussed, and we discussed the sensitivity, slope, accuracy, and biological error of the biological assay. The assay of aloe vera must be fast, simple, and accurate so that it can act as a "fingerprint" for aloe. A proposed chemical-biological assessment of aloe vera was presented to the IASC. The mechanism of action of aloe vera in reference to wound healing, inflammation, and analgesia was presented. We concluded that the many components in aloe make it possible to attack a wide spectrum of irritants. Aloe reduces pain by blocking the synthesis of bradykinin and prostaglandin. The dose-response curves for wound healing, inflammation, and analgesia had good sensitivity and accuracy to evaluate aloe vera.

References

1. D. C. Gowda, B. Neelisiddaiah, and Y. V. Anjaneyalu, "Structural Studies of Polysaccharides from Aloe Vera," *Carbohydrate Research* 72 (1979): 201.
2. T. A. Waller, F. M. Strickland, and R. P. Pelley, "Quality Control and Biological Activity of Aloe Barbadensis Extracts Useful in the Cosmetic Industry," in *Cosmetic Toiletries Manufacturing Worldwide* (London: Martin Caine, Aston Publishing Group, 1994).
3. R. Pelley, Y. T. Wang, and T. A. Waller, "Current Status of Quality Control of Aloe Barbadensis Extracts," *SOFW Journal* 119 (1993): 255.
4. K. F. Swingle, M. J. Reitor, and D. H. Schwartzmiller, "Comparison of Croton Oil and Cantharidin Induced Inflammation of Mouse Ear and Their Modification by Topically Applied Drugs," *Archive of International Pharmacodynamics* 254 (1987): 186.
5. R. H. Davis, K. Y. Rosenthal, L. R. Cesario, and G. R. Rowe, "Processed Aloe Vera Administered Topically Inhibits Inflammation," *Journal of the American Podiatric Medical Association* 79 (1989): 395.
6. I. Danhof, *Aloe through the Ages,* vol. 1 (Grand Prairie, TX: Omnimedicus Press, 1987).
7. H. A. Platt, D. K. Moonka, and R. H. Davis, "Inhibition of Gelatin-Induced Inflammation in Mice by Amino Acids and RNA," *Inflammation* 3 (1978): 225.
8. R. H. Davis, "A Natural Influence on Adjuvant-Induced Arthritis in Rats," *Pennsylvania Academy of Science* 56 (1982): 112.
9. B. E. Meyers, D. K. Moonka, and R. H. Davis, "The Effect of Selected Amino Acids on Gelatin-Induced Inflammation in Adult Male Mice," *Inflammation* 3 (1979): 225.
10. R. H. Davis, *Influence of Nutrition on the Growth and Survival of Cortisone Maintained Adrenalectmized Rats,* Ph.D. thesis, Rutgers University, 1958.
11. Meyers, Moonka, and Davis, "The Effect of Selected Amino Acids," 225.
12. L. McGowan, R. H. Davis, D. B. Stein, S. Bebon, and P. Vaskelis, "The Cytology of the Pelvic Peritoneal Cavity in Normal Women," *American Journal of Clinical Pathology* 49 (1968): 506.
13. R. Davis, and N. Maro, "Aloe Vera and Gibberellin," *Journal of the American Podiatric Association* 79 (1989): 24.
14. Davis and Maro, "Aloe Vera," 24; R. Davis, M. Leitner, J. Russo, and M. Byrne, "Anti-Inflammatory Activity of Aloe Vera against a Spectrum of Irritants," *Journal of the American Podiatric Medical Association* 79 (1989): 263; R. H. Davis, M. Leitner, J. M. Russo, and M. E. Byrne, "Wound Healing: Oral and Topical Activity of Aloe Vera," *Journal of the American Podiatric Medical Association* 79 (989): 559.
15. K. J. Williams, "The Action of Anti-Inflammatory Drugs on Skin Blood Vessels," in C. Hensby and N. J. Lowe, eds., *Non Steroidal Anti-Inflammatory Drugs* (New York: Basel, Karger, 1989).
16. B. C. Coats, *The Silent Healer: A Modern Study of Aloe Vera* (Garland, TX: self-published, 1979).
17. K. Fuijita, R.Teradaira, and T. Nagatsu, "Bradykinase Activity of Aloe Extract," *Biochemical Pharmacology* 25 (1976): 205.
18. L. A. Hart, P. H. Van Enckevort, H. Van Dijk, et al., "Two Functionally and Chemically Distinct Immunomodulatory Compounds in the Gel of Aloe Vera," *J. Ethnopharmacology* 23 (1988): 61.

19. Williams, "The Action of Anti-Inflammatory Drugs," 1989.
20. D. C. Hanley, W. A. Solomon, B. Saffran, and R. H. Davis, "The Evaluation of Natural Substances in the Treatment of Adjuvant Arthritis," *Journal of the American Podiatric Medical Association* 72 (1982): 275; R. H. Davis, E. Shapiro, and P. S. Agnew, "Topical Effect of Aloe Vera with RNA and Vitamin C on Adjuvant Arthritis," *Journal of the American Podiatric Medical Association* 75 (1985): 229.
21. Coats, *The Silent Healer.*
22. R. H. Davis, J. M. Kabbani, and N. P. Maro, "Aloe Vera and Wound Healing," *Journal of the American Podiatric Medical Association* 77 (1987): 165.
23. R. H. Davis, J. J. DiDonato, G. M. Hartman, and R. C. Haas, "Growth Factors in Aloe Vera," *Pennsylvania Academy of Science* 66 (1993): 181.

12

The Conductor-Orchestra Concept of Aloe Vera

The Model for Aloe

The modern symphony orchestra combines instruments from strings, woodwinds, brass, and percussion to form an ensemble capable of beautiful varied musical expression. Although the instrument arrangements vary, they can be grouped together in such a way as to concentrate and blend the sounds into a given tone color. The most beautiful sound in the world is the sound of an orchestra tuning up. Out of this musical chaos come the miracles of Mozart and the grandeur of Beethoven. A conductor may go through many aspects of music and the orchestra in his development. He might be a pianist, an arranger, or an orchestrator. This experience gives the conductor the strength of character that no magic wand can produce. The conductor knows what is expected musically from the orchestra players. He is in charge and is responsible to the orchestra so that the players are happy and compatible. Real talent takes a long time to mature and bring character into sound. The orchestra players are nothing without an orchestra leader, and the conductor can do nothing without the talented orchestra players.

Aloe Function

The relationship that exists within aloe vera we have called the "conductor-orchestra concept" (figure 12.1) The aloe vera molecule is the conductor that leads a symphony of over 200 biologically active substances. It is a polysaccharide molecule in which mannose molecules join together through a beta 1–4 linkage to form a chain.

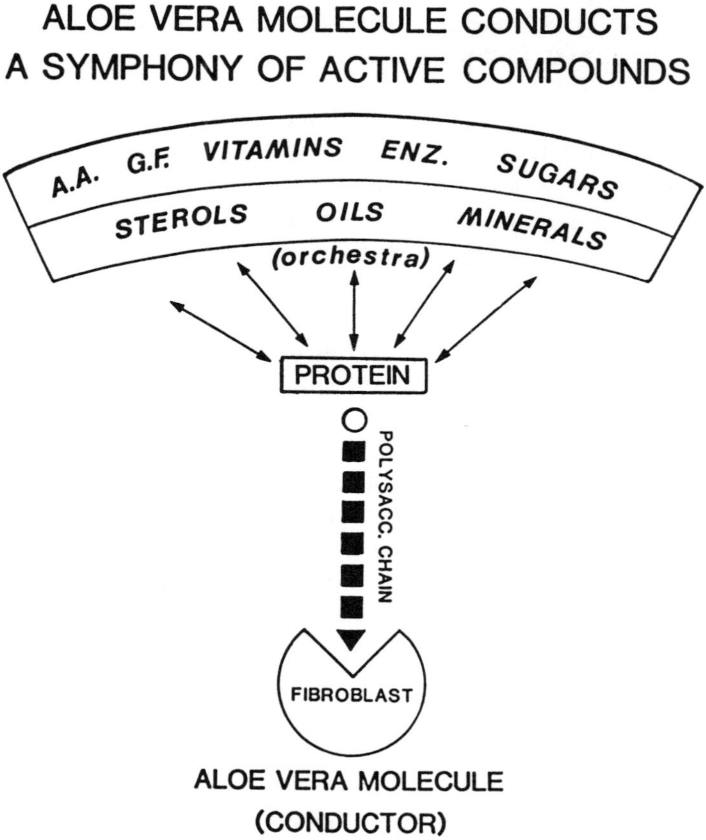
ALOE VERA MOLECULE CONDUCTS
A SYMPHONY OF ACTIVE COMPOUNDS
A.A.
G.F.
VITAMINS
ENZ.
SUGARS
STEROLS
OILS
MINERALS
(orchestra)
PROTEIN
POLYSACC. CHAIN
FIBROBLAST
ALOE VERA MOLECULE
(CONDUCTOR)

Fig. 12.1.

The polysaccharide is the conductor that modulates the biological activity between the surrounding orchestra molecules so that they work together synergistically. The compounds are the orchestra that works with the conductor (polysaccharide) to produce an infinite array of biological activities. The protein at one end helps to direct the mannose phosphate at the end of the polysaccharide into the insulin-like growth factor receptor of the fibroblast, which produces collagen and proteoglycans to improve wound healing. The polysaccharide can stimulate the macrophage to produce a variety of important biologically active substances. The aloe vera molecule can recognize the receptors on cell surfaces but can also recognize the individual biological players in the orchestra. Thus, in an indirect way, the biological compounds help the conductor produce the biological response at the cell receptor. In the union with the fibroblast or macrophage, the aloe vera molecule leads an orchestra of compounds to synergize with each other to produce a symphony of biologically therapeutic effects. To suggest that the conductor—the polysaccharide—works alone in this wonderful creation of God is presumptive. The relationship of these compounds with the aloe vera molecule explains the synergy of activity over a wide biological spectrum such that it is unwise to search for a "magic bullet." This is not to say that we should not isolate biological compounds and activity. Also, we should mention that the polysaccharide has biological activity, but not of the order obtained by synergizing with the surrounding biological compounds. The length of the polysaccharide chain determines the strength and type of biological activity.

The Role of Water in Aloe

A good orchestra player must be subordinate to the perfection of the whole. When you put two hundred musicians together someone must be in control who is respected and who can maintain control. The music must be transmitted in such a way that it does not reveal the personality of the conductor, but of the one who wrote the music. This is true for aloe vera. The important question remains to be answered. How does the polysaccharide (the conductor) communicate and relate to the 200 biologically active compounds in the orchestra? Aloe vera is composed of 99.5 percent water and 0.5 percent solids. The water can, of course, be removed by lyophilization to give us a nice light powder. Water, however, must be added to recover the biological activities characteristic of aloe. Water seems rather commonplace, but it is no innocent bystander in the chemistry of living things. Water is not just a solvent for the organic molecules and the polysaccharide, but plays a major role in the interaction of the polysaccharide with the 200 compounds. Water helps to produce therapeutic activity. The interaction between the conductor and the orchestra arises from water's polarity. The water molecules in aloe vera have large oxygen atoms that draw electrons from two hydrogen atoms imparting positive and negative charges to the ends of the molecule. This polarity enables water to dissolve the active agents and to mold complex molecules. The orchestra molecules as well as the conductor polysaccharide possess both polar and non-polar parts. The polar parts react well with water, whereas the non-polar or hydrophobic parts avoid water. The polarity of water molecules causes them to align their negative ends with the positive ends of other molecules, and vice versa. These water molecule chains can connect the polysaccharide to the orchestra molecules such as amino acids, vitamins, and sterols in such a way that the conductor polysaccharide can communicate and relate to the 200 compounds to produce a beautiful synergy of biological activity. Information can be given back to the conductor in a similar way to influence the polysaccharide's control over the biological influences.

The Standard for Aloe Vera

The conductor-orchestra theory has been adopted as the standard and direction in which Aloecorp operates. An aloe vera unit must be based upon a measured amount of biological-chemical activity of aloe vera. To select a certain component of aloe vera as the "magic bullet" and use it as the standard is unwarranted and not good science. This does not mean that we will not try to fractionate aloe vera to obtain identifiable active compounds. We also wish to obtain as much data as possible about the polysaccharide in aloe vera. The entire picture of aloe vera is important to us. We feel that it is the whole aloe which packs the punch to fight off disease and keep the body in a healthy physiological state. The aloe vera plant takes the energy from the sun to make ATP for work, and from the soil it obtains water and chemicals to produce many biological compounds that can be used to combat disease.

The Yin-Yang Theory and Aloe

Yin-yang is a term used in Chinese culture and philosophy to indicate the active and passive principles of the universe. It proposes a balance based on the elements of yin and yang. The yang or male force represents the light, active generative essences, whereas the yin or female force represents the dark, passive receptive essence. From the interaction of these two forces all things come into existence. Yin is cold and dark, whereas yang is heat and light. Foods can be grouped as yin and yang—hot and cold, sweet and sour.The balance between yin and yang in our foods is necessary for good health. Fevers and infections are yang conditions and are treated with yin foods such as fruits and vegetables. Colds and cancer are yin conditions and are treated with warm foods. This idea of yin and yang was used to express the status of the blood, the body's strength, and natural illnesses. As a result, a whole tradition of food therapies has been employed to treat disease. Certain things build up the body's defense or the immune system, and other things do not.[1]

Aloe vera has been called a modulator in that it brings biological systems into balance. We have demonstrated that aloe vera has an inhibitory system that blocks inflammation as well as a stimulatory system that improves growth and wound healing.[2] R. P. LaBadie has shown the aloe vera fractions can modulate antibodies,[3] whereas our laboratory and the Carrington people have shown that aloe or the polysaccharide can modulate cellular immunity.[4] Aloe vera can inhibit the infiltration of polymorphonuclear leukocytes into a site of irritation. This represents a block on leukotrienes. A normalizing influence of aloe vera can be demonstrated in adjuvant arthritic rats. The anti-inflammatory components such as amino acids and sterols are balanced by growth factors such as gibberellins and auxins. Components in aloe have the capability of increasing as well as decreasing blood sugar.[5] In aloe vera, there appear always to be two components that act in such a way (yin, yang) as to produce a beneficial therapy.

They act to normalize or produce a balance in a biological system. This assumes that the aloe vera preparation was made in the best possible way as close to the leaf gel as possible.

The Toxicity of Aloe Vera

The concept has been proposed that no chemical or group of chemicals is entirely safe. In fact, all chemicals produce undesirable effects on a biological mechanism if a sufficiently great concentration of the chemical is used. The single most important factor that determines the potential harmfulness or safety of a compound is the relationship between the concentration of the chemical and the effect it produces on a biological mechanism.[6]

Plants used as medication or food supplements make up about 25 percent of today's pharmacopoeia. Herbs are being used as therapeutic alternatives to traditional medicine. Many modern drugs are either derivatives of plants or modifications of known plant chemical products. W. M. Busey found that rats exposed to high doses of aloe vera for fourteen days had an acute oral LD_{50} of 22 gm/kg.[7] This is an extremely high dose. The maximum acute oral dose over fourteen days for dogs was greater than 32 gm/kg. Application to skin at 10 gm/kg produced only minimal dermal irritation. M. H. Grossman and H. Cobble found no attributable toxicity in rabbits at high doses. Vital organs, muscle and skin showed negligible toxicity.[8] Hundreds of physician reports in thousands of cases also verify the lack of toxicity. Most of us who have been working with aloe vera at effective dose levels have not recorded toxicity. These early studies could be used as the basis for an acute and chronic toxicity study in mice and rats in preparation as a basis for talks with the FDA.

The dose of aloe vera relative to the cumulative percentage of animals showing a response (such as death) is the basis for the LD_{50}. The dose can be increased by a multiple of 2 until 100 percent of the animals die. The LD_{50} is the dose that kills 50 percent of the animals. A subcutaneous route of administration in adult mice would be an excellent test animal. The 95 percent confidence limits can be obtained using the Litchfield and Wilcoxon method or the Miller and Tainter procedure. Basically, the LD_{50} is obtained from the curve by drawing a horizontal line from the 50 percent mortality point on the ordinate to where it intersects the curve. At the point of intersection, a vertical line is drawn, and where this line intersects the abscissa is the LD_{50}. The slope of the dose-response curve is an index of the margin of safety. The ratio of LD_{50} to ED_{50} represents the therapeutic index.

A chronic toxicity is done on animals receiving daily doses over a year or more to demonstrate the absence of toxicity when the doses involved represent some practical level. One dose level should be 100 times the contemplated dose for humans. The nature and duration of chronic toxicity tests are predicated on the nature of the intended use. No method can be universally applied to establish the duration of the chronic toxicity test. When studies are done on rats, three test groups plus one control group are used. Thirty males and females can be used in each test group, with sixty males and females in the control group. A low-, intermediate-, and high-dose schedule is used. End points include: behavior, symptoms, food and water intake, body weight, blood chemistry and counts. Tissue sections should be taken for histology.[9]

One possible objective of a prolonged toxicity test is an attempt to demonstrate some form of toxicity at least in the high-dose group. If severe toxicity occurs, the dose schedule is in error. Toxicity testing is so well done today that the results are acceptable to most toxicologists. The extent to which a compound is tested depends on the intended use of the compound. Acute and chronic toxicity studies need to be done on aloe vera, since the preparations made in the last few years are so much better than those prepared twenty years ago.

Years ago we use to administer biological agents into test animals over a short period of time at relatively high doses to see if we could obtain leads as to which agent had biological activity. This was called a "Magic Assay." Whole-leaf aloe vera was administered subcutaneously daily for thirteen days at 100 and 300 mg/kg to adult male mice. The relative organ weights of testis, seminal vesicle, spleen, adrenal, and thymus were recorded. Body weight was not significantly altered by whole-leaf aloe vera. Testis, seminal vesicle, spleen, and adrenal weights were not significantly altered, but the relative thymus weight was significantly decreased by the 100 and 300 mg/kg doses of aloe vera (table 12.1). Possibly the release of lymphocytes from the thymus (CD_4 cells) by aloe vera could have produced this effect. We are aware that aloe vera is an immune

THE MAGIC ASSAY FOR WHOLE LEAF ALOE VERA

RELATIVE ORGAN WT. (MG/100g.)	SALINE CONTROLS	ALOE DOSE (MG/KG X 13)	
		100	300
Body Wt.	38.7 ± 0.5	41.0 ± 5.9	39.8 ± 9.1
Testis	721.4 ± 40.6	689.0 ± 41.9	623.6 ± 64.7*
Sem. Ves.	443.1 ± 29.8	454.6 ± 23.4	371.1 ± 52.9*
Spleen	338.6 ± 12.5	373.6 ± 28.5*	471.2 ± 51.6*
Adrenal	28.4 ± 2.5	24.3 ± 1.4	29.5 ± 2.7
Thymus	135.8 ± 9.9	95.7 ± 3.9**	101.3 ± 5.3**

8 - 9 Mice/Group; S.Q. ADM.; *P > 0.1; **P < 0.001

Table 12.1.

modulator particularly in regard to T-cells that play a major role in cellular immunity. T-lymphocytes have receptor molecules that recognize foreign peptides on the surface of cells. This recognition secretes chemical signals called lymphokines that mobilize other components of the immune system. Aloe vera can stimulate macrophages to release growth factors, which can stimulate fibroblasts to produce collagen and proteoglycans for wound healing. This work with aloe vera provides a scientific framework for examining living systems and how they integrate information on how an organism functions.

The ability of an organism to activate the wound-healing process effectively and promptly is essential for its survival. Wound healing, a necessary safeguard against long-term infection and subsequent death, has three major phases: inflammation, proliferation, and remodeling. After injury, fibroblasts migrate toward the wound site, where they proliferate and produce collagen, elastin, and proteoglycans.[10] Proteoglycans form the ground substance in which collagen and other connective tissue fibers are embedded.[11] These substances remodel the connective tissue (figure 12.2). The movement of individual fibroblasts within the extracellular matrix produces the forces for tissue contraction and therefore wound healing.[12] An increase in fibroblast proliferation by platelet and mononuclear phagocyte products improves wound healing.[13]

Aloe vera is a complex plant containing many biologically active substances.[14] Evidence has shown that aloe is effective in wound healing and inflammation reduction.[15] This is attributed to a growth factor–like substance in aloe that activates the wound-healing and inflammation reduction process.

One of the important considerations is to determine whether mannose-6-phosphate (M-6-P) is an active ingredient in aloe for wound healing and anti-inflammation. It is important to understand the role of mannose-6-phosphate (a major constituent of the aloe leaf) and if linkage to a protein is necessary to initiate a growth response. Is wound healing a solitary event of mannose phosphate or a combined effort with other cellular substances in aloe such as glucose phosphate? Proposing a mechanism to explain how aloe affects wound healing and inflammation will be instrumental in determining the most efficient way to use aloe as a growth factor–like substance.

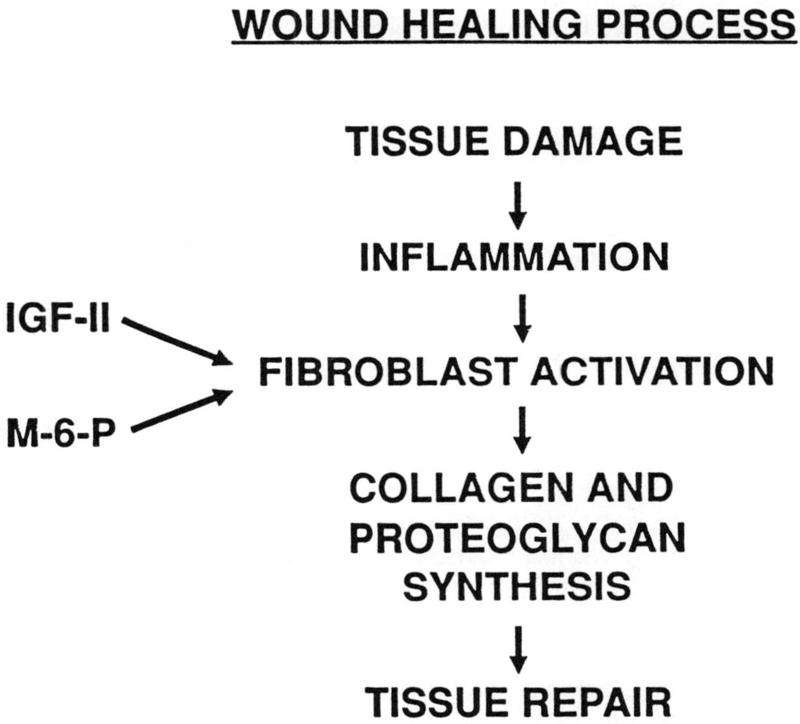
WOUND HEALING PROCESS
TISSUE DAMAGE
INFLAMMATION
IGF-II
FIBROBLAST ACTIVATION
M-6-P
COLLAGEN AND PROTEOGLYCAN SYNTHESIS
TISSUE REPAIR

Fig. 12.2.

Cells in a wound communicate with each other through substances known as growth factors.[16] Growth factors are polypeptide hormones that are stored by most cells and are secreted into local tissues. Once the growth factor has been attracted to the wound area it binds to a cell surface receptor, usually that of a fibroblast.This sequence initiates the biological response: wound healing. The recent experiments by Huang and Huang (1988) have recognized that the intracellular interaction of growth factors with their receptors may be important in generating the biological effects of these growth factors.[17] Vladsky makes the link between the IGF-II receptor and fibroblast growth factor stimulation.[18] Evidence reveals that IGF-II and mannose-6-phosphate bind to different binding sites of the same receptor on the fibroblast.[19] This relationship makes key the stimulation of the fibroblast surface receptor by the mannose-6-phosphate located at the end of the mucopolysaccharide of the aloe plant. This evidence offers a possible link between mannose-6-phosphate and growth factor stimulation of the fibroblast.

Wound Healing

On day 7, control animals receiving saline demonstrated an average decrease in wound diameter of 2.8 mm (42.1 percent). The group receiving 30 mg/kg of mannose-6-phosphate had an average wound decrease of 3.1 mm (43.8 percent), while animals injected with 150 mg/kg had a wound diameter decrease of 3.7 mm (47.3 percent). Neither response is considered significantly different from the control group ($p>0.10$). Mice receiving a dose of 300 mg/kg of the mannose-6-phosphate had an average decrease of 4.3 mm (50.7 percent). This is considered significant ($p<0.01$). Animals that received the 150 mg/kg of glucose-6-phosphate had an average decrease of 3.1 mm (40.3 percent), which is not significant ($p>0.10$). These values are summarized in table 12.2.

Inflammation

The average ear weight difference between the treated right ear and the control left ear of the saline control group was observed to

EFFECT OF MANNOSE-6-PHOSPHATE ON WOUND HEALING AND TOPICAL CROTON OIL INDUCED INFLAMMATION OVER 7 DAYS

	DOSES (MG/KG x 7)	WOUND HEALING MM	WOUND HEALING % Dec.	EDEMA MG	EDEMA % Dec.
Saline	10	2.8 ± 0.2	42.1 ± 2.0	7.3 ± 0.8	———
Glucose-6-PO_4	150	3.1 ± 0.2	40.3 ± 1.7	7.0 ± 0.8	4.1 ± 0.5
Mannose-6-PO_4	30	3.1 ± 0.2	43.8 ± 1.9	6.7 ± 1.0	8.2 ± 1.2
	150	3.7 ± 0.3	47.3 ± 2.4	5.6 ± 0.7	23.3 ± 2.9
	300	4.3 ± 0.2	50.7 ± 1.6*	5.5 ± 0.7	24.7 ± 3.1**

* $p < 0.01$ ** $p = 0.05$

Table 12.2.

be 7.3 mg. The glucose-6-phosphate group had an ear weight difference of 7.0 mg. The groups that were administered mannose-6-phosphate at doses of 30, 150, and 300 mg/kg were observed to have differences of 6.7, 5.6, and 5.5 mg, respectively. The group that received the dose of 300 mg/kg is the only group considered to be significantly different from the control group ($p=0.05$).

Mannose-6-phosphate is an important constituent of the polysaccharide chain in aloe. Our experiments have shown that mannose-6-phosphate demonstrates wound healing and anti-inflammatory activity in a dose-response fashion (figures 12.3 and 12.4). Furthermore, we concluded that glucose-6-phosphate (a control) does not improve wound healing or reduce inflammation. Therefore, our evidence suggests that mannose-6-phosphate is a major structural constituent that stimulates wound healing and anti-inflammation. Our data may implicate a structural blueprint of the mucopolysaccharide in aloe vera (figure 12.5). This figure is a possible representation of a lock and key mechanism between the IGF-II/M-6-P receptor on the fibroblast and the active polysaccharide chain in aloe.

Gowda has reported that there is approximately a six-to-one ratio of mannose to glucose in the aloe polysaccharide chain.[20] We believe that the protein is non-covalently attached to the polysaccharide chain via a glucose-binding site. The polysaccharide can dissociate from the protein in the same manner as it dissociates from the IGF-II/M-6-P receptor.

Current theory suggests that mannose-6-phosphate needs to be protein-linked in order to yield a wound-healing or an anti-inflammatory response.[21] Our data demonstrate that free mannose-6-phosphate effectively reduces inflammation and heals wounds. Our laboratory has previously shown aloe vera extract improves wound healing and reduces inflammation.[22] A comparison of data would suggest that mannose-6-phosphate linked to a protein (thus forming a mucopolysaccharide) may yield even greater wound healing and inflammation reduction.

A Possible Mechanism of Action of M-6-P in Aloe

It is well established that IGF-II and M-6-P bind to the same receptor on the fibroblast.[23] These two ligands bind at separate binding sites within the IGF-II/M-6-P receptor.[24] However, the exact effect

EFFECT OF MANNOSE-6-PHOSPHATE ON WOUND HEALING

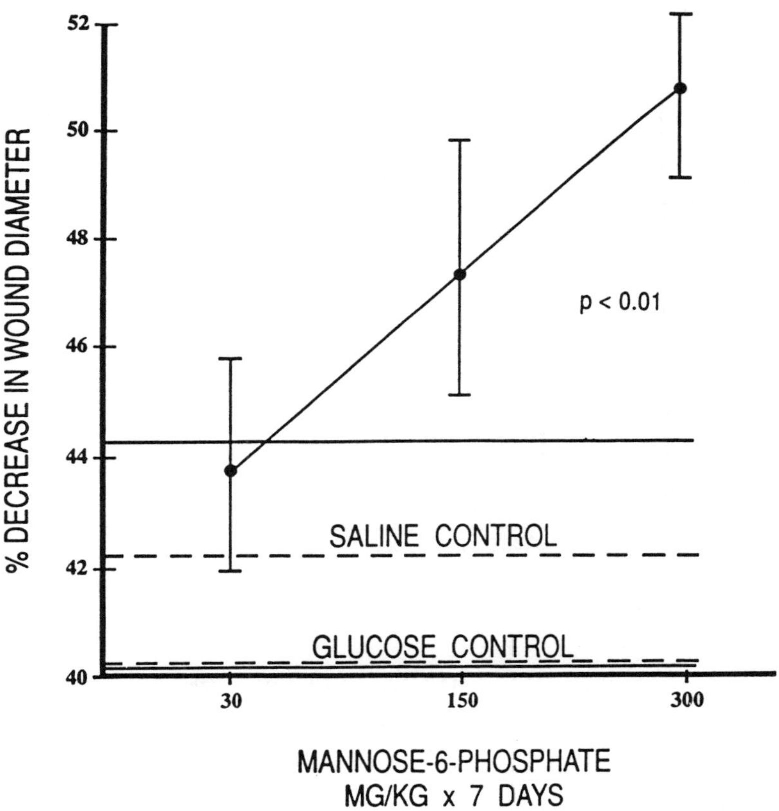

Fig. 12.3.

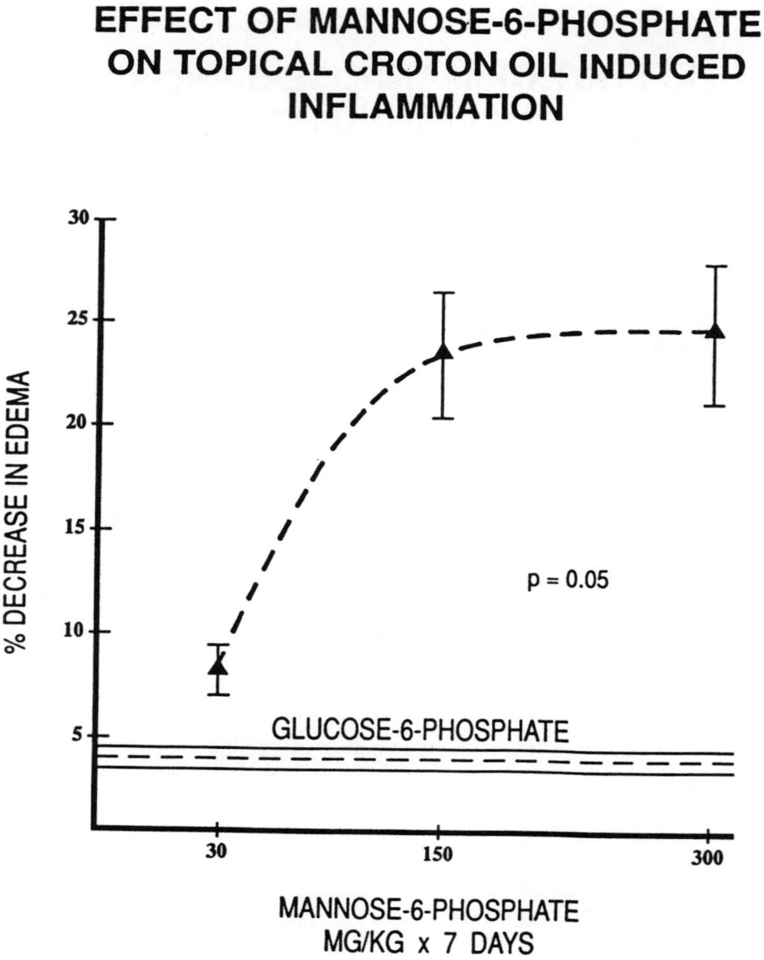

EFFECT OF MANNOSE-6-PHOSPHATE
ON TOPICAL CROTON OIL INDUCED
INFLAMMATION
30
25
20
15
10
5
% DECREASE IN EDEMA
p = 0.05
GLUCOSE-6-PHOSPHATE
30
150
300
MANNOSE-6-PHOSPHATE
MG/KG x 7 DAYS

Fig. 12.4.

MANNOSE-6-PHOSPHATE OF ALOE VERA ACTIVATES THE INSULIN-LIKE GROWTH FACTOR II/ MANNOSE-6-PHOSPHATE RECEPTOR

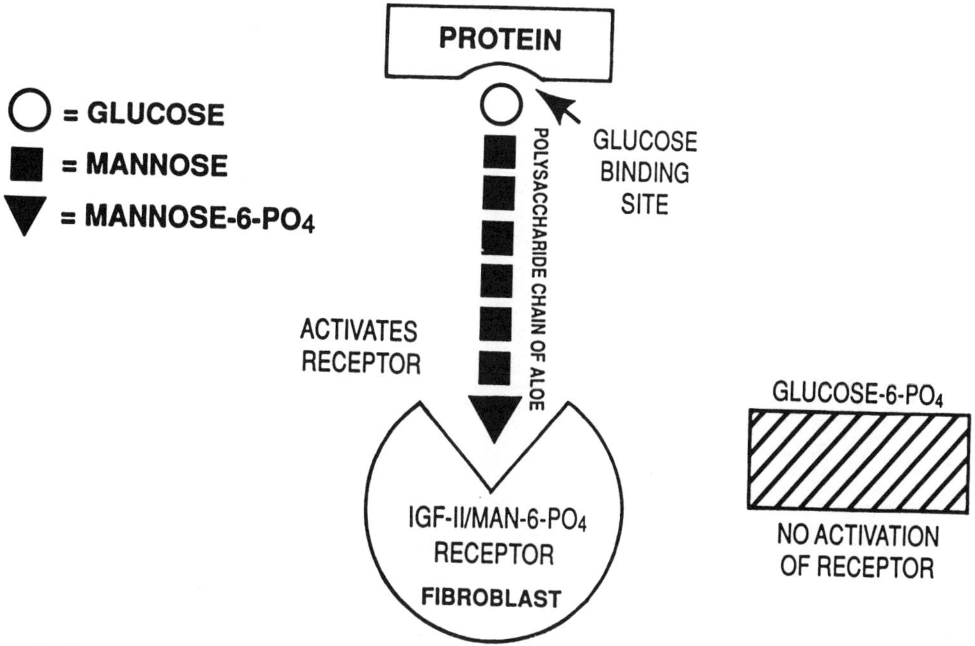

Fig. 12.5.

of these ligands binding to their individual binding sites is still unclear. There are several possible mechanisms of action of these ligands. One possible theory is that the binding of either ligand is capable of activating fibroblast proliferation. This would indicate that free M-6-P is a growth substance capable of yielding the same response as IGF-II. In aloe, M-6-P is part of the polysaccharide chain that is attached to a protein. This may be important in understanding how aloe produces its wound-healing and anti-inflammatory activity.

Another possible theory of fibroblast activation by the binding of the ligands is that they work together. Nolan reports that the binding of a ligand at one binding site is capable of influencing ligand binding at the other binding site of the same receptor.[25] It is therefore possible that the binding of M-6-P to its binding site preferentially increases the affinity of IGF-II to its binding site.[26] This would increase the rate of endocytosis of IGF-II. In this manner, IGF-II is delivered at a higher rate to the cells and thereby increases fibroblast activity and the wound-healing response.

Further experiments are required to clarify the exact mechanism of the IGF-II/M-6-P receptor in yielding fibroblast activation. One possible experiment would utilize an antibody against the IGF-II binding site. In the past, research using a receptor antibody has been unable to identify the exact mechanism of ligand binding.

P. Nissley's group used an antibody that blocked the entire IGF-II/M-6-P receptor.[27] This not only blocked the binding of IGF-II to the receptor, but it also blocked M-6-P binding as well. They reported no decrease in autocrine growth. Nissley then concluded that the IGF-II/M-6-P receptor is not involved in autocrine growth. This experiment failed to clarify the IGF-II/M-6-P receptor mechanism for two reasons. First, the entire receptor was blocked and not the individual IGF-II binding site. Therefore, M-6-P was also blocked from binding to the receptor. Second, IGF-II is apparently capable of binding to cell surface binding proteins other than its receptor. Nolan reports this phenomenon.[28] C. Nolan and his associates found that cells lacking the IGF-II/M-6-P receptor still bound sufficient levels of IGF-II to yield a growth response. This may be the reason that Nissley found no reduction in autocrine growth.

An important experiment may be to produce an antibody specific for the IGF-II binding site within the IGF-II/M-6-P receptor. This antibody should also be specific for the cell surface binding proteins.

If this antibody is successful in blocking all IGF-II binding sites, the exact role of M-6-P will become clear. If a growth response still occurs with M-6-P treatment, then M-6-P alone is capable of stimulating the fibroblasts and M-6-P is a growth substance. If no growth response is observed, then M-6-P functions only to increase IGF-II binding and does not directly stimulate fibroblast activation.

References

1. R. R. Watson, *Nutrition and AIDS* (Boca Raton: CRC Press, 1994).
2. R. H. Davis, W. L. Parker, R. T. Samson, and D. P. Murdoch, "A Stimulatory System in an Extract of Aloe," *Journal of the American Podiatric Medical Association* 81 (1991): 473.
3. L. A. Hart, P. H. Van Enckevort, H. Van Dijk, R. Zaat, K. T. D. DeSilva, and R. P. LaBadie, "Two Functionally and Chemically Distinct Immunomodulatory Compounds in the Gel of Aloe Vera," *Journal of Ethnopharmacology* 23 (1988): 61.
4. D. Womble and J. H. Helderman, "The Impact of Acemannan on the Generation and Function of Cytotoxic T-Lymphocytes," *Immunopharmacology and Immunotoxicology* 14 (1992): 63; R. H. Davis, P. S. Agnew, and E. Shapiro, "Effect of Aloe, Vitamin C and RNA on Adjuvant Arthritis," *Pennsylvania Academy of Science* 58 (1994): 114.
5. H. Hiroshi, T. Michiko, M. Murakami, et al., "Isolation and Hypoglycemic Activity of Arborans A and B: Glycans of Aloe," *International Journal of Crude Drug Research* 24 (1986): 183.
6. T. A. Loomis, *Essentials of Toxicology*, 3d ed. (Philadelphia: Lea and Febiger, 1978).
7. W. M. Busey, M. D. Powers, and R. Vollker, "Acute Oral (Rats), Acute Oral Dose Range (Dogs), Acute Dermal Application (Rabbits)," *Stabilized Aloe Vera* 1 (1968): 137.
8. M. H. Grossman and H. Cobble, "Acute Oral (Rats), Acute Oral Dose Range (Dogs), Acute Dermal Application (Rabbits)," *Stabilized Aloe Vera* 1 (1966): 124.
9. A. J. Lehman, "Appraisal of Safety of Chemicals in Food, Drugs and Cosmetics," in *Association of Food and Drug Officials of the United States* (Baltimore: Association of Food and Drug officials of the United States, 1959).
10. I. Cohen, R. Dieglemann, and W. Lindblad, *Wound Healing/Biochemical and Clinical Aspects,* 1st ed. (Philadelphia: W. B. Saunders, 1992).
11. J. Darnell, H. Lodish and D. Baltimore, *Molecular Cell Biology* (New York: Scientific American Books, 1986); L. Stryer, *Biochemistry,* ed ed. (San Francisco: W. H. Freeman, 1981).
12. Cohen, Dreglemann, and Lindblad, *Wound Healing.*
13. Ibid.
14. R. Davis, "Inhibitory and Stimulatory Systems in Aloe Vera," *Aloe Today,* Winter 1991–92, 6–8.
15. R. Davis, "Aloe Vera: A Natural Approach for Treating Wounds, Edema and Pain in Diabetes," *Journal of the American Podiatric Medical Association* 78

(1987): 60; R. Davis, W. Parker, and D. Murdoch, "Aloe Vera as a Biologically Actie Vehicle for Hydrocortisone Acetate," *Journal of the American Podiatric Medical Association* 81 (1991): 1; R. Davis and N. Maro, "Aloe Vera and Gibberellin," *Journal of the American Podiatric Medical Association* 79 (1989): 24.

16. B. Davis, R. Dulbecco, H. Eisen, and H. Ginsberg, *Micro-Biology*, 3d ed. (Hagerstown: Harper & Row, 1980).
17. C. Nolan, J. Kyle, H. Wantanabe, and W. Sly, "Binding of Insulin-Like Growth Factor II (IGF-II) by Human Cation-Independent Mannose-6-Phosphate/IGF-II Receptor Expressed in Receptor-Deficient Mouse L Cells," *Cell Regulation* 1 (1990): 197.
18. Ibid.
19. T. Braulke, S. Tippmer, H. Chao, and K. Von Figura, "Insulin-Like Growth Factors I and II Stimulate Endocytosis but Do Not Affect Sorting of Lysosomal Enzymes in Human Fibroblasts," *Journal of Biological Chemistry* 265 (1990): 6650; C. Polychronakos, H. Guyda, U. Janthly, and B. Posner, "Effects of Mannose-6-Phosphate on Receptor Mediated Endocytosis of Insulin-Like Growth Factor-II," *Endocrinology* 127 (1990): 1861; M. Zhongmin, J. Grubb, and W. Sly, "Cloning, Sequencing and Functional Characterization of the Murine 46-kDa Mannose-6-Phosphate Receptor," *Journal of Biological Chemistry* 266 (1991): 10589; B. Westlund, N. Dahms, and S. Kornfeld, "The Bovine Mannose-6-Phosphate/IGF II Receptor," *Journal of Biological Chemistry* 266 (1991): 23233; D. Morgan, J. C. Edman, D. N. Standring, V. A. Fried, M. C. Smith, R. A.Roth, and W. J. Rutter, "Insulin-Like Growth Factor II Receptor as a Multifunctional Binding Protein," *Nature* 329 (1987): 301.
20. D. Gowda, B. Neelisiddaiah, and Y. Anjaneyalo, "Structural Studies of Polysaccharides from Aloe Vera," *Carbohydrate Research* 72 (1979): 201.
21. V. Grey, C. Rouyer-Fessard, S. Gammeltoft, M. Bourque, C. Morin, and M. Laburthe, "Insulin-Like Growth Factor II/Mannose-6-Phosphate Receptors Are Transiently Increased in the Rat Distal Intestinal Epithelium after Resection," *Molecular and Cellular Endocrinology* 75 (1991): 221.
22. Davis, "Aloe Vera," 60; Davis, Parker, and Murdoch, "Aloe Vera," 1; Davis and Maro, "Aloe Vera," 24.
23. Braulke, Tippmer, Chao, and Von Figura, "Insulin-Like Growth Factors," 6650; Polychronakos, Guyda, Janthly, and Posner, "Effects," 1861; Zhongmin, Grubb, and Sly, "Cloning," 10589; Westlund, Dahms, and Kornfeld, "The Bovine Mannose-6-Phosphate/IGF II Receptor," 23233; Morgan, Edman, Standring, Fried, Sith, Roth, and Rutter, "Insulin-Like Growth Factor II Receptor," 301.
24. Nolan, Kyle, Wantanable, and Sly, "Binding of Insulin-Like Growth Factor II," 197.
25. Ibid.
26. Grey, Rouyer-Fessard, Gammeltoft, Bourque, Morin, and Laburthe, "Insulin-Like Growth Factor II/Mannose-6-Phosphate Receptors," 221; R. MacDonald, "Mannose-6-Phosphate Enhances Cross-Linking Efficiency between IGF-II and IGF-II/M-6-P Receptors in Membranes," *Endocrinology* 128 (1991): 413; R. Roth, "Structure of the Receptor for Insulin-Like Growth Factor–II: The Puzzle Amplified," *Science* 239 (1988): 1269.
27. P. Nissley, L. Lilly, and K. Wieland, "Evidence against a Role for Insulin-Like

Growth Factor II in the Autonomous Growth of Rat 18, 54 SF Cells,'' *Molecular and Cellular Endocrinology* 75 (1991): 213.
28. Nolan, Kyle, Wantanable, and Sly, "Binding of Insulin-Like Growth Factor II," 192.

13
General Summary

The aloe plant exhibits radial arrangement of four rows of leaves alternately arranged. The inner leaves are "pup leaves," which receive nourishment from the outer leaves. We observed that long tubes that run from the leaf tip to the base play a major role in carrying nourishment to the "pup leaves." Wind moves the leaves and provides a movement of the gel inward. Wind movement of gel increases the production of aloe vera in the leaf. Big fans could be strategically placed around an aloe plant field so that the plants were moved by the fans and the production of aloe vera would be increased as a result. The outer epidermis of the leaf contains stomata through which CO_2 enters the leaf. Carbon dioxide combines with water in the presence of chlorophyl and light to form an active carbon. The active carbon forms carbohydrates, proteins, fatty acids and vitamins. The xylem transports water, minerals, and nitrogen from the roots, and the phloem transports synthesized materials to other parts of the leaf. The vascular bundles connect with the long tubes running lengthwise in the leaf. Mucilage is formed under the rind and has good wound-healing activity. The mucilage and the aloe gel play a role in the sealing off of a wound in the leaf.

The aloe vera cell was seen by the electron microscope. The nucleus was clearly visible and surrounded by two cell membranes that contained mucopolysaccharides. The mucopolysaccharides are transferred into the cell lumen for storage. We measured the metabolic activity of fresh aloe vera leaf gel and obtained a good dose-response curve on O_2 consumption and CO_2 production. This assay could be used to evaluate anti-bacterial and anti-fungal activity of aloe vera. Mucilage stimulates fibroblasts and epidermal cells for growth and repair. The occlusive nature of mucilage increases wound healing from a mechanical and endocrine viewpoint. The transformation of mucilage from a sol to a gel we call a sol-gel transformation.

An attempt was made to transfer this transformation from the leaf to an animal wound. A fast, economical, and easy-to-perform aloe leaf assay was developed to measure the increased production of aloe vera. Beginning in 1935 with the work of Collins and Collins, aloe vera was placed on a more solid foundation, as investigators moved from simple observation to good experimental design. We now have good scientific evidence that aloe vera works. No longer can it be said that aloe is a myth or magic. When one can establish good dose-response curves for each effect in aloe vera, one can say that aloe vera works. We know that aloe vera is effective on wound healing, anti-inflammation, and analgesia and is bacteriocidal. Applications have been made in general medicine, surgery, dentistry, veterinary medicine, and microbiology. We have a good idea about the dose of aloe vera that should be used. Stabilization of aloe and the route of administration have received some attention. However, more effort must be made in the transition from basic research to clinical science. Significant research reports were presented to show the growth and development of aloe vera.

From an evaluation of the biologically active components in aloe vera, the total biological activity comes from a synergistic modulation of the compounds involved rather than from a single component. Water plays a major role in the relationship between the polysaccharide and the many biologically active ingredients in aloe. We asked the question, "What is good aloe?" It is aloe in which all the active components are preserved with all their biological benefits. The chemical composition of aloe with its biological activity was presented as well as the two major processing procedures used by the aloe industry. Adulteration is a major concern to the industry because it reduces the biological benefits causing the consumer to lose confidence in aloe vera. The IASC has developed a certification process that guarantees the purity of aloe vera and can now guarantee good aloe and, at the same time, warn the consumer of fraudulent claims. A complete fact sheet on aloe vera is the result of both good research and encouragement by the industry. The Food, Drug, and Cosmetic Act assures the consumer that foods are pure and safe to eat and were produced under sanitary conditions. This law tells us we must make good aloe. Aloe vera must be processed in the best way to provide maximum benefit to a person's health.

Our view is that pharmacological agents of both oil and water solubilities can be placed in aloe and carried through the skin to blood vessels. We have defined a biological vehicle as one that acts as a physical carrier for active biological agents and adds biological activity to the test compound. It is a physical carrier plus added aloe vera activity. Aloe vera can add its biological activity to most test agents. Hydrocortisone fails to penetrate the skin stratum corneum and is wasted. Aloe enhances penetration and adds to the biological activity of hydrocortisone. Aloe vera increases the penetration of skin by water hydration, occlusiveness, and increasing compound solubility. The trypan blue penetration assay was used to prove how aloe vera increases the penetration through the skin. Aloe vera is a good vehicle for estrogen. Whole-leaf aloe vera increased the uterotropic effect of estradiol benzoate in ovariectomized mice even though it had no estrogenic activity by itself. Aloe vera synergizes with testosterone proprionate. The combined treatment of aloe plus testosterone was greater than the sum of the aloe and androgen treatments. Aloe vera, which has no androgenic activity, provided a synergistic relationship with testosterone proprionate. Aloe vera appeared to antagonize pituitary gonadotropin, as evidenced by the fact that ovarian hypertrophy did not occur in our experimental design. We speculated that the high dose of aloe blocked the releasing hormone or the tropic hormone by interleukin. Aloe vera stimulates the release of interleukin from macrophages. Possibly low doses of aloe given to normal mice increase ovarian weight, in which case one must consider the possibility that aloe vera modulates the hypothalamic-pituitary control over the ovaries. Aloe vera also antagonizes chorionic gonadotropin. This antagonism was recorded on uterine weight but not on ovarian weight. Since aloe vera was not responsive at the ovarian level but was at the uterine level (inhibitory), one must consider the possibility that aloe vera antagonizes the HCG at the controversial uterine receptor, because aloe vera normally enhances the estrogenic response. The stimulatory and inhibitory influence of aloe vera verifies the modulation and vehicle effect. Much work needs to be done on the biological vehicle effect of aloe vera in regard to hormones and pharmacological agents. The biological vehicle effect will reduce the amount of test agent needed to produce the therapeutic response.

Dr. D. C. Gowda gave us important structural studies of polysaccharides from aloe vera. The polysaccharide was considered to be a linear (1–4) linked glucomannan having a glucose-to-mannose ratio of 1:2.8. Dr. Gowda gave us a detailed study of the chemical nature of aloe vera and how to precipitate the polysaccharide with 50 percent ethanol. From this Gowda separated by dialysis a coarse white fibrous powder that was composed of glucose and mannose in a molar ratio of 1:6. Methylation studies showed the glucose and mannose are beta 1–4 linked in the polysaccharide. Much of the present-day chemical research is based on the Gowda experiment. Aloe vera has many biologically active components such as amino acids, vitamins, growth factors, aspirin-like substances, sterols, and immune mechanisms. Some ingredients antagonize each other to produce a masking effect, while others synergize with each other. Some components are stimulators, and others are inhibitors. The balance between the stimulation and inhibition in aloe help us to understand the miracles in the aloe plant. This balance involves compounds, mediators, and immune mechanisms. One component stimulates immunity, whereas another inhibits an immune mechanism. We performed a study in which we compared the wound-healing and the anti-inflammatory activities from a 50 percent ethanol extract of aloe vera. Most of the anti-inflammatory activity (78 percent) was present in the supernatant, as compared to 32 percent recorded in the precipitate. No wound-healing activity was recorded for the supernatant (0 percent), but as much as 160 percent activity was present in the precipitate. Possibly the supernatant was masking some of the wound-healing activity in the precipitate. Many components in aloe vera contribute to the total biological activity, so that it is difficult, if not impossible, to postulate that the activity is coming from a single ingredient. The carrageenan-inflamed synovial pouch response to aloe vera confirms our biological results based on the Gowda experiment. The fibroblast stimulation activity of aloe vera recorded in wound healing was observed in this study. The fibroblast response in the air pouch was not a chronic inflammation but rather a growth-repair response. Our work suggests that aloe vera is a modulator of the immune response, wound healing, and inflammation. Future chemical and biological studies must be done to further understand aloe vera, but these studies must have a basis in the Gowda experiment.

Mucilage in the presence of aloe gel hardens and acts as a Crazy Glue. When this is applied to the surface of two wooden sticks, it requires a force of 1228 gm to pull the sticks apart. It is this mechanism that sealed the animal wounds to which we have applied an aloe leaf successfully. Aloe stimulates the fibroblast to increase wound tensile strength. We speculate that it may stimulate glucosamine to form collagen and proteoglycans, but zinc and vitamin C must be present. A review of the mechanical properties of skin shows similarities to plant elements. Many factors affect wound tensile strength such as anemia, water content of wounds, protein depletion, and availability of vitamin C. Zinc deficiency has an adverse effect on wound healing by inhibiting epithelialization, tensile strength, and collagen. Aloe vera contains vitamin C, zinc, water, growth factors, and protein needed for wound healing. Diluting aloe gel with water reduces gelation. Aloe vera is hydroscopic—that is, it picks up water. Aloe with mucilage causes water to move away from aloe. This shows the occlusive nature of mucilage. When a 1:1 mixture of mucilage–aloe vera gel was placed on an open wound for three days, wound healing was improved fourfold, as compared to untreated controls. The topical effect of whole-plant aloe combined with mucilage in a 1:1 ratio at 1 and 5 percent dose in petrolatum over four days with 0.5 aloe pulp produced a dramatic effect on wound tensile strength. The 1 percent dose increased wound tensile strength 18 percent, whereas the 5 percent dose produced a 60 percent increase in tensile strength over controls. Adding 0.5 percent aloe pulp to the 5 percent aloe–mucilage increased the wound tensile strength still further to 131 percent. This is the strongest preparation for wound healing we have seen thus far. The combination of mucilage and aloe forms an excellent bandage for open wounds.

Gibberellin is a plant growth factor present in aloe vera that plays a major role in growth. Even though it is a growth factor in plants, no one has shown that it has anti-inflammatory and wound-healing activity in animals. Gibberellin and related compounds may offer an alternative therapy for managing inflammation and wounds even under an abnormal physiological state such as diabetes. Gibberellin produces the wound-healing effect in a dose-response manner. Gibberellin blocks hydrocortisone acetate inhibition on wound healing much as aloe vera does. Cells in a wound communicate with each other through substances known as growth factors such as gibberellin. These substances bring order to the healing of wounds. Gibberellin may be an active acute anti-inflammatory ingredient in aloe, but it does not reduce granuloma tissue around a foreign substance under the skin. Our data show that aloe vera and gibberellin have parallel activity on inhibiting polymorphonuclear leukocyte migration into an area of inflammation. Possibly aloe and gibberellin block leukotrienes. Gibberellin stimulates open wound healing in a dose-response manner. Since gibberellin blocks hydrocortisone acetate inhibition on wound healing much as aloe does, gibberellin in aloe may act as a buffer against powerful sterols having anti-inflammatory activity. Gibberellin makes it possible for aloe to have both anti-inflammatory and wound-healing activity at the same time. Gibberellin enhances wound tensile strength, and when it is put in aloe vera, the aloe has an additive vehicle effect.

We have reviewed the current background of the AIDS virus and have asked the question whether or not aloe vera has a place in AIDS therapy. There are a number of observations that do not fit the current theory about AIDS. For example, can one be exposed to HIV without developing AIDS? An alternative was presented for explaining AIDS. Synthetic drugs have not solved the problem, but a nutritional (alternative) approach seems to shed light on how to fight AIDS. Two approaches toward how to use the immune system to fight disease were discussed. Acemannan is an active polysaccharide that increases the immune response to an antigen. Aloe vera can prevent and regress the development of adjuvant-induced arthritis. This condition involves both antibody and cellular immunity. Aloe vera can act as an adjuvant to enhance the immune response to an antigen. In fact, immunomodulatory compounds have been obtained from aloe gel. The worldwide AIDS epidemic appears to be out of control because of complacency and a lack of leadership. The world is not responding because there is no effective treatment to the AIDS crisis. Aloe vera, at the very least, could act as a "biological vehicle" in treatment of the global AIDS syndrome.

Some 37 million Americans suffer from some form of inflammatory disease for which no cure exists. Most drugs treat the pain and inflammation, but no drug can reverse the progress of arthritis. Ascorbic acid, RNA, and aloe extract were found to have good anti-inflammatory and anti-arthritic activity. At 5 percent concentration, the combination in cream regressed adjuvant arthritis 45 percent and the inflammation was inhibited 39 percent. Vitamin C decreased the swelling of an arthritic paw of a lab animal by "mopping up" reactive oxygen radicals. Ribonucleic acid was effective in both preventing and regressing adjuvant arthritis. The immunosuppressive action by RNA was evident in the arthritis model. All the known amino acids and three sterols are present in aloe vera. Decolorized aloe vera reduces edema and inflammation in normal rats. In the diabetic model aloe was effective in healing wounds and reducing edema as well as pain. Aloe blocked irritants such as gelatin, kaolin, carrageenan, mustard, and croton oil. Since steroids inhibit wound healing, aloe vera's positive influence on wounds and circulation makes it a natural vehicle for corticosteroids. Aloe vera, hydrocortisone, and sterol influence on wound tensile strength and anti-inflammation was presented. We asked the question, "If aloe vera contains these growth inhibitors, why does the whole-plant aloe promote growth so significantly?" Aloe vera contains strong growth factors that buffer the powerful anti-inflammatory components so that it has wound healing and anti-inflammatory activity simultaneously. A thorough discussion of the role of sterols in aloe vera was presented.

The role of aspirin in preventing heart attacks is its strongest credential as a therapeutic. People who take aspirin have fewer heart attacks than people who seldom take aspirin. Aspirin works by preventing prostaglandin synthesis throughout the body. Pain, fever, and inflammation are symptoms that aspirin best relieves. It relieves the red, swollen, painful joints of arthritis. Two aspirins every four hours give maximum benefit. However, side effects such as ulcers, irritation, allergy, and drug interaction are problems at the higher doses. Since aspirin blocks prostaglandin, it reduces stickiness of platelets to prevent formation of clots that stop blood flow. In a clinical study, we showed that aloe vera increased peripheral blood flow 85 percent, possibly by increasing the local metabolic substances that cause vasodilation of small blood vessels to increase foot blood flow. The combination of aspirin and aloe vera exhibited an additive topical anti-inflammatory effect. An additive response was also recorded for systemic anti-inflammation. These data prove that aloe vera is a good biological vehicle for aspirin whereby the dose of aspirin can be reduced so as to eliminate side effects. We discussed the influence of aspirin on the cardiovascular system, fever, and inflammation.

The mechanism of action of aspirin was discussed so as to better understand the influence of aloe vera. The relationship between prostaglandin and aspirin helps us to interpret how analgesic agents work. Aloe vera can increase the analgesic activity of aspirin by: protecting its half-life in the blood; increasing its availability to the tissues; increasing its mechanism of action; and synergistically combining with the analgesic activity of aspirin. Our data prove that aloe vera enhances the analgesic and anti-inflammatory activity of aspirin and is a good vehicle for salicylates. The dose of aspirin can be reduced to get the therapeutic effect with reduced toxicity.

We have described some of the biological assays that can be used to standardize aloe vera. A biological reference standard was recommended so that an aloe unit could be obtained for each activity exhibited by aloe. In most of our assays, we tested aloe vera in the living organism so that its biological activity was assessed among a variety of tissues and cells. The assay is made at the multicellular level in an attempt to model the human condition. When the biological and chemical assays on aloe vera agree, this is strong evidence for specific aloe vera activity. The best biological, active preparation can be obtained for anti-inflammation, analgesia, wound healing, and immunity so that one can obtain a unit for each activity. Each standard preparation can be called a reference standard. Unknown fractions of aloe vera can be compared to the appropriate reference standard. The slopes of each dose-response curve must be parallel in order to make a comparison of biological activity. One cannot "fool" the sensitivity, slope, and plateau of a dose-response curve for specific activity of aloe vera. A well-defined unit of specific aloe vera activity provides a good standardization for aloe vera. We have submitted to the IASC a proposed chemical-biological assessment of aloe vera. If the IASC adopts this procedure, we feel certain that it would be impossible to "fool" this certification agency as to whether a preparation is aloe or a fraudulent substance that looks like aloe vera. We have presented our best explanation of the mechanism of action of aloe vera. This explanation attempts to clarify how the many components in aloe vera can attack a wide variety of irritants, injuries, and insults. We have developed a fine open wound assay as well as a wound tensile strength assay. Both assays could be used to standardize aloe vera. The analgesia assay has good sensitivity and accuracy to evaluate aloe vera.

The relationship that exists within aloe vera we have called the "conductor-orchestra concept." The polysaccharide molecule is the conductor that leads a symphony of over two hundred biologically active substances. It contains mannose molecules joined together through beta 1–4 linkages to form a chain. The conductor modulates the biological activity between the surrounding orchestra molecules so that they work together synergistically. The protein at one end of the chain helps to direct the mannose phosphate at the other end of the polysaccharide to fit into the insulin-like growth factor receptor of the fibroblast, which produces collagen and proteoglycans for wound healing. The conductor can recognize the receptors on cell surfaces but can also recognize the individual biological players in the orchestra. Water plays a major role in the polysaccharide communicating with the active compounds in the orchestra. Water helps to produce therapeutic activity. The interaction between the conductor and the orchestra arises from water's polarity. The orchestra molecules, as well as the conductor polysaccharide, possess both polar and non-polar parts that relate with the polarity of water to form a water communication chain. Aloe vera has been called a modulator in that it brings biological systems into balance. We have demonstrated this normalizing influence of aloe vera in many instances. Aloe vera appears always to have two components that act in a yin-yang fashion so as to produce a beneficial therapy. Aloe vera acts to produce a balance in a biological system. One of the ways aloe vera produces communication between cells so as to produce balance is through growth factors. For example, gibberellin blocks the sterol activity so that there is always the balance between wound-healing and anti-inflammatory activity. This balance or modulation of therapeutic activity is usually never seen with one compound but is part of the miracle of aloe vera. The conductor-orchestra concept is an attempt to explain how aloe vera works, and this concept has been generally received by the entire aloe industry.

Index

Absorption, 50
Acemannan, 172
Acetylsalicylic acid, 1
Adulteration, 36
AIDS, 6
Air pouch, assay, 97
Amino acids, 273
Analgesia, 57, 278
Androgen, 69
Anthraquinone, 32
Anti-fibrosis, 200
Applications, 30
Arachadonic acid, 228
Arthritis, 141
Aspirin, 226
AZT, 169

Bayer, 227
B-cells, 164
Beta-sitosterol, 34
Bioavailability, 53
Biological error, 265
Blood flow, 231
Bone glue, 122
Bradykinin, 227, 242

Cardiovascular, 230
Carrageenan, 101, 240
Castration, 70
Cell, 13
Co-factors, 167
Components, 89
Conductor-orchestra, 264, 290
Connective tissue, 110
Cotton pellets, 195
Crazy Glue, 109
Croton oil, 55, 194, 268
Cushing's, 2
Cyclo-oxygenase, 228

Decolorized aloe, 194
Dermatitis, 194
Diabetes, 87, 121
Dilemma, 202
Dose-response, 195
Drugs, 250

Electron microscope, 16
ELISA test, 164
Estrogen, 56, 60

Fern reaction, 14
Fillet method, 35
Fingerprint, 37
Fisher ratio, 146

Gibberellin, 6, 132, 147, 313
Glycoprotein, 36
Gold, 246
Gonadotropin, 73, 78
Gowda, 85
Granuloma, 197, 236
Growth factors, 136

Helper T-cell, 162
Histamine, 114
Hot plate method, 255
Hydrocortisone, 5, 56, 57, 155, 209
Hydroxyproline, 120

IASC, 2
Ibuprofen, 2

IGF receptor, 272
Immature mice, 74
Immunosuppressive, 188
In vivo assay, 264
Indole acetic acid, 132, 150
Indomethacin, 245
Inhibition assay, 73
Interleukin, 73, 171
Irritant, 275

Jess F. Clarke, 232
Jesus burial, 110
Joint, 99

Kaolin, 194
Kaplan, 209
Kaposi's sarcoma, 165
Killer T-cell, 165

Law, 42
Leaf, 10
Least square, 18
Leukocytes, 214
Leukotrienes, 3
LH, 60
Lupeol, 204
Lyophilization, 293

Macrophage, 135, 155
Magic assay, 296
Magic bullet, 39, 86
Malic acid, 8
Mannose, 5
Mast cells, 100
Mediators, 38, 39
Miracle foot repair, 232
Modulation, 86
Mopping-up, 4
Mucilage, 14
Mustard, 195

Nerve ending, 250
Neurogenic, 252
Normal rats, 203
NSAIDS, 248
Nutrition, 164, 168, 177

Objective, 202, 209
Open wound healing, 145
Ovariectomized, 60, 61
Oxygen radicals, 4, 175

Pain, 189
Penetration, 48, 49
Periodic acid, 9
Phenylalanine, 192
Phloem, 12
Pituitary, 74
PMN assay, 141
Polysaccharide, 173
Prostaglandin, 3, 226
Proteoglycans, 109
Punch biopsy, 19
Pup leaves, 8, 268

Quantification of PMNs, 195

Regulation, 40, 41
Remodeling, 135
Rheumatoid arthritis, 183
Rind, 20
RNA, DNA, 32
Ruthenium red, 9

Salicylic acid, 34, 227
Skin, 111
Sol-gel, 16
Standardization, 263
Steroid effect, 192
Sterols, 33, 209
Stomata, 12
Synergism, 68
Synthesis of aloe, 11

Temperature, 16, 125
Tensile strength, 112
Testosterone, 66
Topical anti-inflammatory, 53
Transmission, 161
Trauma, 194
Tritiated thymidine, 135
Trypan blue assay, 49
Tryptophane, 192

Ultraviolet light, 229
Unilateral ovaryx, 76
Unit, 38, 272
Uterotropic effect, 64

Vaginal smear, 62
Vascularity, 97
Vehicle effect, 47, 49
Viscosity, 123
Vitamins, 9, 47

Warburg, 279
Wasting syndrome, 177
Water, 12, 22
Whole leaf, 35
Wind, 21
Wound diameter, 91
Wound healing, 92, 95
Wound tensile strength, 113

X brand, 271
Xylem, 10

Y = a + bx, 281
Yin-Yang theory, 294

Zinc, 34, 111, 313